ISBN 0-8373-5094-8
94 ADMISSION TEST SERIES

New RUDMAN'S QUESTIONS AND ANSWERS ON THE...

GMC

GMC APPRENTICE PROGRAM BATTERY TESTS

How to qualify for admission into General Motors Corporation Apprentice Program!

Intensive preparation for the examination including...

- Reasoning and Logic
- Mathematics
- Mechanical Comprehension

NLC
NATIONAL LEARNING CORPORATION

COPYRIGHT NOTICE

National Learning Corporation

212 Michael Drive, Syosset, NY 11791
(516) 921-8888 • www.passbooks.com
E-mail: info@passbooks.com

PUBLISHED IN THE UNITED STATES OF AMERICA

PASSBOOK SERIES®

THE *PASSBOOK SERIES®* has been created to prepare applicants and candidates for the ultimate academic battlefield—the examination room.

At some time in our lives, each and every one of us may be required to take an examination—for validation, matriculation, admission, qualification, registration, certification, or licensure.

Based on the assumption that every applicant or candidate has met the basic formal educational standards, has taken the required number of courses, and read the necessary texts, the *PASSBOOK SERIES®* furnishes the one special preparation which may assure passing with confidence, instead of failing with insecurity. Examination questions—together with answers—are furnished as the basic vehicle for study so that the mysteries of the examination and its compounding difficulties may be eliminated or diminished by a sure method.

This book is meant to help you pass your examination provided that you qualify and are serious in your objective.

The entire field is reviewed through the huge store of content information which is succinctly presented through a provocative and challenging approach—the question-and-answer method.

A climate of success is established by furnishing the correct answers at the end of each test.

You soon learn to recognize types of questions, forms of questions, and patterns of questioning. You may even begin to anticipate expected outcomes.

You perceive that many questions are repeated or adapted so that you gain acute insights, which may enable you to score many sure points.

You learn how to confront new questions, or types of questions, and to attack them confidently and work out the correct answers.

You note objectives and emphases, and recognize pitfalls and dangers, so that you may make positive educational adjustments.

Moreover, you are kept fully informed in relation to new concepts, methods, practices, and directions in the field.

You discover that you are actually taking the examination all the time: you are preparing for the examination by "taking" an examination, not by reading extraneous and/or supererogatory textbooks.

In short, this PASSBOOK®, used directedly, should be an important factor in helping you to pass your test.

MECHANICAL APTITUDE

Mechanical aptitude involves the ability to comprehend mechanical principles governing the actions of mechanism in motion and pertaining to the use of various mechanical devices.

Mechanical aptitude forms one of the basic components of various technical, vocational, aptitude, achievement, and classification examinations. It is also used to indicate a distinct, separate sector of intelligence.

Mechanical aptitude is divided into two major phases. TOOL RECOGNITION AND USE *and* MECHANICAL COMPREHENSION. MECHANICAL COMPREHENSION is specifically treated in this section.

MECHANICAL COMPREHENSION

CONTENTS

MECHANICAL APTITUDE

Mechanical aptitude involves the ability to comprehend mechanical principles governing the actions of mechanism in motion and pertaining to the use of various mechanical devices.

Mechanical aptitude forms one of the basic components of various technical, vocational, aptitude, achievement, and classification examinations. It is also used to indicate a distinct, separate sector of intelligence.

Mechanical aptitude is divided into two major phases. TOOL RECOGNITION AND USE *and* MECHANICAL COMPREHENSION. TOOL RECOGNITION AND USE is specifically treated in this section.

Tool Recognition and Use

CONTENTS

ABSTRACT REASONING

SPATIAL RELATIONS/TWO DIMENSIONS

EXAMINATION SECTION

CONTENTS

ABSTRACT REASONING

CONTENTS

NUMBER SERIES PROBLEMS

CONTENTS

GMC APPRENTICE PROGRAM BATTERY TESTS

INTRODUCTION

PURPOSE

The purpose of the apprentice program is to train men and women in those areas of skilled trades where such training is available and thereby equip those persons to master all of the operations performed by journeymen.

APPLICATION

In the part of the application under "*List the Skilled Trades for which you are applying for apprenticeship*", if you only want to be considered for one trade, list only that trade, leaving the other choices blank. To aid you in making your decision, a short description of the trades under consideration is given on the application form.

HIGH SCHOOL AND OTHER SCHOOLING TRANSCRIPTS

The transcript of your high school records (grades 9 through 12), *not a diploma*, must be submitted. It is necessary to use the transcript to establish your qualifications for the program and to calculate the number of points awarded in the selection process. If you received your high school diploma through the G.E.D. program, you *must* submit an official copy of the numerical results. Also, transcripts are required for other courses taken at trade schools, Vocational-Technical, College, etc., so that credit for applicable courses can be awarded in the selection process.

The above-noted transcripts or any other information you wish to submit for consideration; i.e., military records of courses, must be submitted to the Apprentice Committee, Human Resources Development Department.

INTERVIEWS

Interviews for qualified applicants will be conducted by the local Apprentice Committee as soon as possible after completion of the testing. This will be done on the applicant's own time and you will be notified when and where to report.

LENGTH OF TRAINING PROGRAM

The apprentice training program is normally four (4) years in length, but is based on the number of hours actually worked - the program being divided into eight (8) periods of 916 hours each, or a total of 7,328 hours of shop work. Training will be done on all three shifts for varying lengths of time.

RELATED TRAINING

Apprentices shall be required during the period of their apprenticeship to become proficient in mathematics, science, drawing and technical information related to their jobs by satisfactorily completing related and supplemental classroom instruction not to exceed 576 hours. Classes will be taken at various schools in the area and may be either day or evening classes opposite the shift they are working. Time spent in related training will be paid at the apprentice's straight-time rate, and General Motors will also pay registration fees and/or tuition required.

TESTS

Those who qualify will be notified of the test dates, so please be sure you show a correct address and phone number on your application. Those applicants who have been previously tested at GM locations may retest if desired. Applicants will be tested on their own time.

Applicants who submitted all transcripts in a timely manner and qualify will be given a battery of tests in the following areas:

1. Reasoning and logic;
2. Mathematics, including Algebra and Geometry; and
3. Mechanical comprehension.

HOW TO TAKE A TEST

You have studied hard, long, and conscientiously.

With your official admission card in hand, and your heart pounding, you have been admitted to the examination room.

You note that there are several hundred other applicants in the examination room waiting to take the same test.

They all appear to be equally well prepared.

You know that nothing but your best effort will suffice. The "moment of truth" is at hand: you now have to demonstrate objectively, in writing, your knowledge of content and your understanding of subject matter.

You are fighting the most important battle of your life — to pass and/or score high on an examination which will determine your career and provide the economic basis for your livelihood.

What extra, special things should you know and should you do in taking the examination?

BEFORE THE TEST

YOUR PHYSICAL CONDITION IS IMPORTANT

If you are not well, you can't do your best work on tests. If you are half asleep, you can't do your best either. Here are some tips:

1. Get about the same amount of sleep you usually get. Don't stay up all night before the test, either partying or worrying — DON'T DO IT.
2. If you wear glasses, be sure to wear them when you go to take the test. This goes for hearing aids, too.
3. If you have any physical problems that may keep you from doing your best, be sure to tell the person giving the test. If you are sick or in poor health, you really cannot do your best on any test. You can always come back and take the test some other time.

AT THE TEST

EXAMINATION TECHNIQUES

1. Read the *general* instructions carefully. These are usually printed on the first page of the examination booklet. As a rule, these instructions refer to the timing of the examination; the fact that you should not start work until the signal and must stop work at a signal, etc. If there are any *special* instructions, such as a choice of questions to be answered, make sure that you note this instruction carefully.

2. When you are ready to start work on the examination, that is as soon as the signal has been given, read the instructions to each question booklet, underline any key words or phrases, such as *least*, *best*, *outline*, *describe*, and the like. In this way you will tend to answer as requested rather than discover on reviewing your paper that you *listed without describing*, that you selected the *worst* choice rather than the *best* choice, etc.

3. If the examination is of the objective or so-called multiple-choice type, that is, each question will also give a series of possible answers: A, B, C, or D, and you are called upon to select the best answer and write the letter next to that answer on your answer paper, it is advisable to start answering each question in turn. There may be anywhere from 50 to 100 such questions in the three or four hours allotted and you can see how much time would be taken if you read through all the questions before beginning to answer any. Furthermore, if you come across a question or a group of questions which you know would be difficult to answer, it would undoubtedly affect your handling of all the other questions.

4. If the examination is of the essay-type and contains but a few questions, it is a moot point as to whether you should read all the questions before starting to answer any one. Of course if you are given a choice, say five out of seven and the like, then it is essential to read all the questions so you can eliminate the two which are most difficult. If, however, you are asked to answer all the questions, there may be danger in trying to answer the easiest one first because you may find that you will spend too much time on it. The best technique is to answer the first question, then proceed to the second, etc.

5. Time your answers. Before the examination begins, write down the time it started, then add the time allowed for the examination and write down the time it must be completed, then divide the time available somewhat as follows:

   a. If 3 ½ hours are allowed, that would be 210 minutes. If you have 80 objective-type questions, that would be an average of about 2 ½ minutes per question. Allow yourself no more than 2 minutes per question, or a total of 160 minutes, which will permit about 50 minutes to review.

   b. If for the time allotment of 210 minutes, there are 7 essay questions to answer, that would average about 30 minutes a question. Give yourself only 25 minutes per question so that you have about 35 minutes to review.

6. The most important instruction is *to read each question* and make sure you know what is wanted. The second most important instruction is to *time yourself properly* so that you answer every question. The third most important instruction is to *answer every question.* Guess if you have to but include something for each question, Remember that you will receive no credit for a blank and will probably receive some credit if you write something in answer to an essay question. If you guess a letter, say "B" for a multiple-choice question, you may have guessed right. If you leave a blank as the answer to a multiple-choice question, the examiners may respect your feelings but it will not add a point to your score. Some exams may penalize you for wrong answers, so in such cases *only*, you may not want to guess unless you have some basis for your answer.

7. Suggestions

   a. Objective-Type Questions

      (1) Examine the question booklet for proper sequence of pages and questions.

      (2) Read all instructions carefully.

      (3) Skip any question which seems too difficult; return to it after all other questions have been answered.

      (4) Apportion your time properly; do not spend too much time on any single question or group of questions.

      (5) Note and underline key words—*all, most, fewest, least, best, worst, same, opposite.*

      (6) Pay particular attention to negatives.

      (7) Note unusual option, e.g., unduly long, short, complex, different or similar in content to the body of the question.

      (8) Observe the use of "hedging" words—*probably, may, most likely, etc.*

      (9) Make sure that your answer is put next to the same number as the question.

      (10) Do not second guess unless you have good reason to believe the second answer is definitely more correct.

      (11) Cross out original answer if you decide another answer is more accurate; do not erase, *until* you are ready to hand your paper in.

      (12) Answer all questions; guess unless instructed otherwise.

      (13) Leave time for review.

b. Essay-Type Questions

(1) Read each question carefully.

(2) Determine exactly what is wanted. Underline key words or phrases.

(3) Decide on outline or paragraph answer.

(4) Include many different points and elements unless asked to develop any one or two points or elements.

(5) Show impartiality by giving pros and cons unless directed tu select one side only.

(6) Make and write down any assumptions you find necessary to answer the question.

(7) Watch your English, grammar, punctuation, choice of words.

(8) Time your answers; don't crowd material.

8. Answering the Essay Question

Most essay questions can be answered by framing the specific response around several key words or ideas. Here are a few such key words or ideas:

M's: manpower, materials, methods, money, management

P's: purpose, program, policy, plan, procedure, practice, problems, pitfalls, personnel, public relations

a. Six basic steps in handling problems:

(1) preliminary plan and background development

(2) collect information, data and facts

(3) analyze and interpret information, data and facts

(4) analyze and develop solutions as well as make recommendations

(5) prepare report and sell recommendations

(6) install recommendations and follow up effectiveness

b. Pitfalls to Avoid

(1) *Taking Things for Granted*
A statement of the situation does not necessarily imply that each of the elements is necessarily true; for example, a complaint may be invalid and biased so that all that can be taken for granted is that a complaint has been registered

(2) *Considering only one side of a situation*
Wherever possible, indicate several alternatives and then point out the reasons you selected the best one.

(3) *Failing to indicate follow up*
Whenever your answer indicates action on your part, make certain that you will take proper follow-up action to see how successful your recommendations, procedures, or actions turn out to be.

(4) *Taking too long in answering any single question*
Remember to time your answers properly.

EXAMINATION SECTION

EXAMINATION SECTION

TEST 1

DIRECTIONS: Each question or incomplete statement is followed by several suggested answers or completions. Select the one that BEST answers the question or completes the statement. *PRINT THE LETTER OF THE CORRECT ANSWER IN THE SPACE AT THE RIGHT.*

1. A gap of several thousandths of an inch between two parts is MOST accurately measured with a 1. ...
   A. divider B. feeler gage
   C. vernier caliper D. gage block

2. For a very high speed reduction the type of gear generally used is the 2. ...
   A. worm and gear B. spur gear
   C. bevel gear D. herringbone gear

3. The spiral flutes on a twist drill are provided to 3. ...
   A. remove the chips B. form a clearance hole
   C. prevent the drill from wobbling D. save material

4. The tool whose size is specified by weight is a 4. ...
   A. cold chisel B. hammer
   C. wrench D. pair of pliers

5. Ball bearings are USUALLY made of 5. ...
   A. steel B. brass C. cast iron D. babbit

6. An item which has the LEAST value in promoting general shop safety is 6. ...
   A. plenty of overtime B. safety posters
   C. skilled employees D. expensive equipment

7. It would be MOST necessary to provide a metal cover for a container used for 7. ...
   A. machine shop scrap B. floor sweepings
   C. oily rags and waste D. broken glass

8. A helper is NOT expected to assume much responsibility. This means that 8. ...
   A. he should not report defective equipment unless asked
   B. his superiors have a low opinion of his ability
   C. he never does important work
   D. generally other employees are assigned to make the decisions

9. A sheet metal screw differs from an ordinary machine screw in that it 9. ...
   A. requires a special nut
   B. always requires a special screw driver
   C. is self-tapping
   D. is made only in short lengths

10. In moving heavy equipment or materials with an overhead travelling crane, a good procedure is to have the crane operator take operating signals from only a single designated person on the floor. This is important because it 10. ...
   A. avoids the necessity of more than one person knowing the signals
   B. prevents overloading the crane with too much load
   C. requires fewer men
   D. avoids the danger of conflicting signals

11. Protective goggles should NOT be worn when 11. ...
   A. descending a ladder after finishing a job
   B. dusting off machinery
   C. chipping concrete
   D. sharpening a cold chisel on a grinding wheel

12. The GREATEST danger in the use of ladders, stairways, floors and platforms made of iron is that they 12. ...
   A. are difficult to maintain
   B. are slippery when greasy and wet
   C. have sharp edges causing injuries
   D. are too rigid and cause fatigue

13. Compressed air should NOT be used directly from a hose for dusting off work clothing MAINLY because 13. ...
   A. the air may contain considerable moisture
   B. the dust may blow into machinery
   C. it may cause personal injury
   D. it is too noisy

14. The term which CORRECTLY refers to a machine screw is 14. ...
   A. 8-24 B. #2 head C. 10-penny D. 1/2 by 3/4

15. Artificial respiration is applied when an accident has caused 15. ...
   A. broken limbs B. scalding
   C. breathing difficulties D. loss of blood

16. Lock washers are used PRINCIPALLY with 16. ...
   A. wood screws B. lag screws
   C. self-tapping screws D. machine screws

17. All employees receive a copy of the book of "Rules and Regulations." The MOST likely reason for issuing this book is to 17. ...
   A. give the answers to all technical questions
   B. relieve management of responsibility for accidents that may occur
   C. improve the employees' skills
   D. acquaint employees with their duties and responsibilities

18. If, when you are using an extension light with a long cord, the light should go out unexpectedly, you should FIRST 18. ...
    A. inspect the cord for a broken wire
    B. replace the bulb with a new one
    C. check the fuses in the supply circuit
    D. check if the plug is still in the outlet

19. The MOST common danger in working around rotating machinery is from 19. ...
    A. the suction effect created
    B. static electricity
    C. flying particles
    D. catching clothing on the moving parts

20. Acetylene is COMMONLY used 20. ...
    A. in cutting steel with a torch
    B. as a rust remover
    C. for extinguishing fires
    D. as a solvent for cleaning instruments

21. In drilling a hole which is to be tapped for a 3/8" screw the twist drill size is 21. ...
    A. 1/8" B. 5/16" C. 3/8" D. 7/16"

22. The material which is an alloy is 22. ...
    A. aluminum B. tin C. zinc D. bronze

23. Cold chisels with "mushroomed" heads are repaired by 23. ...
    A. cutting with hacksaw B. turning
    C. grinding D. hammering

24. In a first aid kit, you would NOT expect to find 24. ...
    A. bandages B. absorbent cotton
    C. splints for a broken leg D. band-aids

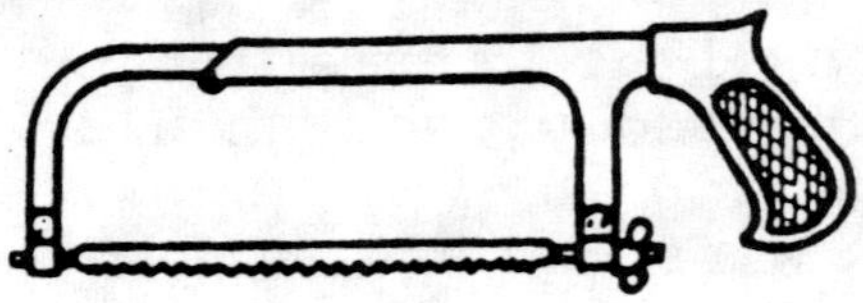

Fig. 1

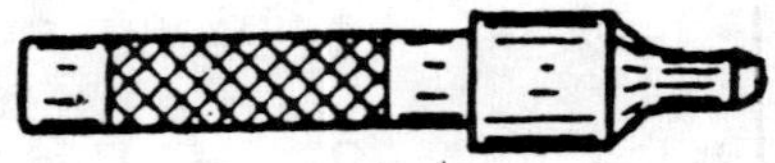

Fig. 2

Fig. 3

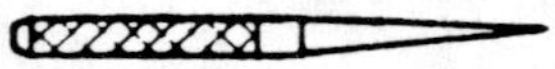

Fig. 4

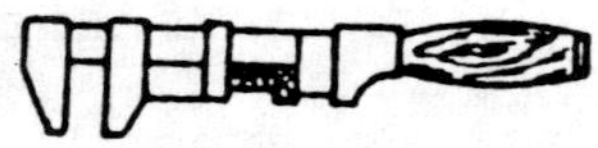

Fig. 5

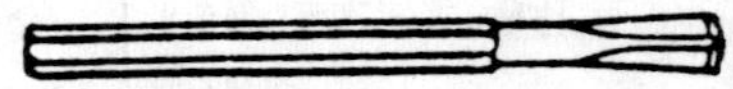

Fig. 6

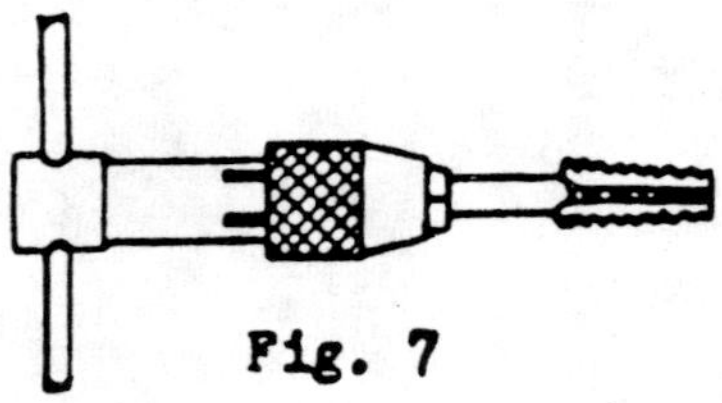

Fig. 7

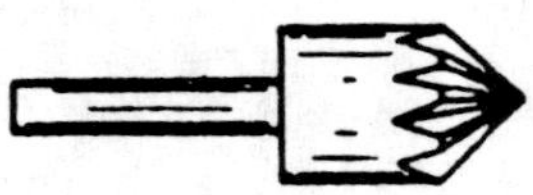

Fig. 8

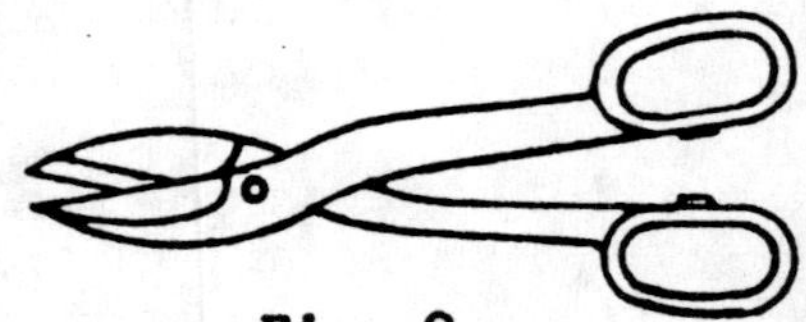

Fig. 9

Questions 25-33.

DIRECTIONS: Questions 25 to 33 inclusive refer to the figures above.

25. To thread a rod the tool to use is that shown in Figure
    A. 3 B. 6 C. 7 D. 8

26. The tool shown in Figure 9 ordinarily would NOT be used to cut a
    A. sheet of aluminum B. sheet of copper
    C. sheet of paper D. tin plate

27. In Figure 5 there is shown a(n)
    A. monkey wrench B. stillson wrench
    C. strap wrench D. open end wrench

28. The PROPER use for the tool shown in Figure 4 would be as a
    A. center punch B. drift pin
    C. pick D. scriber

29. The tool shown in Figure 7 is used in
    A. broaching B. drilling C. tapping D. reaming

30. The tool shown in Figure 8 is used in
    A. reaming B. countersinking
    C. counterboring D. cutting concrete

31. A star drill is shown in Figure
    A. 2 B. 6 C. 7 D. 8

32. The number "18" shown on the tool of Figure 3 indicates
    A. type of thread B. size of opening
    C. depth of opening D. threads per inch

33. The tool to use to PROPERLY flare one end of copper tubing is shown in Figure
    A. 2 B. 4 C. 6 D. 8

34. In treating injuries it is MOST important that any bandages used be 34. ...
A. clean B. damp C. large D. waterproof

35. The instrument COMMONLY used to measure speed of rotation is called a 35. ...
A. manometer B. tachometer
C. chronometer D. planimeter

36. When making a piping installation, the steel pipe is BEST turned by a 36. ...
A. monkey wrench B. adjustable open end wrench
C. alligator wrench D. stillson wrench

37. The MAIN purpose of periodic inspections and tests made on equipment which is in constant use is to 37. ...
A. familiarize the operating men with the equipment
B. keep the maintenance men busy during otherwise slack periods
C. discover minor faults before they develop into serious breakdowns
D. encourage the men to take better care of the equipment

38. A large oil storage tank has several manholes for easy access to the interior for periodic cleaning. You would NOT expect any of the manhole cover plates to be fastened to the tank by means of 38. ...
A. hinges and bolts B. rivets
C. studs and nuts D. swing bolts and nuts

39. Compound used on threaded pipe joints should be applied on 39. ...
A. the piece that is threaded on the outside
B. the joint edge after tightening
C. both threaded pieces
D. the piece that is threaded on the inside

40. When installed on moving machinery or shafting, set screws are often recessed so that no part of the screw sticks up above the surface MAINLY for 40. ...
A. strength B. appearance C. balance D. safety

41. When using a portable extension cord and lamp, an important safety precaution to take is to make sure that the cord 41. ...
A. is not too long B. does not kink
C. does not create a tripping hazard D. does not lie in dirt

42. If a machine screw does NOT turn easily with the screwdriver you are using, you should try one with a 42. ...
A. sharper tip B. wider tip
C. longer blade D. thicker handle

43. The presence of lubricating oil on shop floors is 43. ...
A. good because it lays the dust
B. bad because it causes accidents
C. good because it absorbs moisture and prevents dampness
D. bad because it injures cement floors

44. The fastening at the points marked "X" in the steel drum shown, is MOST commonly done with
    A. rivets B. machine screws
    C. lag screws D. bolts

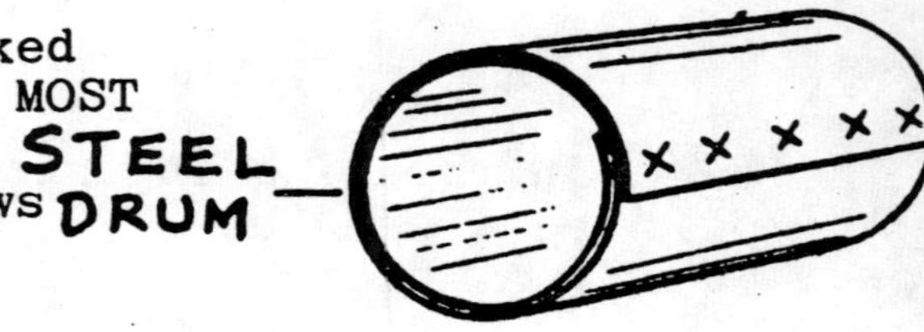

45. A piece is to be cut out of the angle iron in order to make the right angle bracket shown. Angle "X" should be
    A. 30 degrees B. 45 degrees
    C. 60 degrees D. 90 degrees

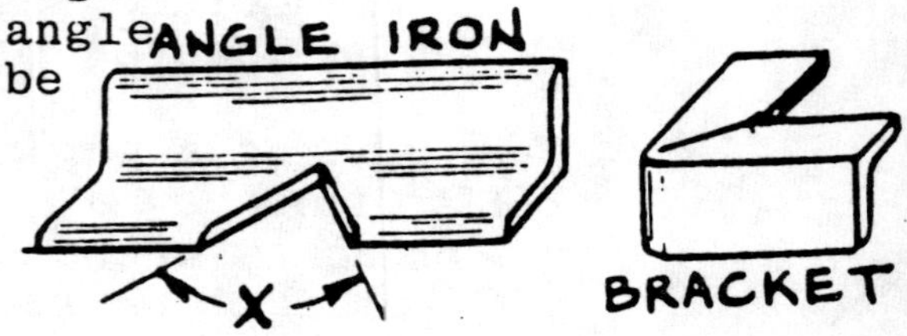

46. A screwed fitting by-pass is shown without valves. In making up this by-pass the gap would be occupied by a standard
    A. coupling B. expansion joint
    C. close nipple D. union

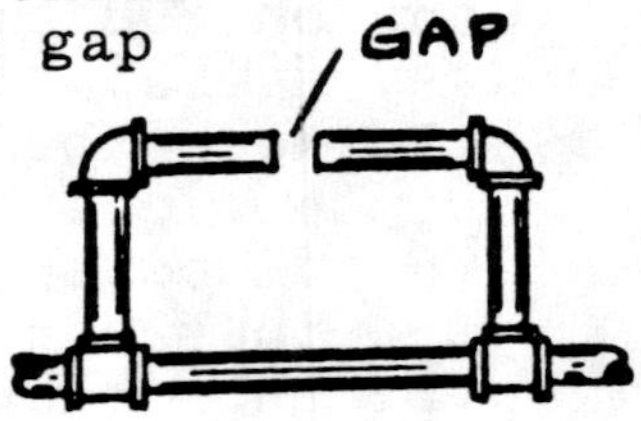

47. The 2" pipe run shown has a pitch of ¼" per foot. The total rise in 25' is
    A. 4¼" B. 5¼" C. 6¼" D. 8¼"

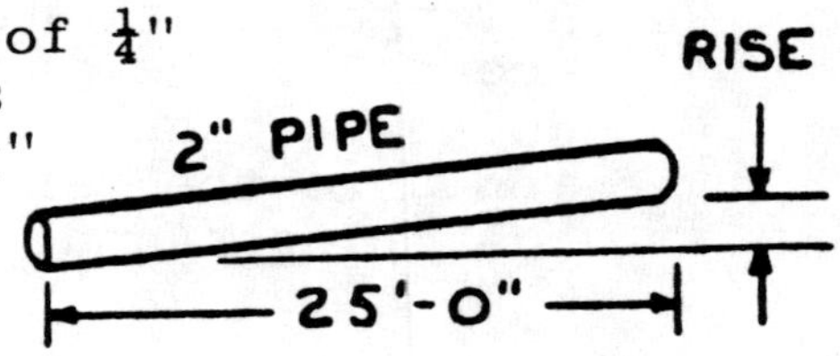

48. The pitch (or distance between centers) of the evenly spaced tubes is
    A. 2½" B. 1½" C. 1" D. 3/4"

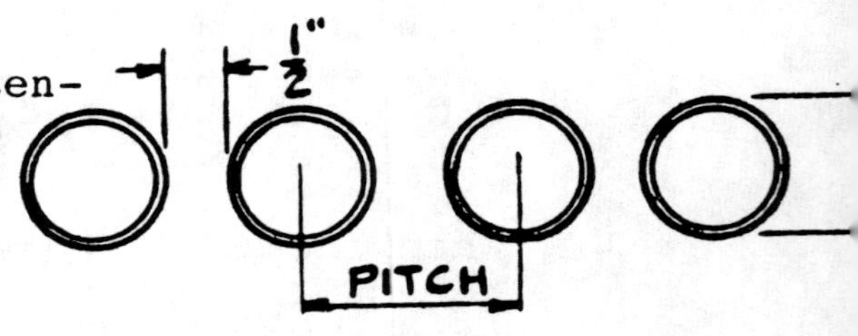

49. The flange bolts should be pulled up with a pair of
    A. monkey wrenches B. stillson wrenches
    C. strap wrenches
    D. open end wrenches

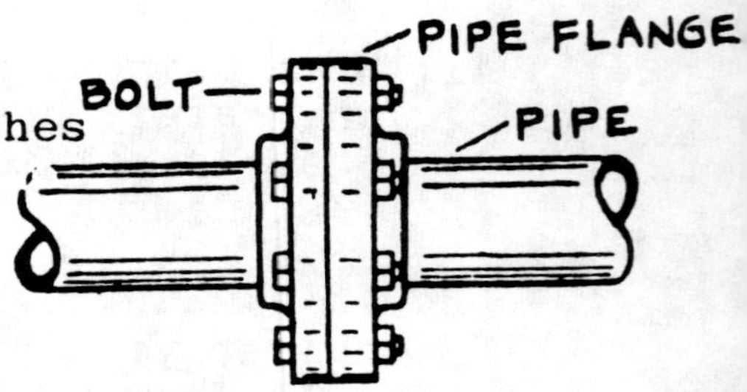

50. The distance "X" between the centers of the two end holes is
    A. 3 3/4" B. 3½"
    C. 3" D. 2 3/4"

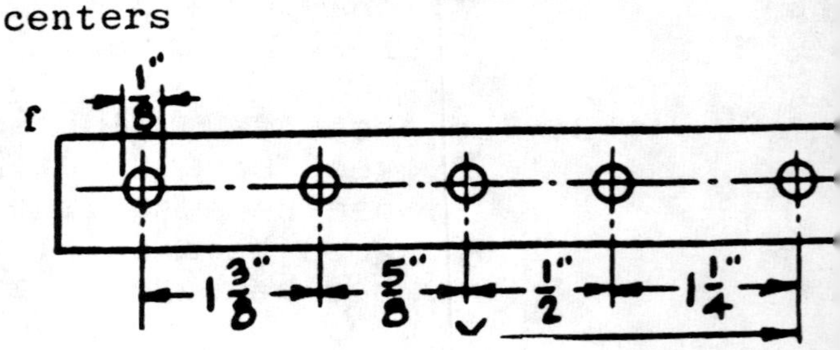

51. Accident reports SHOULD be based on 51. ...
A. conclusions B. facts C. opinions D. theories

52. The jaws of a vise close 3/16 of an inch for each turn of the screw. If the vise is open 6 inches, the number of turns required to close the jaw is 52. ...
A. 8 B. 16 C. 32 D. 64

53. Bolts are USUALLY designated by 53. ...
A. diameter and length
B. weight and diameter
C. number per pound
D. weight of each

54. To polish a steel rod the BEST material to use would be 54. ...
A. sand paper
B. emery cloth
C. terry cloth
D. crocus cloth

55. Alcohol is COMMONLY used as a(n) 55. ...
A. anti-freeze
B. lubricant
C. paint thinner
D. ruse remover

56. On a piece of round stock turning in a lathe it is POOR practice to use a file 56. ...
A. at all
B. without a handle
C. that has sharp teeth
D. when the lathe is turning fast

57. Holes are USUALLY countersunk for 57. ...
A. carriage bolts
B. lag screws
C. flat head screws
D. square nuts

58. If the inside diameter of a pipe is 3/8 of an inch and the wall thickness is .091 inches, the outside diameter of the pipe is 58. ...
A. .193 inches
B. .284 inches
C. .466 inches
D. .557 inches

59. A tapered thread is used on water pipe. The advantage of using a tapered thread is that 59. ...
A. it is easier to cut
B. it helps make a tight joint
C. no joint compound need be used
D. it reduces the weight of the piping

60. The teeth of a hacksaw are generally set so as to make a cut wider than the saw blade. This is done MAINLY to 60. ...
A. permit easy movement of the blade
B. strengthen the teeth
C. prevent dulling the blade
D. cool the blade

61. A hole has been drilled in a piece of metal and it is necessary to enlarge it by 0.010 of an inch to an exact size. The PROPER tool to use is a 61. ...
A. countersink
B. drill
C. reamer
D. rat tail file

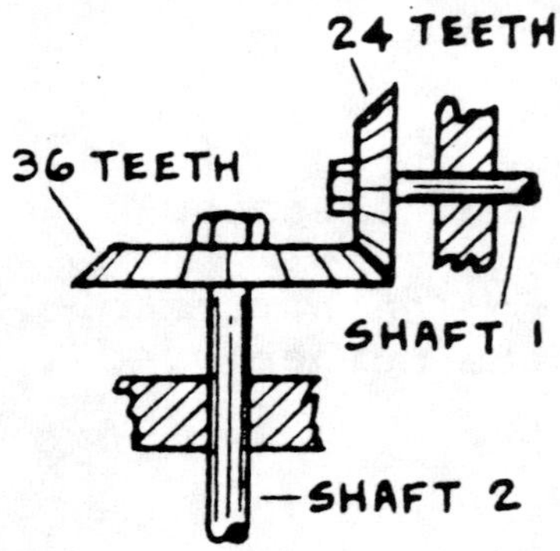

Fig. 1

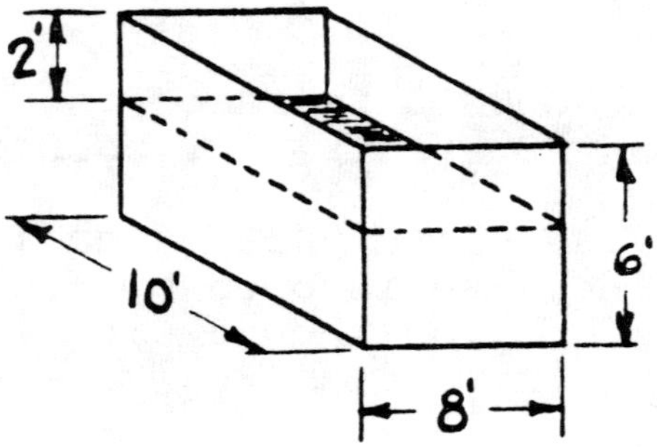

Fig. 2

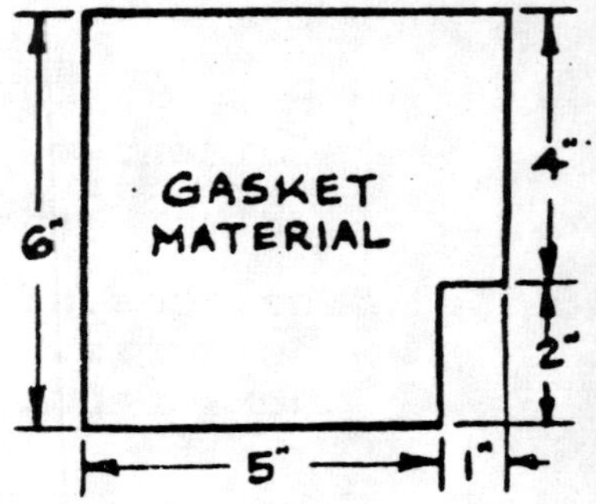

Fig. 3

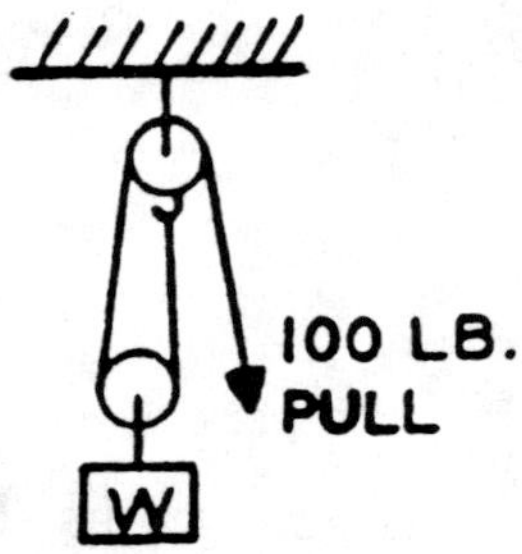

Fig. 4

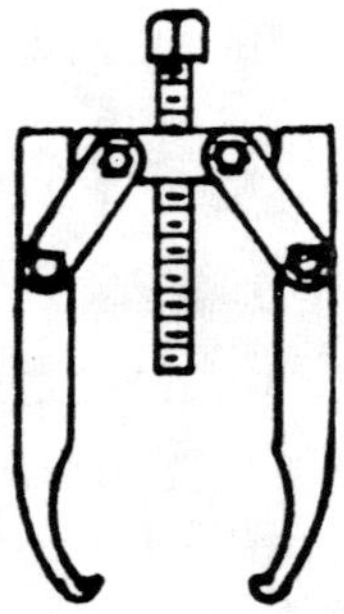

Fig. 5

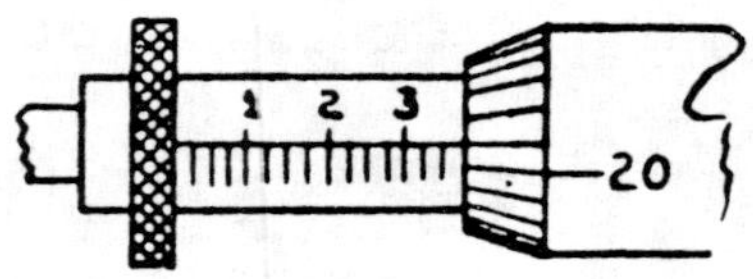

Fig. 6

Questions 62-73.
DIRECTIONS: Questions 62 to 73 inclusive refer to the Figures above

62. In Figure 1 are shown two
    A. spur gears   B. herringbone gears
    C. worm gears   D. bevel gears

63. In Figure 1 when shaft 2 revolves at 150 rpm, shaft 1 revolves a
    A. 225 rpm   B. 150 rpm   C. 100 rpm   D. 60 rpm

64. The TOTAL capacity of the partly filled tank in Figure 2, in cubic feet, is
    A. 160   B. 240   C. 320   D. 480

65. The tank in Figure 2, as shown, is
    A. 1/3 full   B. 1/2 full   C. 2/3 full   D. 3/4 full

66. The diameter of the LARGEST circular gasket that may be cut from the gasket material in Figure 3 is
    A. 2"   B. 4"   C. 5"   D. 6"

67. The area in square inches of the gasket material in Figure 3 is
    A. 28   B. 32   C. 34   D. 36

68. The perimeter in inches of the gasket material in Figure 3 is
    A. 18   B. 24   C. 30   D. 36

69. In Figure 4 the MAXIMUM weight "W" that can be lifted as shown with a pull of 100 lbs. is 69. ...
A. 50 lbs. B. 100 lbs. C. 200 lbs. D. 300 lbs.

70. The device shown in Figure 5 is used 70. ...
A. to remove a pulley from the end of a shaft
B. for punching holes in sheet metal
C. as a jog in drilling
D. to extract broken taps

71. In Figure 5 to turn the bolt you would NOT use a 71. ...
A. stillson wrench B. monkey wrench
C. box wrench D. an adjustable open end wrench

72. In Figure 6 there is shown a 72. ...
A. vernier caliper B. snap gauge
C. micrometer caliper D. thread gauge

73. The reading on the instrument shown in Figure 6 is 73. ...
A. 0.322" B. 0.361" C. 0.369" D. 0.371"

74. If it is necessary for you to make some adjustment with your hands under a piece of heavy equipment, while a fellow worker lifts up and holds one end of it by means of a pinch bar, one important precaution you should take is to 74. ...
A. insert a temporary block to support the piece
B. watch the bar to be ready if it slips
C. wear gloves
D. work as fast as possible

75. If a measurement scaled from a drawing is one inch, and the scale of the drawing is 1/4 inch to the foot, then the one inch measurement would represent an actual length of 75. ...
A. 4 feet B. 2 feet C. 1/4 of a foot D. 4 inches

76. A circular disc is divided into 18 equal segments, each segment will have an angular section of 76. ...
A. 10° B. 15° C. 20° D. 24°

77. A lathe collar is BASICALLY a 77. ...
A. drill B. chuck C. mandrel D. knurling tool

78. Babbitt hammers are used in machine shops PRINCIPALLY to 78. ...
A. protect workmen from flying chips
B. prevent sparks
C. prevent marring the work
D. reduce noise

79. A protractor is an instrument for measuring 79. ...
A. angles B. area
C. the depth of drilled holes
D. the thickness of sheet metal

80. A ladder which is painted is a safety hazard MAINLY because the paint 80. ...
A. is slippery after drying
B. may conceal weak spots in the rails and rungs
C. causes the wood to crack more quickly
D. peels and the wood starts to decay

81. The MAIN reason for imbedding steel rods in concrete is to 81. ...
A. prevent the rods from rusting
B. decrease the density of the concrete
C. increase the strength of the concrete
D. increase the weight of the concrete

82. A department rule prohibits indulgence in intoxicating liquor, or being under its influence, while on duty. This rule is rigidly enforced in order to 82. ...
A. prevent an employee from endangering himself or others
B. help promote temperance
C. enable an employee to save money
D. eliminate absenteeism

83. Standard forms frequently call for entries on them to be printed. The MAIN reason for this practice is that printing, as compared to writing, is GENERALLY 83. ...
A. more compact
B. more legal
C. more legible
D. easier to do

84. The instrument COMMONLY used to measure the diameter of a piece of work in a lathe is a 84. ...
A. micrometer caliper
B. pair of outside calipers
C. vernier caliper
D. pair of dividers

85. The MOST important reason for roping off the work area when repairs are made is to 85. ...
A. prevent delays to the public
B. protect the repair crew
C. prevent distraction of the crew by the public
D. protect the public

86. Copper liners are often put on the jaws of a vise to 86. ...
A. protect the jaws of the vise
B. protect the work
C. decrease noise
D. grip the work tighter

87. If a co-worker is in contact with a high-voltage circuit, the FIRST action taken should be to 87. ...
A. call a doctor
B. use a resuscitation method on him
C. call the foreman
D. cut off power

88. By the gauge of sheet metal is meant the sheet's 88. ...
AA. width B. thickness C. length D. area

89. When used in reference to pipe the abbreviations I.D. and O.D. refer to the pipe 89. ...
A. density B. diameters C. length D. weight

90. The BEST immediate first aid for a scraped knee is to 90. ...
A. apply plain vaseline
B. apply an ice pack
C. apply heat
D. wash it with soap and water

91. Of the sizes of sandpaper given, the FINEST is 91. ...
A. 1/2 B. 0 C. 00 D. 000

92. Powdered graphite is a good 92. ...
A. abrasive
B. adhesive
C. insulator
D. lubricant

93. A particular casting will be LIGHTEST in weight if made of 93. ...
A. cast iron
B. aluminum
C. brass
D. steel

94. To prevent an ordinary steel nut from working loose under vibration the BEST device to use is a 94. ...
A. cotter pin
B. drop of solder
C. fibre washer
D. lock washer

95. The head of a small rivet is readily formed with a 95. ...
A. ballpeen hammer
B. claw hammer
C. center punch
D. nail set

96. The machine used to bend sheet metal is called a 96. ...
A. brake B. miller C. planer D. router

97. The word "plan" when used on a blueprint indicates 97. ...
A. a side elevation view
B. a top view
C. a front elevation view
D. the order of assembly

98. Drilling must be done with special care when using any one of the very small size twist drills because the 98. ...
A. drill speed may be too fast
B. the drill is apt to break
C. cut material will clog the drill
D. drill may overheat

99. A parting tool is USUALLY used for work in a 99. ...
A. planer
B. milling machine
C. lathe
D. shaper

100. Diagonal pliers are PROPERLY used to 100. ...
A. cut pipe
B. flatten steel tubing
C. turn hexagonal nuts
D. cut wire

KEY (CORRECT ANSWERS)

1.	B	21.	B	41.	C	61.	C	81.	C
2.	A	22.	D	42.	D	62.	D	82.	A
3.	A	23.	C	43.	B	63.	A	83.	C
4.	B	24.	C	44.	A	64.	D	84.	B
5.	A	25.	A	45.	D	65.	C	85.	D
6.	A	26.	C	46.	D	66.	C	86.	B
7.	C	27.	A	47.	C	67.	C	87.	D
8.	D	28.	D	48.	B	68.	B	88.	B
9.	C	29.	C	49.	D	69.	C	89.	B
10.	D	30.	B	50.	A	70.	A	90.	D
11.	A	31.	B	51.	B	71.	A	91.	D
12.	B	32.	D	52.	C	72.	C	92.	D
13.	C	33.	A	53.	A	73.	C	93.	B
14.	A	34.	A	54.	D	74.	A	94.	D
15.	C	35.	B	55.	A	75.	A	95.	A
16.	D	36.	D	56.	B	76.	C	96.	A
17.	D	37.	C	57.	C	77.	B	97.	B
18.	D	38.	B	58.	D	78.	C	98.	B
19.	D	39.	A	59.	B	79.	A	99.	C
20.	A	40.	D	60.	A	80.	B	100.	D

TEST 2

DIRECTIONS: Each question or incomplete statement is followed by several suggested answers or completions. Select the one that BEST answers the question or completes the statement. *PRINT THE LETTER OF THE CORRECT ANSWER IN THE SPACE AT THE RIGHT.*

1. A drill gauge is used for measuring drill 1. ...
   A. length B. diameter C. hardness D. pitch

2. The wrench which is LEAST likely to slip off a nut of standard size is a(n) 2. ...
   A. "S" wrench
   B. box wrench
   C. monkey wrench
   D. adjustable open-end wrench

3. Wing nuts are especially useful when 3. ...
   A. the nut is to be removed frequently
   B. space is limited
   C. vibration effects must be counteracted
   D. the nut is never to be removed

4. Gauge blocks are used for checking the accuracy of 4. ...
   A. micrometers
   B. levels
   C. dividers
   D. spring calipers

5. The proper shop machine to use in order to plane flat steel stock is a 5. ...
   A. shaper B. lathe C. brake D. boring mill

6. On a lathe, a face-plate is sometimes used instead of a 6. ...
   A. compound rest
   B. tool post
   C. chuck
   D. saddle

7. Of the following, it would be MOST difficult to hand file 7. ...
   A. brass
   B. stainless steel
   C. copper
   D. lead

8. A screw which USUALLY has a square head is a 8. ...
   A. lag screw
   B. Phillips head screw
   C. fillister head screw
   D. thumb screw

9. Of the following, the BEST precaution to take when removing a broken tap by using a hammer and punch is to 9. ...
   A. wear gloves
   B. wear goggles
   C. use a soft hammer
   D. lubricate the punch

10. Speed and feed CANNOT be varied independently of each other when 10. ...
    A. drilling
    B. tapping
    C. boring
    D. reaming

11. Of the following, the dimension which calls for the HIGHEST accuracy and provides for the LEAST tolerance is   11. ...
A. 3.05" ± .01"   B. 3.020" ± .005"
C. 3.010" ± .002"   D. 3.025"

12. An oilstone would be LEAST likely to be used to sharpen a   12. ...
A. scraper   B. chisel   C. knife   D. saw

13. It would be POOR practice to use a flat cold chisel to   13. ...
A. cut thin sheet metal
B. cut a semi-circular groove in a steel block
C. split a nut
D. cut a rivet

14. A hole drilled in a shaft would PROBABLY be reamed to fit a   14. ...
A. cotter pin   B. cap screw
C. taper pin   D. carriage bolt

15. A soft-face hammer would NOT have a pounding surface made of   15. ...
A. copper   B. babbitt
C. lead   D. steel

16. V-blocks are ESPECIALLY useful for holding   16. ...
A. square pieces   B. circular bars
C. flat plates   D. hexagonal pieces

Questions 17-24.

DIRECTIONS: Questions 17 to 24 inclusive are based on the description of the Subway Car Air Compressor System given below. Read this information carefully before answering these questions.

SUBWAY CAR AIR COMPRESSOR SYSTEM

A two-stage, motor-driven air compressor having a large low pressure cylinder and a smaller high pressure cylinder is used. The low pressure cylinder, fitted with an air intake filter, performs the first stage of compression and discharges through an intercooler into the high pressure cylinder where the second stage of compression is performed. An unloader valve insures that compression does not begin until the motor has reached its full speed. An aftercooler is located between the compressor discharge and a compressor reservoir. An automatic drain valve located on the compressor reservoir automatically discharges precipitated moisture from the reservoir whenever the compressor governor functions to cut in power or shut off power to the compressor motor. The governor operates to stop the compressor when the reservoir air pressure reaches 140 lbs. and to start the compressor when the reservoir air pressure drops to 125 lbs. A safety valve set at 150 lbs. is connected to the compressur reservoir.

17. The number of air cooling devices provided in the compressor system is   17. ...
A. 1   B. 2   C. 3   D. 4

18. When the motor is starting up, it is protected by the 18. ...
    A. safety valve B. governor
    C. drain valve D. unloader valve

19. The intake filter is MOST likely designed to screen out 19. ...
    A. dirt B. water C. oil D. heat

20. The air pressure is LOWEST in the 20. ...
    A. small cylinder B. large cylinder
    C. compressor reservoir D. aftercooler

21. The automatic drain valve is triggered by the 21. ...
    A. governor B. unloader valve
    C. safety valve D. intercooler

22. The motor should stop running when the reservoir air pressure reaches 22. ...
    A. 125 lbs. B. 130 lbs. C. 135 lbs. D. 140 lbs.

23. Water automatically drains from the 23. ...
    A. low pressure cylinder B. high pressure cylinder
    C. air reservoir D. intercooler

24. Compression begins with the motor 24. ...
    A. off B. at low speed
    C. at intermediate speed D. at full speed

25. A steel rod having a diameter of 2 1/8 inches is to be discarded when worn more than .005 inches. The MINIMUM diameter permissible for this rod is 25. ...
    A. 2.125" B. 2.120" C. 2.075" D. 1.625"

26. Incorrect use of a machinist's hammer frequently results in uneven face wear. To properly recondition the face of the hammer, it would be BEST to use a 26. ...
    A. milling machine B. shaper
    C. grinder D. file

27. A stubby screwdriver is ESPECIALLY designed for turning screws 27. ...
    A. having a damaged screw slot
    B. which are jammed tight
    C. inaccessible to a longer screwdriver
    D. with stripped threads

28. Allen-type wrenches are USUALLY L-shaped. This shape 28. ...
    A. is only for distinguishing it from other wrenches
    B. is used to make the wrench sturdier
    C. permits a higher leverage with the short end inserted in a screw to be tightened
    D. permits a higher leverage with the long end inserted in a screw to be tightened

29. On a lathe, when a fixed cut is made at right angles to the axis of the work, the operation is known as 29. ...
A. straight turning
B. taper cutting
C. boring
D. reaming

30. The MOST important reason for dipping a chisel into cold water when it is being ground is to 30. ...
A. provide lubrication for the grinding process
B. keep the chisel clean
C. preserve the temper of the chisel
D. reduce the wear on the grinding wheel

31. To determine the taper per inch of a piece of work by using a steel scale, the number of dimensions to be measured if the piece is a cone, is a MINIMUM of 31. ...
A. one
B. two
C. three
D. four

32. A drilled hole is spotfaced 32. ...
A. only if it is to be threaded
B. to provide a smooth seat for a nut or cap screw head
C. to bring the hole diameter to exact dimensions
D. to strengthen the material around the hole

33. Open end wrenches with small openings are generally made shorter in overall length than open end wrenches with larger openings. The MOST important reason for this is to 33. ...
A. provide compactness
B. save material
C. provide correct leverage
D. prevent cracking of the wrench

34. A tool used to remove taper shank drills from a drilling machine spindle is known as a 34. ...
A. drift
B. dinking punch
C. pin punch
D. center punch

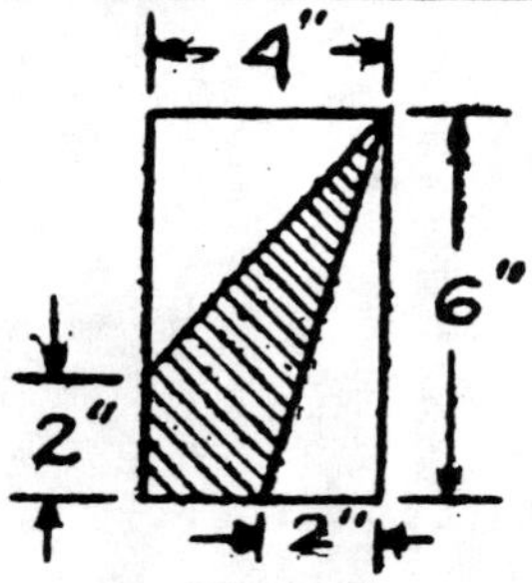

Fig. 1

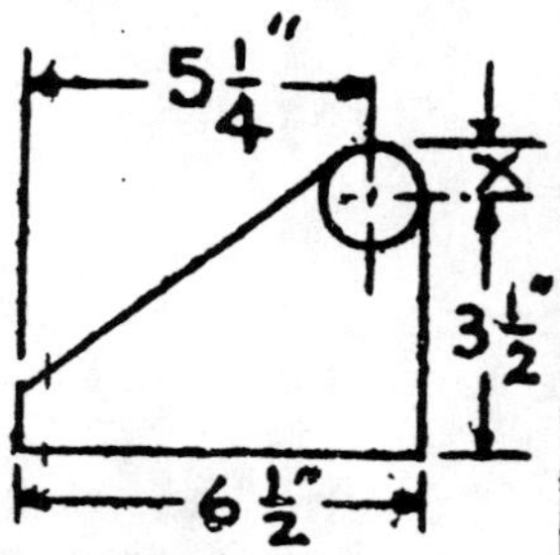

Fig. 2

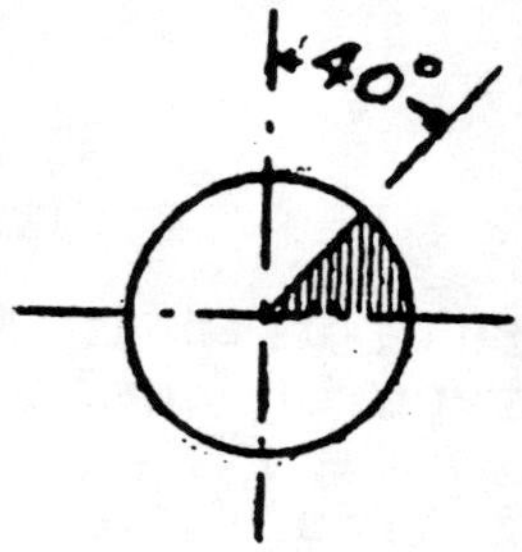

Fig. 3

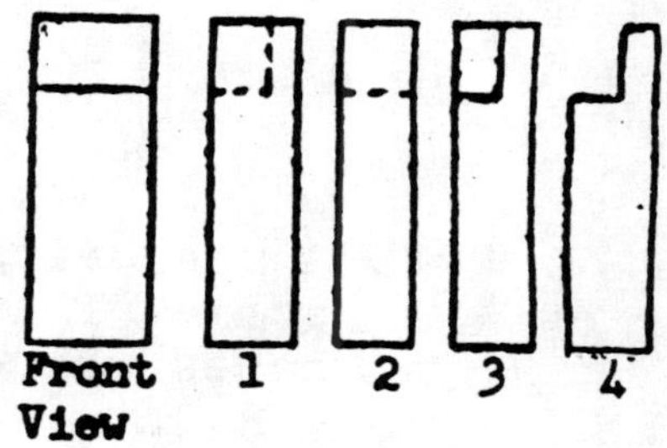

Fig. 4

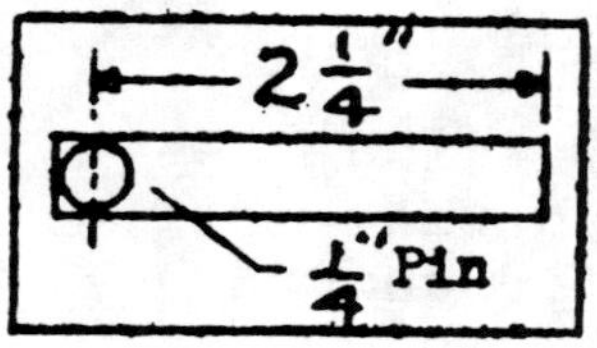

Fig. 5

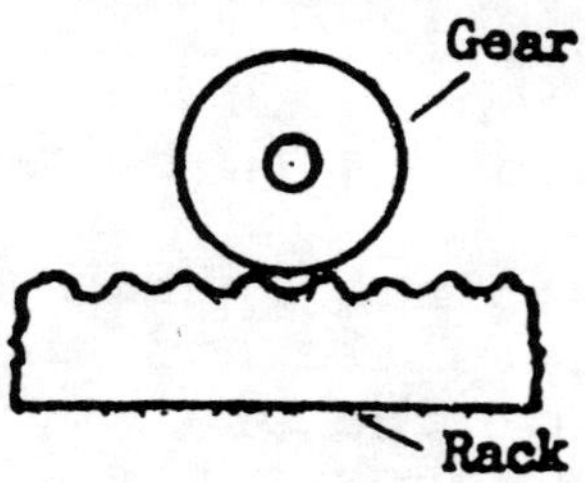

Fig. 6

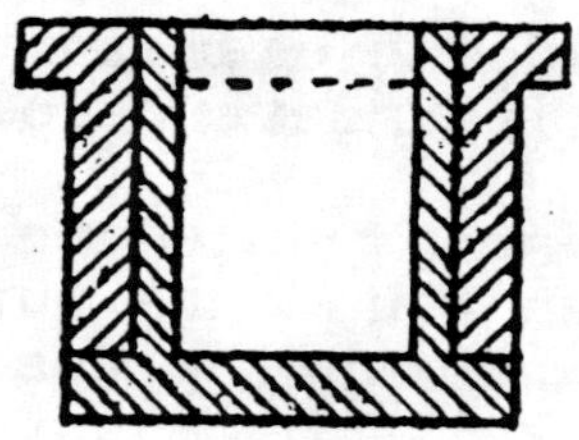

Fig. 7

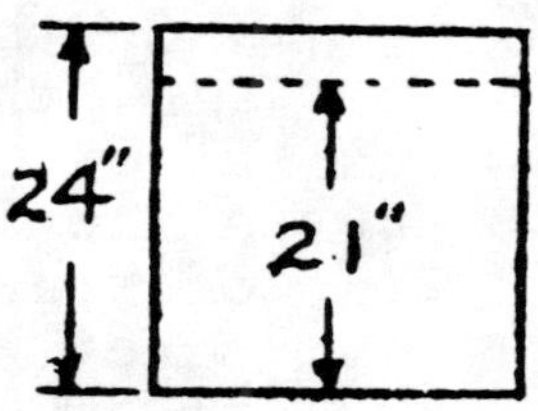

Fig. 8

Questions 35-42.

DIRECTIONS: Questions 35 to 42 inclusive refer to the figures above. Each question gives the proper figure to use with that question.

35. In Figure 1, the area in square inches of the shaded portion of the rectangle is
    A. 28 B. 24 C. 14 D. 10

36. In Figure 2, dimension "X" is
    A. 1.25" B. 1.75" C. 2" D. 2.5"

37. Figure 3 shows a shaded sector on a circular metal sheet. The MAXIMUM number of such sectors which can be cut from the sheet is
    A. 7 B. 8 C. 9 D. 10

38. Figure 4 shows a front view of a steel piece. The CORRECT side view is
    A. No. 1 B. No. 2 C. No. 3 D. No. 4

39. Figure 5 shows a circular pin which slides horizontally in a slotted rigid steel block. The MAXIMUM distance the pin can move, going from left to right is
    A. $2\frac{1}{2}$" B. 2 3/8" C. 2 1/8" D. 2"

40. In Figure 6, a gear with 30 teeth is turned by a gear rack having 20 teeth per inch. If the rack moves 3/4" horizontally, the gear will revolve
    A. $\frac{1}{2}$ turn B. 2/3 of a turn C. $1\frac{1}{2}$ turns D. 2 turns

41. In Figure 7 is a cross-section of an assembly. The number of separate pieces is
    A. 1 B. 2 C. 3 D. 4

42. Figure 8 shows a water tank having a total capacity of 120 gallons, which is partially filled. If 40 gallons are drained, the new water level will be
    A. 16" high B. 13" high C. 10" high D. 8" high

43. A measuring rule used in special cases is a hooked scale. This type of scale would be MOST useful in cases where 43. ...
A. it is difficult to see if the edge of the rule is even with the edge from which the measurement is to be made
B. the depth of a blind hole is to be measured
C. the inside diameter of a hole is to be measured
D. the circumference of a rod is to be measured

44. A machine shop procedure is to rub a thin application of prussian blue on a surface plate and then rub the piece of work being tested on the plate. This procedure is MOST likely to be used to check a steel block which has been 44. ...
A. scraped B. drilled
C. hacksawed D. reamed

45. Rubber tubing deteriorates MOST rapidly when in contact with 45. ...
A. water B. air C. oil D. soapsuds

46. Ordinarily when using a file, pressure is applied on the forward stroke only. One exception to this rule is when filing 46. ...
A. lead B. steel C. cast iron D. nickel

47. The PROPER file to use for enlarging a hole would be a 47. ...
A. flat file B. rat-tail file
C. square file D. mill file

48. The diameter of a hole required to be 3.254" should be checked with 48. ...
A. an inside vernier caliper
B. dividers and a steel scale
C. calipers and a steel scale
D. a micrometer depth gauge

49. When using a hacksaw, it is GOOD practice to 49. ...
A. tighten the blade in the frame by using pliers on the wing nut
B. use heavy pressure on both the forward and return strokes
C. slow the speed of cutting when the piece is almost cut through
D. use very short, very rapid strokes

50. With the standard measuring micrometer, starting with a zero reading, three complete revolutions of the sleeve will give a reading of 50. ...
A. 0.75" B. .06" C. .03" D. .003"

51. A NO-GO ring gauge fits loosely over a circular rod which is being checked. This would mean that the 51. ...
   A. rod is satisfactory
   B. rod must be scrapped
   C. diameter of the rod must be reduced
   D. rod is too long

52. A screw driver bit and brace has an advantage over an ordinary screw driver MAINLY because 52. ...
   A. more leverage can be applied to tighten a screw
   B. the screw driver bit cannot slip in a screw slot
   C. fewer turns are required to tighten a screw
   D. the bit is shorter than a screw driver blade

53. The PROPER way to clean a file which has been used on soft material is to use a 53. ...
   A. piece of emery cloth B. file card
   C. sharp scriber D. bench brush

54. When hand reamers are used the amount of metal to be removed is in the range of 54. ...
   A. millionths of an inch B. thousandths of an inch
   C. hundredths of an inch D. tens of an inch

55. If a drill makes a hole larger than its diameter, a LIKELY cause would be 55. ...
   A. too low a drill speed
   B. too sharp a drill
   C. that the drill has been ground out of center
   D. that the drill has cutting edges of equal length

56. A counterbored hole is designed to take a(n) 56. ...
   A. fillister head screw B. flat head screw
   C. oval head screw D. Phillips head screw

57. A slight coating of rust on small tools is BEST removed by 57. ...
   A. applying a heavy coat of vaseline
   B. scraping with a sharp knife
   C. rubbing with kerosene and fine steel wool
   D. rubbing with a dry cloth

58. If a co-worker becomes caught in a running machine, the FIRST thing to do is to 58. ...
   A. try to pull him out
   B. call the foreman
   C. call the shop physician
   D. shut the power off the machine

59. From a safety standpoint, the LEAST desirable time to wear gloves is when 59. ...
   A. running a lathe
   B. carrying castings
   C. lifting heavy materials with a chain hoist
   D. handling hot objects

60. Before taking apart a mechanical assembly, one or more sets of center punch marks are made on the assembly. This is GENERALLY done in order to 60. ...
   A. show the parts are new
   B. test the hardness of the metal
   C. make accurate reassembly easier
   D. facilitate disassembly

61. Galvanizing is a process used on sheet metal to 61. ...
   A. increase its tensile strength
   B. make it rust-resistant
   C. soften it for drilling
   D. prepare it for welding

62. The MOST important reason for keeping a cold chisel free from oil or grease is to 62. ...
   A. make it cut better
   B. avoid oil splattering from the blows
   C. prevent fire hazard when the tool heats up
   D. prevent the hammer from glancing off the chisel head

63. Cotter pins are MOST generally used with 63. ...
   A. acorn nuts
   B. castellated nuts
   C. knurled nuts
   D. wing nuts

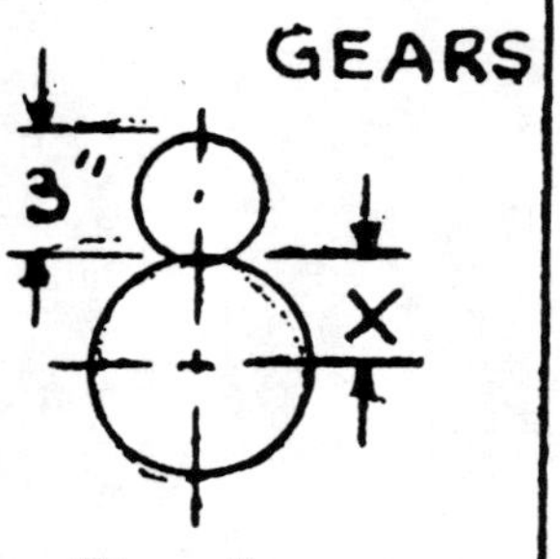

Fig. 1

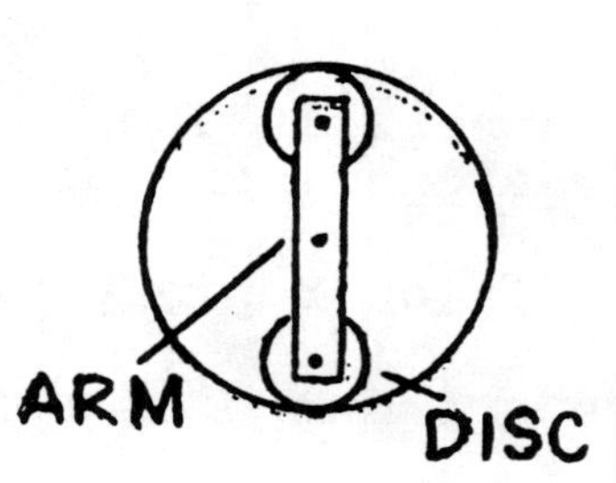

Fig. 2

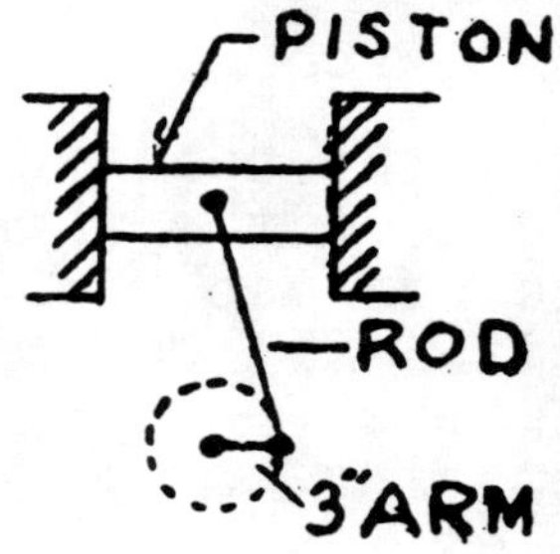

Fig. 3

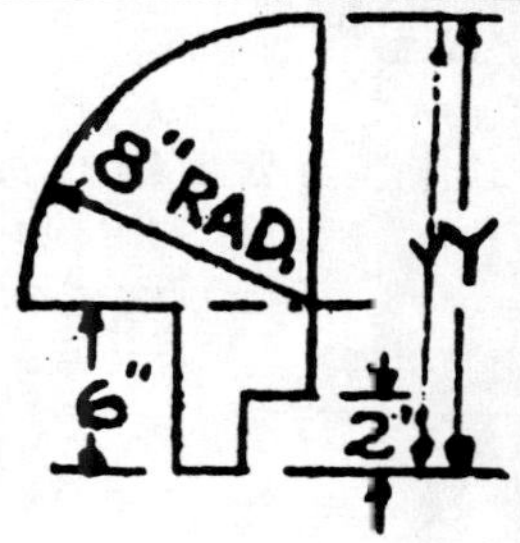

Fig. 4

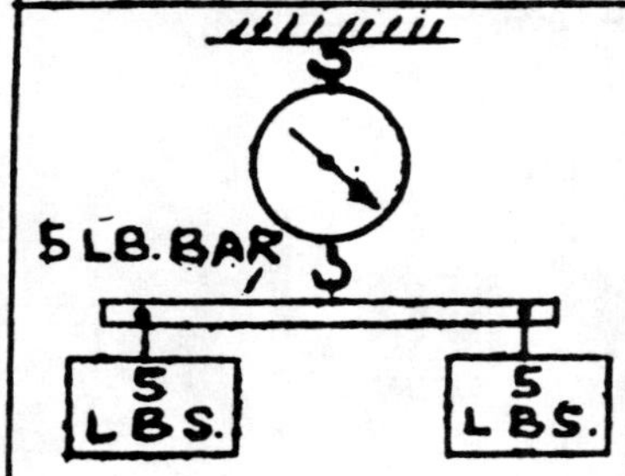

Fig. 5

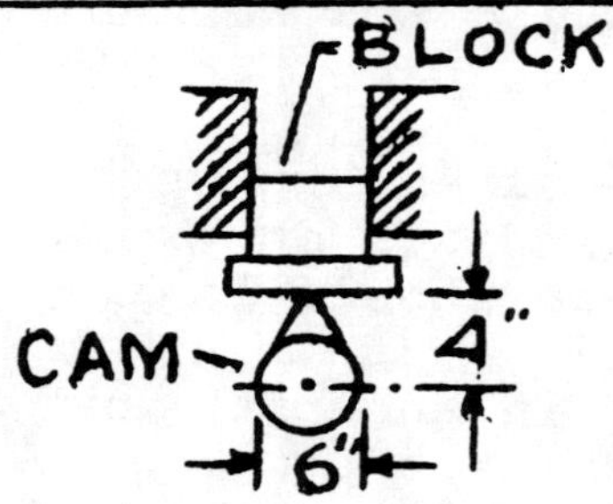

Fig. 6

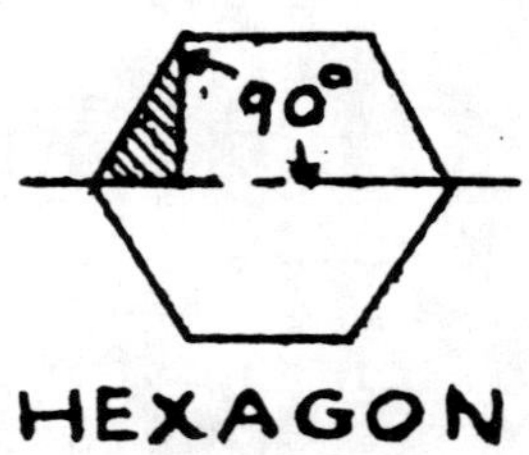

Fig. 7

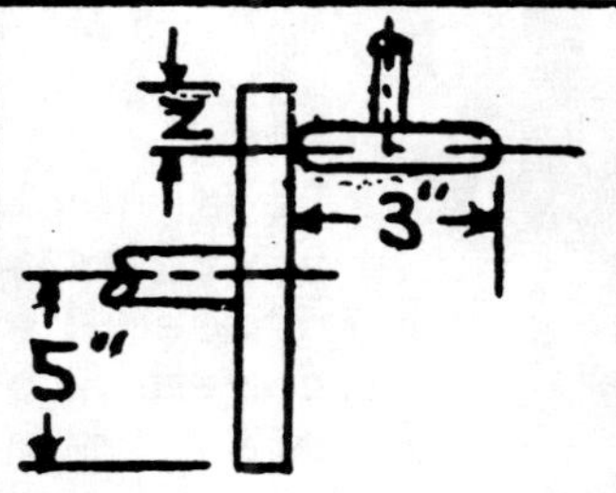

Fig. 8

Questions 64-71.

DIRECTIONS: Questions 64 to 71 inclusive refer to the figures above. Each question gives the proper figure to use with that question.

64. In Figure 1, for the large gear to rotate at 1/4 the speed of the small gear, distance "X" should be
A. 12" B. 9" C. 6" D. 3"

65. In Figure 2, the large circle has a circumference 3 times that of each small disc. The number of revolutions made by a small disc for every ½ turn of the arm is
A. 3 B. 2 C. 1½ D. 1

66. In Figure 3, one revolution of the crank arm will move the piston through a TOTAL distance of
A. 3" B. 6" C. 9" D. 12"

67. In Figure 4, the distance "Y" is
A. 10" B. 12" C. 14" D. 16"

68. In Figure 5, which shows a balanced bar, the weighing scale will read approximately
A. zero B. 5 lbs. C. 10 lbs. D. 15 lbs.

69. In Figure 6, rotation of the cam will permit the block to drop a MAXIMUM of
A. 1" B. 4" C. 6" D. 7"

70. In Figure 7, the TOTAL area of the hexagon will be found by multiplying the area of the shaded segment by
A. 14 B. 12 C. 10 D. 8

71. In Figure 8, both wheels will turn at the same speed when "Z" is
A. 1.5" B. 2" C. 3" D. 3.5"

72. On grinders, the tool rest is generally about 1/8 inch from the face of the wheel. Greater clearance is USUALLY undesirable because 72. ...
A. material will be ground off too rapidly from the work piece
B. the cutting action of the grinder will not be visible
C. the work piece will heat excessively
D. too much clearance may cause the work piece to jam and break the wheel

73. If a newly appointed helper feels he knows how to do a certain job, but his foreman insists on explaining the procedure in detail, the helper should listen to the foreman because 73. ...
A. he may catch the foreman in an error and thus prove he does know how to do the job
B. he can still do the job in his own way after the foreman has left
C. it will be the helper's responsibility to perform the job in the manner required by his foreman
D. he must humor the foreman, even if the foreman is wrong

74. When using a hand file to finish a piece of work held between lathe centers, it is generally BEST to 74. ...
A. do the finishing operation without running the lathe
B. use only one hand to hold and guide the file
C. hold the handle of the file in one hand and use the other hand to help guide the file
D. use a file which has no handle

75. A flat steel bar 2 feet long, which is given a 90° twist at the mid-point will 75. ...
A. increase in overall length
B. still be exactly 2 feet long from end to end
C. be better able to resist a bending force
D. be better able to resist a tension force

76. The dimension "6-inch" when used in connection with a screwdriver refers to the length of the 76. ...
A. handle B. ferrule
C. screwdriver from end to end D. blade

77. When tapping a drilled hole, the tap diameter 77. ...
A. is greater than the hole diameter
B. is smaller than the hole diameter
C. is exactly equal to the hole diameter
D. depends on the depth of the hole

78. A serious safety hazard occurs when a 78. ...
A. soft hammer is used to strike a hardened steel surface
B. hardened steel hammer is used to strike a soft iron surface
C. soft hammer is used to strike a soft iron surface
D. hardened steel hammer is used to strike a hardened steel surface

79. After a piece of work has been set into a lathe for machining, it is good practice to revolve the work one complete revolution by hand, before running the lathe with power on. The MAIN reason for doing this is to 79. ...
   A. make certain the lathe gears are not overloaded
   B. make certain the lathe is running true
   C. see there is ample clearance between work, dog, chuck and carriage
   D. get the feel of the work

80. A non-adjustable wrench which will accommodate different size nuts is a(n) 80. ...
   A. stillson wrench B. monkey wrench
   C. chain wrench D. alligator wrench

81. On your first day on the job as a helper, you are assigned to work with a maintainer. During the course of the work, you realize that the maintainer is about to violate a basic safety rule. In this case, the BEST thing for you to do is to 81. ...
   A. say nothing until he actually violates this safety rule and then call it to his attention
   B. say nothing, but later report this action to the foreman
   C. walk away from him so that you will not become involved
   D. immediately call it to his attention

82. The MAIN reason for using copper tips in soldering irons is because copper is 82. ...
   A. a good electrical conductor
   B. a good heat conductor
   C. has a low melting point
   D. very soft

83. The material discharged by a carbon dioxide fire extinguisher should NOT be handled because it 83. ...
   A. is a poisonous liquid
   B. is highly volatile
   C. is valuable for re-use
   D. can cause a frost-bite

84. In order to cast a number of duplicate parts, it is generally necessary to first make a mold from a 84. ...
   A. template B. fixture C. pattern D. jog

85. There are a few workers who are seemingly prone to accidents and who, regardless of their assigned job, have a higher accident rate than the average worker. If your coworker is known to be such an individual, the BEST course for you to pursue would be to 85. ...
   A. warn him not to make mistakes
   B. provide him with a copy of all rules and regulations
   C. do most of the assigned work yourself
   D. personally check safety precautions on each job

86. In a large shop, helpers are expected to do their work in a definitely prescribed manner because 86. ...
A. good results are more certain with less supervision
B. it insures discipline
C. no other method would work
D. it permits speed-up

87. A new helper is told by an experienced helper that he is not doing a particular job properly. The BEST reason for the new helper to give this advice due consideration is that the other helper 87. ...
A. has the authority to enforce his advice
B. has more experience on the job
C. will be resentful if his advice is not taken
D. will not help the new man again if his advice is not taken

88. A nail set is a tool used for 88. ...
A. straightening bent nails
B. cutting nails to specified size
C. sinking a nail head in wood
D. measuring nail size

89. It is important to make certain a ladle does not contain water before using it to scoop up molten solder since the water may 89. ...
A. cause serious personal injury
B. prevent the solder from sticking
C. cool the solder
D. dilute the solder

90. The device used to locate the center of a hole to be drilled in the same position on a number of identical castings is called a(n) 90. ...
A. circular chaser
B. guide pillar
C. blanking tool
D. jig

91. A new helper trying to complete a job on time finds that he is being delayed by a maintainer who keeps engaging him in conversation concerning sporting activities. It would be BEST for the helper to 91. ...
A. complain about this to the man's foreman
B. simply continue to work and turn his back on the man without answering him
C. converse with the man so that he will not antagonize him and later explain why the job wasn't finished on time
D. tell the man he has no time to talk since he must finish the job on time

92. It is NOT good practice to cut thin-walled copper tubing with an ordinary three-wheel pipe cutter because 92. ...
A. the tubing is likely to collapse
B. too much time is required
C. the tubing end must be reamed after cutting
D. the cutters will be dulled

93. When grinding a weld smooth it is MOST important to avoid 93. ...
    A. grinding too slowly
    B. overheating the surrounding metal
    C. grinding too much of the weld away
    D. grinding after the weld has cooled off

94. Cadmium plating is applied to iron brackets and hangers after the parts have been drilled. The reason for plating after drilling is 94. ...
    A. that the plating makes the metal too hard to drill
    B. to avoid the safety hazard in drilling cadmium plated materials
    C. to save plating material
    D. to protect the inside surfaces of the holes

95. A gouge is a carpenter's tool used for removing material by 95. ...
    A. filing B. grinding C. drilling D. chiseling

96. To make certain two points separated by a vertical distance of 8 feet are in perfect vertical alignment, it would be BEST to use a(n) 96. ...
    A. height gauge B. plumb bob
    C. surface gauge D. protractor

97. Steel helmets give workers the MOST protection from 97. ...
    A. falling objects B. eye injuries
    C. fire D. electric shock

98. A claw hammer is PROPERLY used for 98. ...
    A. driving a cold chisel B. driving nails
    C. setting rivets D. bending steel

99. When mounting and fastening enamel sign plates, care MUST be taken to prevent 99. ...
    A. corrosion B. chipping
    C. electrolysis D. discoloration

100. Employees of the department are cautioned not to use water to extinguish fires caused by high voltage arcing. The MOST likely reason for this rule is that water 100. ...
    A. would cause the fuses to blow in the electrical circuits
    B. will cause corrosion of sensitive electrical parts
    C. coming into contact with a hot electrical arc causes asphyxiating fumes to be generated
    D. may conduct the electrical current and create a shock hazard

---

KEY (CORRECT ANSWERS)

1.	B	21.	A	41.	B	61.	B	81.	D
2.	B	22.	D	42.	B	62.	D	82.	B
3.	A	23.	C	43.	A	63.	B	83.	D
4.	A	24.	D	44.	A	64.	C	84.	C
5.	A	25.	B	45.	C	65.	C	85.	D
6.	C	26.	C	46.	A	66.	D	86.	A
7.	B	27.	C	47.	B	67.	C	87.	B
8.	A	28.	C	48.	A	68.	D	88.	C
9.	B	29.	A	49.	C	69.	A	89.	A
10.	B	30.	C	50.	A	70.	B	90.	D
11.	C	31.	B	51.	B	71.	D	91.	D
12.	D	32.	B	52.	A	72.	D	92.	A
13.	B	33.	C	53.	B	73.	C	93.	C
14.	C	34.	A	54.	B	74.	C	94.	D
15.	D	35.	D	55.	C	75.	C	95.	D
16.	B	36.	A	56.	A	76.	D	96.	B
17.	B	37.	A	57.	C	77.	A	97.	A
18.	D	38.	D	58.	D	78.	D	98.	B
19.	A	39.	C	59.	A	79.	C	99.	B
20.	B	40.	A	60.	C	80.	D	100.	D

TEST 3

DIRECTIONS: Each question or incomplete statement is followed by several suggested answers or completions. Select the one that BEST answers the question or completes the statement. *PRINT THE LETTER OF THE CORRECT ANSWER IN THE SPACE AT THE RIGHT.*

1. When installing a new abrasice wheel on a grinder, it is GOOD practice to 1. ...
   A. force fit the wheel on the spindle
   B. burnish the spindle to insure a snug fit
   C. tighten the spindle nut as tightly as possible and then back it off 1/2 a turn
   D. tighten the spindle nut just enough for the flanges to hold the wheel firmly

2. The points of a steel divider are BEST sharpened 2. ...
   A. with a small hand oilstone moistened with light oil
   B. on a high speed grinder
   C. with a half-round file
   D. on a lathe

3. To repair a machinist's steel chisel which has a mushroomed head, the PROPER procedure is to 3. ...
   A. hacksaw the mushroomed head off
   B. countersink the mushroomed head
   C. soften the chisel and reshape the head on a lathe
   D. grind the head to its original shape and harden the chisel

4. Hand taps for making threads generally come in sets of three, respectively called, taper, second and bottoming taps. When tapping a blind hole in a steel block,the 4. ...
   A. taper tap is used last
   B. bottoming tap is used first
   C. second tap is never used
   D. bottoming tap is used to complete the thread at the bottom of the hole

5. The star drill is a multiple-pointed chisel used for drilling 5. ...
   A. brass B. stone and concrete C. wood D. aluminum

6. Shop employees are required to promptly report when first-aid supplies are used. The MOST important reason for this is to 6. ...
   A. figure the costs of these supplies
   B. prevent theft of these supplies
   C. make certain first-aid supplies are immediately replenished
   D. determine if the first-aid was properly administered

7. Generally all scale, rust and grease are removed from metals before they are welded. This is MAINLY done in order to 7. ...
   A. make the area to be welded clearly visible
   B. prevent the weld from cooling too rapidly
   C. reduce accident hazard
   D. reduce the amount of welding material required

8. One advantage of the ordinary closed-end flat wrench is that 8. ...
   A. it provides a better hand grip than other wrenches
   B. it has no open jaws which tend to spread easily
   C. it is adjustable for various nut sizes
   D. the same wrench can be used for square and hexagon nuts

9. A tool which would NOT be used in an electric drill is a(n) 9. ...
   A. twist drill B. reamer C. auger bit D. flat drill

10. When using a hacksaw, it would be POOR practice to 10. ...
   A. relieve pressure on the back stroke
   B. saw more rapidly when the blade is almost through the cut
   C. saw close to the point where the work is clamped
   D. set the blade in the frame so that the forward stroke will be the cutting stroke

11. The BEST file to use for sharpening a rip saw is a(n) 11. ...
   A. triangular file B. rasp C. round file D. square file

12. A soldering iron should be tinned 12. ...
   A. before soldering B. when cold
   C. only when storing it
   D. only when soldering tin pieces

13. Ordinary solder is made of 13. ...
   A. tin and brass B. lead and copper
   C. tin, lead and copper D. tin and lead

14. The purpose of the compound rest on a lathe is to 14. ...
   A. support the cutting tool in its various positions
   B. hold the live center
   C. hold the dead center
   D. hold the necessary gears for obtaining the various spindle speeds

15. In order to cast a number of duplicate parts, it is GENERALLY necessary to FIRST make a mold from a(n) 15. ...
   A. jig B. template C. pattern D. fixture

16. A holding nut is USUALLY used with a(n) 16. ...
   A. lag screw B. self-tapping screw
   C. drive screw D. stove bolt

17. The abrasive which is NOT commonly available in coarse quality is 17. ...
   A. sand paper B. emery
   C. carborundum D. crocus cloth

18. Spot welding is MOST commonly used to 18. ...
   A. hold structural beams together
   B. fix long deep cracks in heavy castings
   C. fasten light metal sheets together
   D. make long watertight seams

19. A steel rod required to have an initial diameter of 3 1/8 inches is to be discarded when worn more than .005 inches. The MINIMUM diameter permissible for this steel rod is 19. ...
   A. 3.145 inches B. 3.120 inches
   C. 3.065 inches D. 2.755 inches

20. A mitre box is used for 20. ...
   A. holding a saw at a fixed angle to the work
   B. storing sensitive measuring instruments
   C. setting the angle of the cutting tool on a lathe
   D. supporting heavy units

21. A taper on a piece of round stock is MOST usually made on a(n) 21. ...
   A. radial drilling machine B. shaper
   C. planer D. lathe

22. The MAXIMUM number of 65 pound castings which can safely raised, using a hoist having a 1200 pound capacity, is 22. ...
   A. 22 B. 20 C. 18 D. 16

23. The device used on a milling machine to divide the circumference of a piece of work into any number of equal parts is called a(n) 23. ...
   A. taper attachment B. index head
   C. face plate D. dead center

24. Of the following, the MOST accurate measuring device is a 24. ...
   A. folding rule B. cloth tape
   C. machinist's steel rule D. straight wooden rule

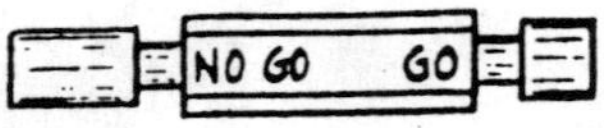

(A)

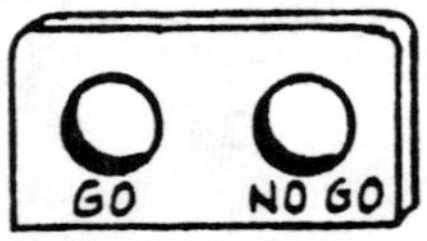

(B)

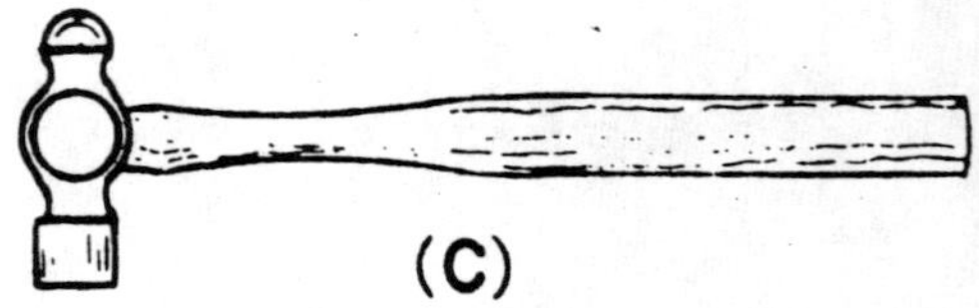

(C)

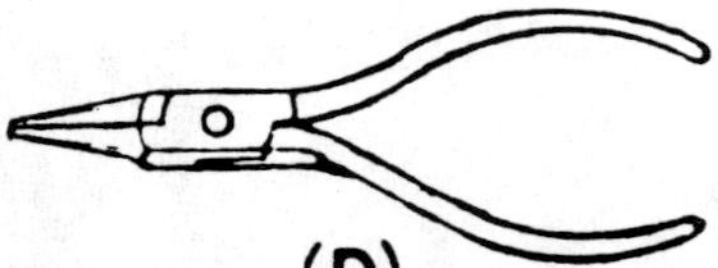

(D)

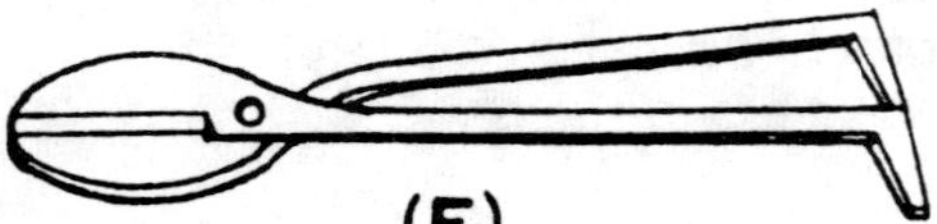

(E)

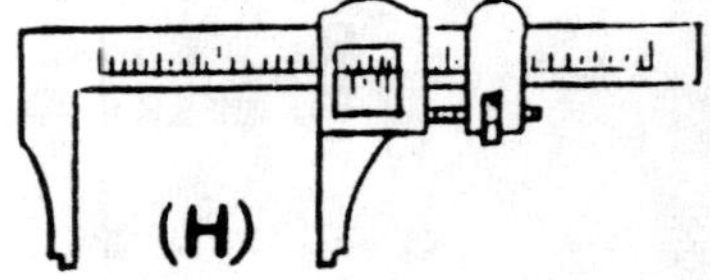

(H)

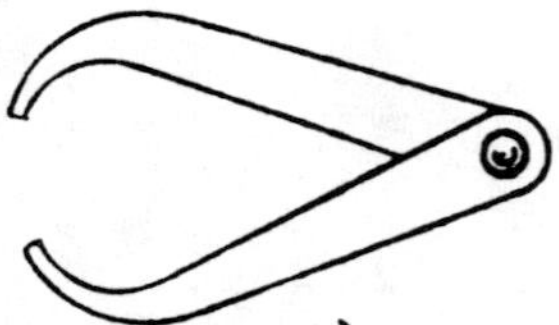

(J)

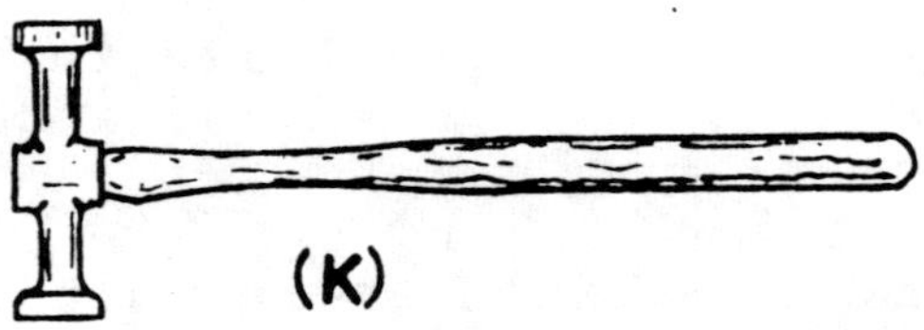

(K)

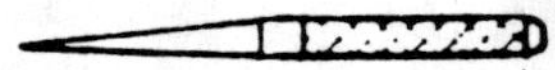

(L)

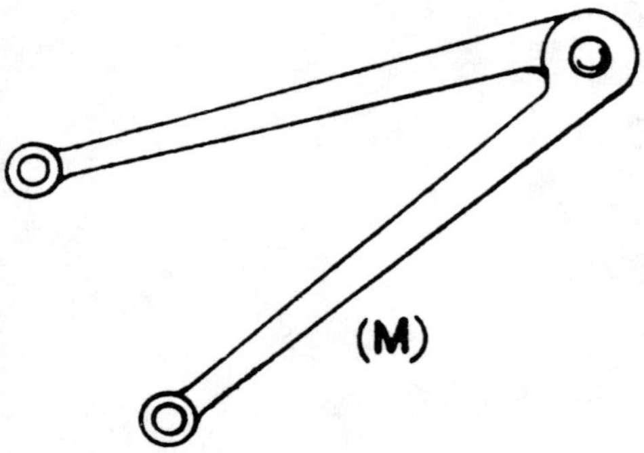

(M)

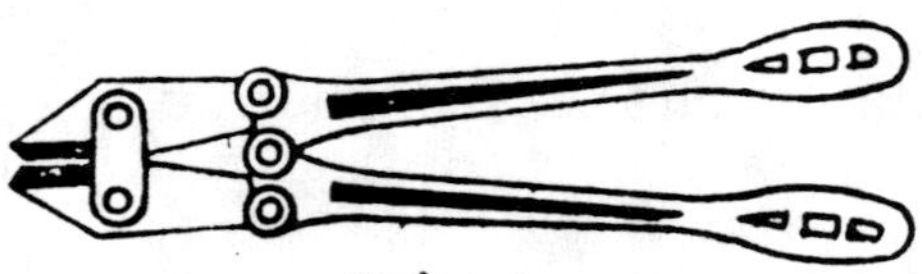

(P)

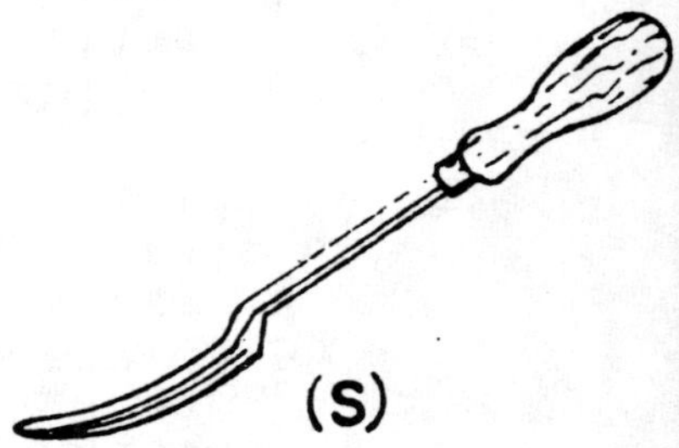

(S)

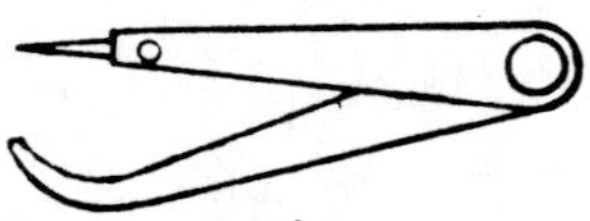

(T)

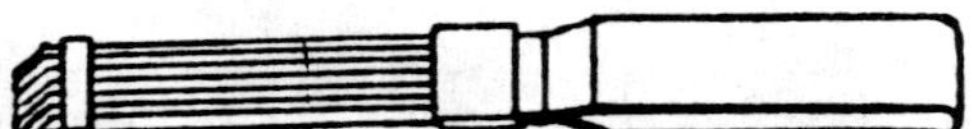

(V)

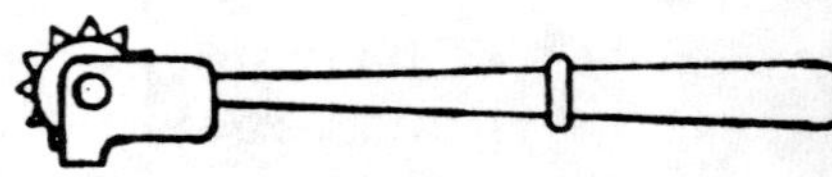

(W)

Questions 25-34.

DIRECTIONS: Questions 25 to 34 inclusive refer to the use of the tools show above. Read the item, and for the operation given, select the proper tool to be used from those shown. PRINT on your answer s in the correspondingly numbered item space, the letter given be your selected tool.

25. Cutting off the head of a 3/16" bolt.
26. Scribing arcs on the end of a piece of round stock to determine the center.
27. Smoothing out a dent in a piece of formed sheet metal.
28. Dressing up the working surface of a grinding wheel.
29. Quickly checking the bore of a quantity of brass bushings for proper tolerance limits.
30. Peening a rivet.
31. Scraping a bearing.
32. Removing a large screw plug having two blind holes on the top circular surface.
33. Determining the exact inside diameter of a metal tube.
34. Scraping carbon off a cylinder head.

Questions 35-42.
DIRECTIONS: Questions 35 to 42 are based on the Edison storage battery maintenance procedure given below. Read this procedure carefully before answering these items.

EDISON STORAGE BATTERY MAINTENANCE PROCEDURE

Take a voltage reading of each cell in the battery with a voltmeter. Any battery with two or more dead or reverse cells is to be removed and sent to the shop. All cell caps are to be opened and the water level brought up to 2 3/4" above the plates. Any battery requiring a considerable amount of water must be called to the foreman's attention. All cell caps must be brushed clean and special Edison battery oil applied to them. No batteries are to remain in service with cell caps broken or missing. The normal specific gravity reading of the solution must not be above 1.230 nor below 1.160. This reading is to be taken only on batteries which are found to be weak. Batteries with specific gravity lower than 1.160 must be sent to the shop. Be careful when disconnecting leads from the battery, since a slight turn of the connecting post will result in a dead cell due to the cell plates becoming short-circuited. When disconnecting leads use a standard Edison terminal puller. When recording defective cells, give the battery number, the car number, and the position of the cell in the battery. No. 1 cell is the cell to which the positive battery lead is connected and so on up to the last cell, No. 26 ,to which the negative lead is connected.

35. A normal specific gravity reading would be 35. ...
A. 1.450 B. 1.294 C. 1.200 D. 1.180

36. Batteries with below normal specific gravity reading MUST 36. ...
A. always have water added
B. be called to the foreman's attention
C. not be given a voltmeter test
D. be sent to the shop

37. The battery leads are disconnected by using 37. ...
A. gas pliers
B. Edison battery oil to free them
C. a screwdriver to pry them off
D. a standard Edison terminal puller

38. To completely record a defective cell 38. ...
A. only one identifying number is required
B. two identifying numbers are required
C. three identifying numbers are required
D. four identifying numbers are required

39. A battery MUST be taken out of service if it has 39. ...
A. one dead cell B. broken cell caps
C. one reversed cell D. a low water level

40. The battery water level should be brought up above the plates by 40. ...
    A. 2.75 inches B. 1.370 inches
    C. 1.264 inches D. 0.600 inches

41. Specific gravity readings are to be taken only on batteries which 41. ...
    A. are removed from service
    B. have missing cell caps
    C. are weak
    D. have a high water level

42. Dead cells are sometimes caused by 42. ...
    A. a slight turn of the connecting post
    B. taking unnecessary gravity readings
    C. adding too little battery oil
    D. adding too much water

43. Using only the balance weights shown, the LEAST number of weights required for a scale to balance with a 3/4 pound load is
    A. 6 B. 5 C. 3 D. 1

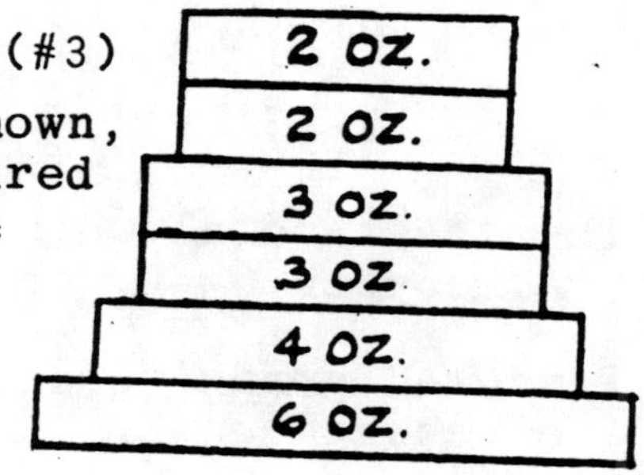

44. One complete turn of the drum crank will move the weight vertically upward a distance of
    A. 4 feet B. $3\frac{1}{2}$ feet
    C. 3 feet D. $1\frac{1}{2}$ feet

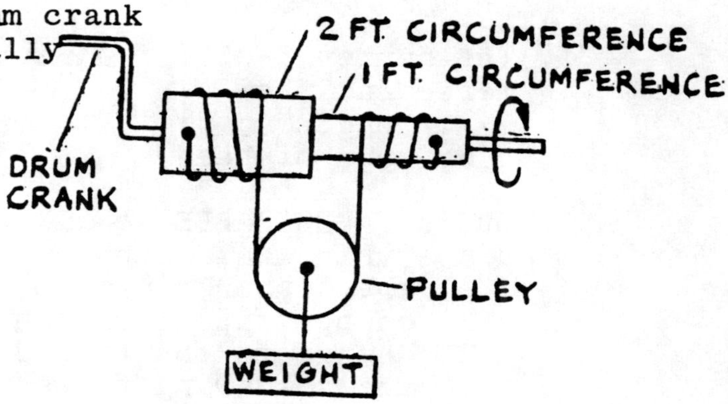

45. The dimension "X" on the plate is
    A. 5" B. 4"
    C. $3\frac{1}{2}$" D. $2\frac{1}{2}$"

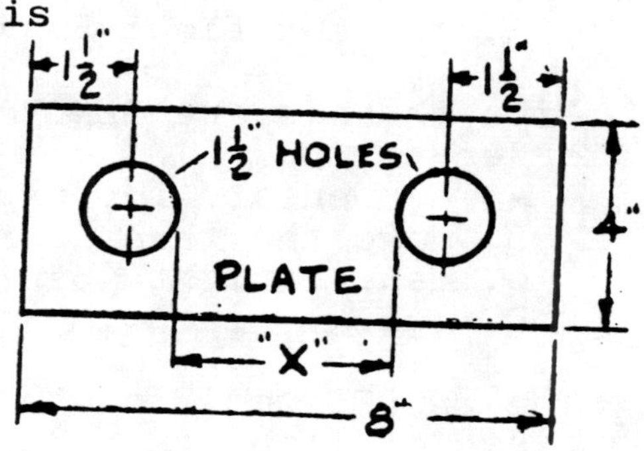

46. In the rectangular sheet shown, the area (in square inches) of the shaded portion is
    A. 38 B. 32
    C. 24 D. 18

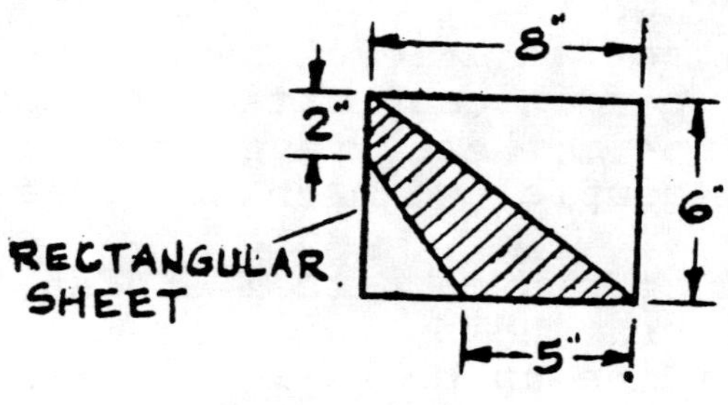

47. If the pinion makes six complete revolutions then the gear rack will move
    A. 24" B. 32"
    C. 44" D. 64"

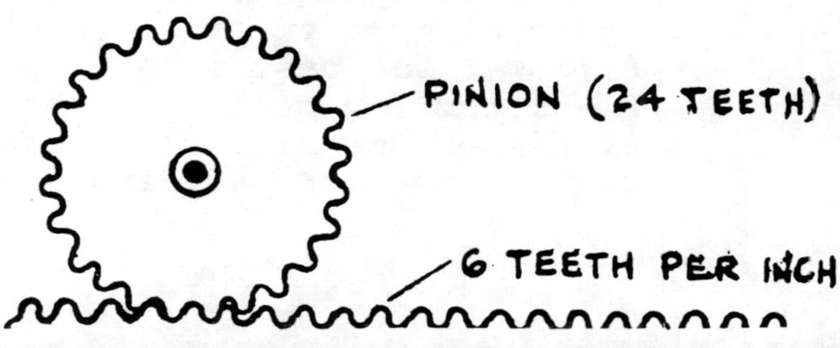

48. The sheet metal which is MOST difficult to solder is 48. ...
A. copper B. brass C. aluminum D. tin

49. Powdered graphite is a good 49. ...
A. abrasive B. lubricant C. adhesive D. insulator

50. The material which is an alloy is 50. ...
A. copper B. brass C. nickel D. silver

51. The number 6-32 for a machine screw specifies the diameter and the 51. ...
A. length
B. number of threads per inch
C. type of head
D. hardness

52. It is UNDESIRABLE to allow a soldering iron to overheat since this would cause 52. ...
A. the copper tip to harden
B. copper tip to soften
C. damage to the tinned surface of the tip
D. the soldering fumes to become poisonous

53. A tachometer is an instrument used to measure 53. ...
A. current flow B. RPM C. water flow D. temperature

54. Pipe threads are GENERALLY coated with white lead in order to 54. ...
A. compensate for expansion and contraction
B. make the threads run easier
C. make a tight joint
D. quickly identify the threaded joints

55. The PROPER tool to use when making a 1/8 inch hole in a piece of light gauge sheet metal is a(n) 55. ...
A. hand drill
B. ratchet brace
C. awl
D. air drill

56. Eyebolts are GENERALLY fastened to the shells of machines in order to 56. ...
A. act as a leveling device
B. permit easy attachment of lifting chains
C. permit easy tagging of equipment
D. couple two machines together

57. A drift pin is a tool GENERALLY used to 57. ...
A. ream holes
B. line up holes in similar superimposed heavy plates
C. countersink holes
D. machine finish a drilled hole

58. The correct speed at which to use a drill is important. In general,good practice requires the drill speed to be 58. ...
A. lower for cast iron than for brass
B. higher for cast iron than for brass
C. higher for mild steel than for brass
D. the same for cast iron, brass and mild steel

9. (#3)

59. With respect to the driving wheel, the driven wheel will rotate at
   A. twice the speed
   B. 2/3 the speed
   C. 1/3 the speed
   D. the same speed

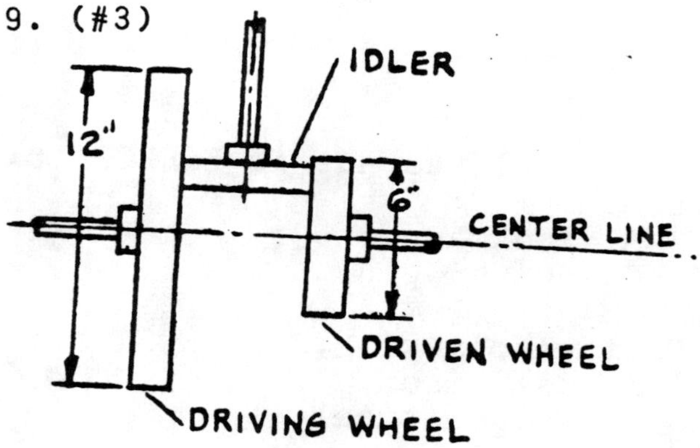

60. In the combination of wheels shown, the rotating speed of wheel W is
   A. 1/4 as much as wheel Y
   B. 3 times that of wheel Y
   C. 4 times that of wheel Y
   D. 5 times that of wheel Y

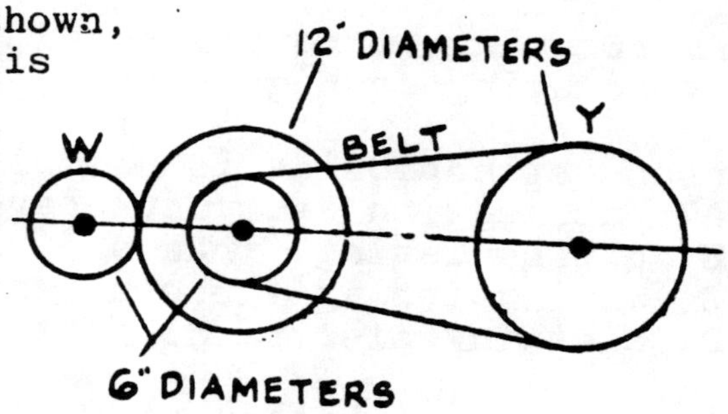

61. The number of complete turns the vise handle MUST make to fully close the jaws is
   A. 6   B. 12   C. 16   D. 24

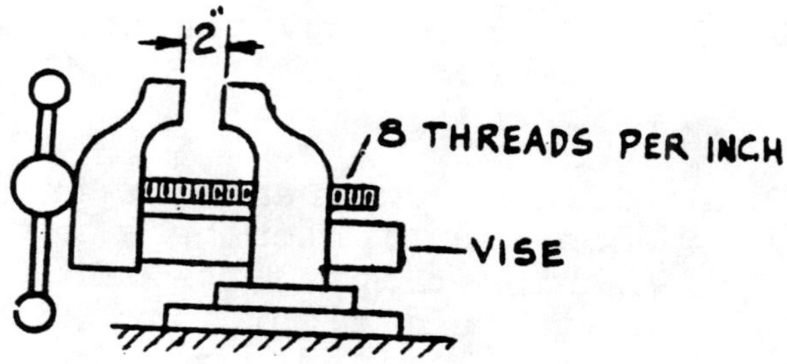

62. The total MAXIMUM number of triangular pieces, equal in area to A or B, which can be cut from the full tin sheet is
   A. 3   B. 5   C. 8   D. 9

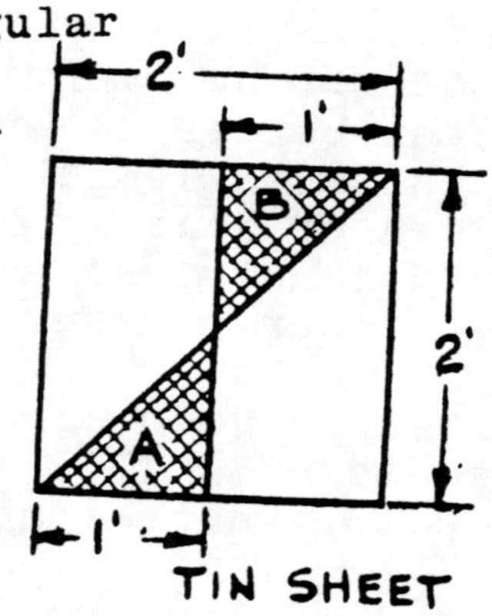

63. The male plug will PROPERLY fit into the receptacle if projection
   A. 9 is lined up with hole 2
   B. 11 is lined up with hole 1
   C. 8 is lined up with hole 1
   D. 7 is lined up with hole 2

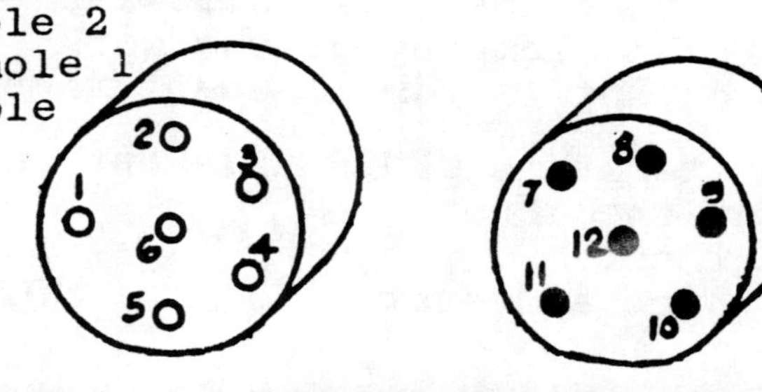

64. A castellated nut is ESPECIALLY designed to accommodate a(n) 64. ...
A. lockwasher
B. acorn cap
C. cotter pin
D. additional lock nut

65. Of the following, the MOST brittle material would be 65. ...
A. cast iron
B. annealed aluminum
C. forged steel
D. rolled steel

66. When checking the diameter of a piece of round stock being turned in a lathe, it is GOOD practice to use a micrometer with the piece 66. ...
A. rotating at normal speed
B. stationary
C. rotating at high speed
D. always out of the lathe

67. Carbon tetrachloride is useful for 67. ...
A. lubrication and rust prevention
B. extinguishing fires and cleaning electrical parts
C. extinguishing fires and rust prevention
D. cleaning electrical parts and rust prevention

68. Copper tubes are often used in preference to steel pipe because the copper tubes are less likely to 68. ...
A. corrode B. freeze C. puncture D. sweat

69. Of the following, the tool which is NOT tempered is a(n) 69. ...
A. center punch
B. hacksaw blade
C. chisel
D. abrasive wheel

70. An offset box wrench is preferable to a straight box wrench for tightening a nut which 70. ...
A. has stripped threads
B. is marred
C. is held tight with a lockwasher
D. has limited space in front of it

71. The PRINCIPAL advantage of using a reversible ratchet socket wrench is that 71. ...
A. nuts cannot be overtightened
B. it gives better leverage than any other type wrench with the same length handle
C. nuts can be quickly loosened and tightened in cases where a complete turn of the wrench is not possible
D. it has fewer parts to wear compared to other wrenches

72. A screwdriver in good condition should have a blade whose bottom edge is 72. ...
A. rounded B. knife-sharp C. chisel-shaped D. flat

73. A POOR procedure when drilling is 73. ...
A. to use cutting oil when drilling metal
B. tilting the drill sidewise to enlarge a hole
C. tight clamping of the work
D. setting the drill shaft tightly into the chuck

74. Micrometers are GENERALLY kept in covered boxes MAINLY to protect them from 74. ...
A. theft
B. humidity changes
C. dirt and dust
D. temperature changes

75. In the mechanical assembly shown, an INCORRECT dimension would be
   A. Y equals $2\frac{1}{2}$" B. X equals $5\frac{1}{2}$"
   C. W equals 3" D. V equals $7\frac{1}{2}$"

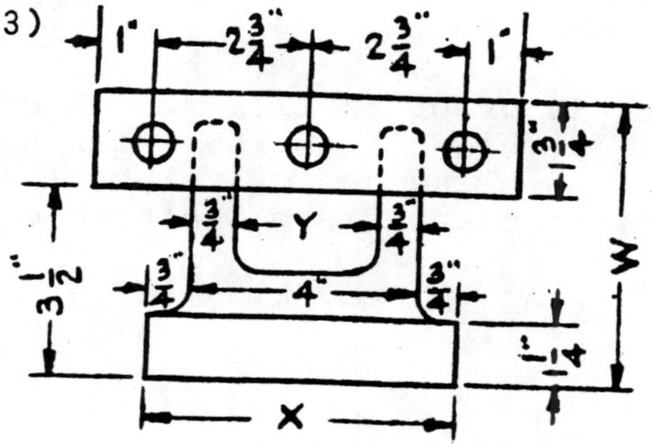

76. In order to properly secure the three metal pieces tightly together by means of the single machine screw a thread should be tapped in piece
   A. 1 and piece 3   B. 3
   C. 1   D. 2

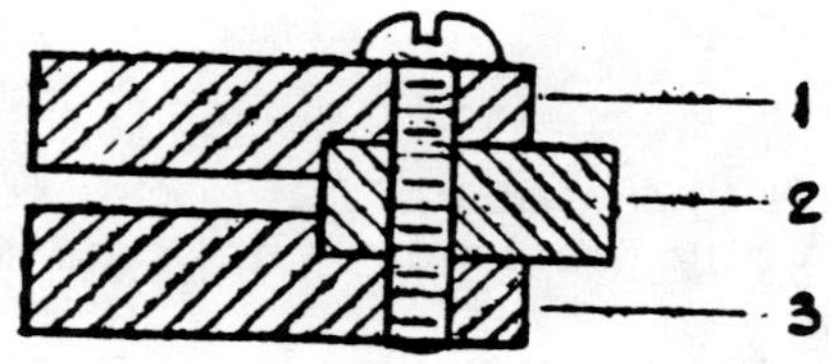

77. If an 8" level indicates 16 quarts of oil in the tank, then the number of quarts of oil to be added to raise the level from 6" to 8" is
   A. 3 quarts   B. 4 quarts
   C. 5 quarts   D. 7 quarts

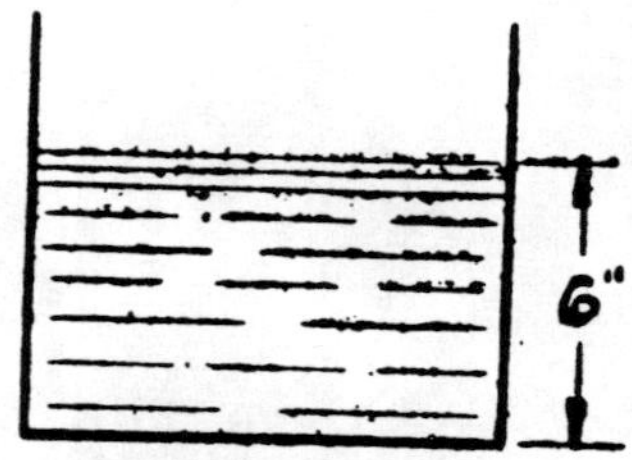

OIL TANK

78. In the pile of timbers shown there are fewer
   A. rectangular timbers than round timbers
   B. round timbers than rectangular timbers
   C. triangular timbers than round timbers
   D. round timbers than triangular timbers

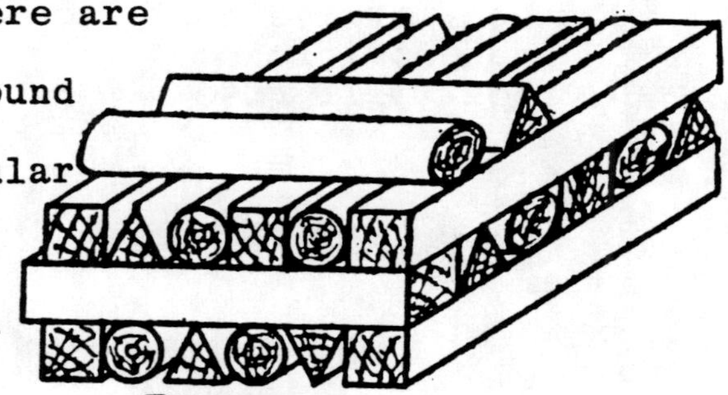
TIMBERS

79. The form shown, which is open at both ends, can be shaped from metal sheet number
   A. 2   B. 3
   C. 1   D. 4

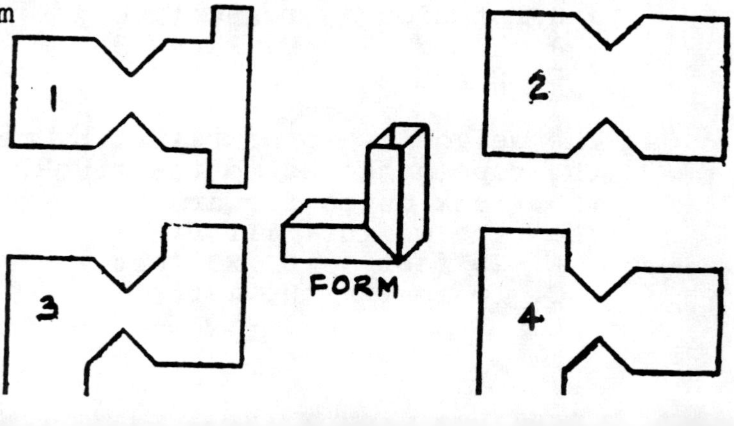

80. In order to fill the three reservoirs with air from the compressor, the LEAST number of valves to be opened or closed from their normal position is
   A. 1 B. 3 C. 4 D. 5

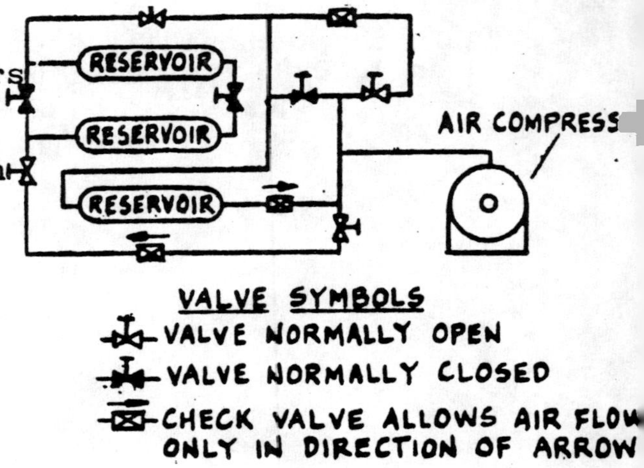

81. If the contacts come together once every second, the cam is rotating at
   A. 30 RPM B. 55 RPM
   C. 65 RPM D. 78 RPM

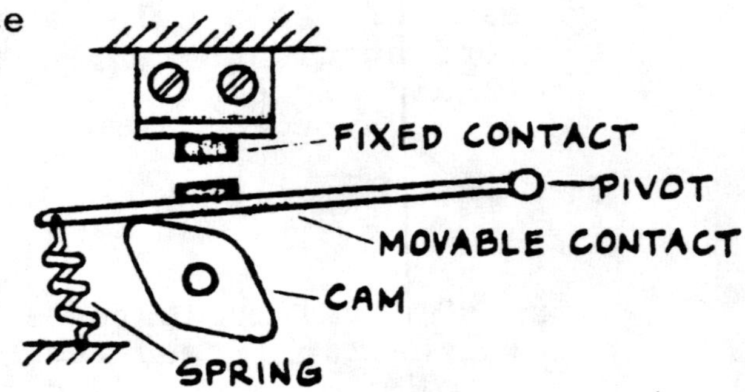

82. If the float in the tank develops a bad leak, then the
   A. flow of fuel will stop
   B. float will stay in the position shown
   C. needle valve will remain in the open position
   D. float will rise

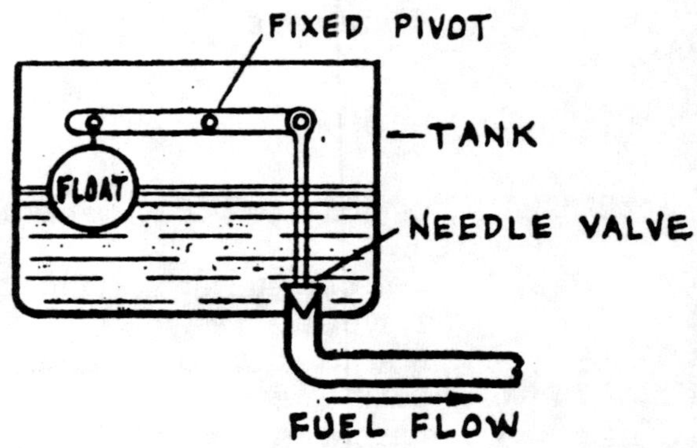

83. A cold chisel is shown in position 1 or 2 and the grinding wheel is shown with directions of rotation 3 or 4. To properly sharpen the cold chisel, the CORRECT combination of position and rotation is, respectively,
   A. 1 and 4 B. 1 and 3
   C. 2 and 4 D. 2 and 3

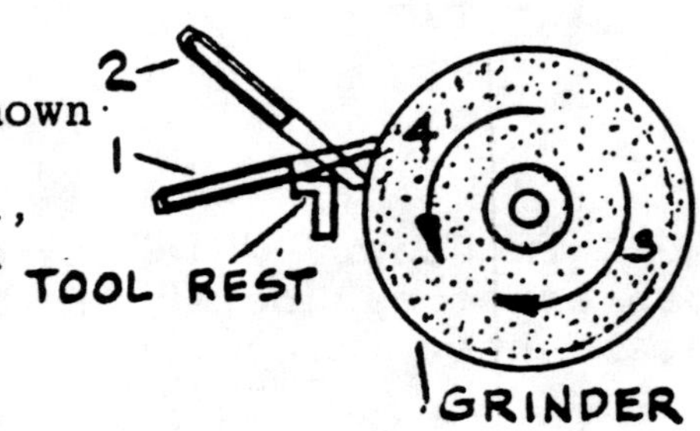

84. The weight is to be raised by means of the rope attached to the truck. If the truck moves forward 20 feet, then the weight will rise
   A. 25 feet B. 20 feet
   C. 10 feet D. 4 feet

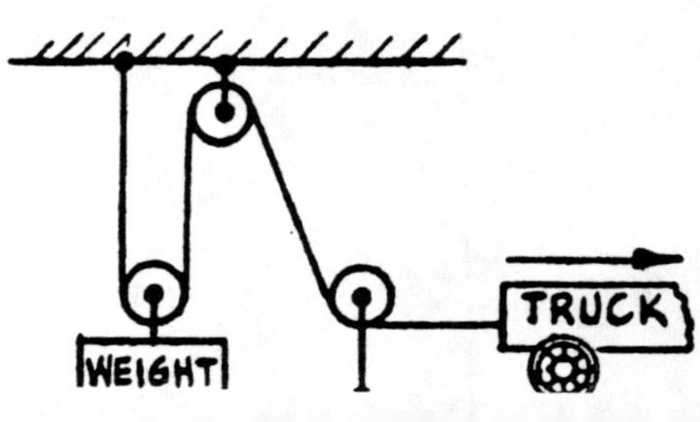

Questions 85-94.
DIRECTIONS: Questions 85 to 94 inclusive in Column I are tools or instruments. The proper use of each tool or instrument is listed in Column II. For each tool or instrument listed in Column I, select the PROPER use from Column II. Print on your answer sheet in the correspondingly numbered item space, the letter given beside your selected use.

COLUMN I (Tool or Instrument)

85. Gage blocks
86. Feeler gage
87. Plumb bob
88. Dial test indicator
89. Pair of V blocks
90. Spirit level
91. Protractor
92. Carpenter's try-square
93. Concentricity gage
94. Scleroscope

COLUMN II (Use)

A. to true up work in a lathe
B. to accurately check measuring instruments
C. to hold cylindrical work in accurate alignment for drilling
D. to test hardness of metals
E. to test alignment of two holes of different diameters
H. to establish a long perpendicular line on a wall surface
J. to check a corner of a piece of work for squareness
K. to horizontally align a piece of work
L. to measure small clearances between adjacent parts
M. to establish and measure angles

85. ...
86. ...
87. ...
88. ...
89. ...
90. ...
91. ...
92. ...
93. ...
94. ...

95. Employees of the department are cautioned not to use water to extinguish fires caused by high voltage arcing. The MOST likely reason for this rule is that water 95. ...
   A. may conduct the electrical current and create a shock hazard
   B. coming into contact with a hot electrical arc causes asphyxiating fumes to be generated
   C. will cause corrosion of sensitive electrical parts
   D. would cause fuses to blow in the electrical circuits

96. From the standpoint of management, the MOST desirable characteristic in a newly appointed helper would be 96. ...
A. the lack of outside personal interests
B. the ability to keep to himself and away from the other employees
C. the ability to satisfactorily perform his assigned duties
D. eagerness to ask questions about all phases of the work

97. There are a few workers who are seemingly prone to accidents and who, regardless of their assigned job, have a higher accident rate than the average worker. If your co-worker is known to be such an individual, the BEST course for you to pursue would be to 97. ...
A. do most of the assigned work yourself
B. refuse to work with this individual
C. provide him with a copy of all rules and regulations
D. personally check all safety precautions on each job

98. The MOST logical method to use in providing shop employees with quick assistance in the case of minor injuries is to 98. ...
A. instruct most of the employees in first-aid techniques
B. have at least two or three doctors always on the premises
C. provide every employee with a first-aid kit
D. have at least two or three nurses always ready to render assistance

99. Tolerances on machine work are USUALLY expressed in 99. ...
A. millionths of an inch
B. thousandths of an inch
C. hundredths of an inch
D. tenths of an inch

100. Goggles are NOT necessary when 100. ...
A. welding
B. burning with an oxy-acetylene torch
C. soldering copper plates
D. grinding a tool on an emergy wheel

KEY (CORRECT ANSWERS)

1.	D	21.	D	41.	C	61.	C	81.	A
2.	A	22.	C	42.	A	62.	C	82.	C
3.	D	23.	B	44.	C	63.	B	83.	A
4.	D	24.	C	44.	D	64.	C	84.	C
5.	B	25.	P	45.	C	65.	A	85.	B
6.	C	26.	T	46.	D	66.	B	86.	L
7.	C	27.	K	47.	A	67.	B	87.	H
8.	B	28.	W	48.	C	68.	A	88.	A
9.	C	29.	A	49.	B	69.	D	89.	C
10.	B	30.	C	50.	B	70.	D	90.	K
11.	A	31.	S	51.	B	71.	C	91.	M
12.	A	32.	M	52.	C	72.	D	92.	J
13.	D	33.	H	53.	B	73.	B	93.	E
14.	A	34.	V	54.	C	74.	C	94.	D
15.	C	35.	C	55.	A	75.	C	95.	A
16.	D	36.	D	56.	B	76.	B	96.	C
17.	D	37.	D	57.	B	77.	B	97.	D
18.	C	38.	C	58.	A	78.	C	98.	A
19.	B	39.	B	59.	D	79.	B	99.	B
20.	A	40.	A	60.	C	80.	A	100.	C

MECHANICAL APTITUDE

EXAMINATION SECTION

TEST 1

MECHANICAL COMPREHENSION

DIRECTIONS: Questions 1 to 4 test your ability to understand general mechanical devices. Pictures are shown and questions asked about the mechanical devices shown in the picture. Read each question and study the picture. Each question is followed by four choices. For each question, choose the one BEST answer (A,B,C,or D). Then *PRINT THE LETTER OF THE CORRECT ANSWER IN THE SPACE AT THE RIGHT.*

1. The reason for crossing the belt connecting these wheels is to 1. ____

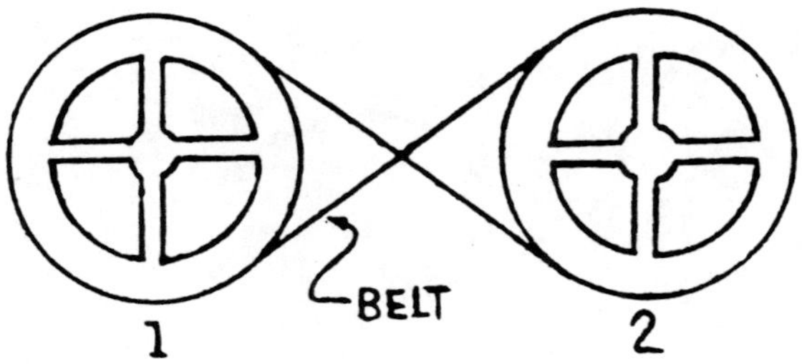

A. make the wheels turn in opposite directions
B. make wheel 2 turn faster than wheel 1
C. save wear on the belt
D. take up slack in the belt

2. The purpose of the small gear between the two large gears is to 2. ____

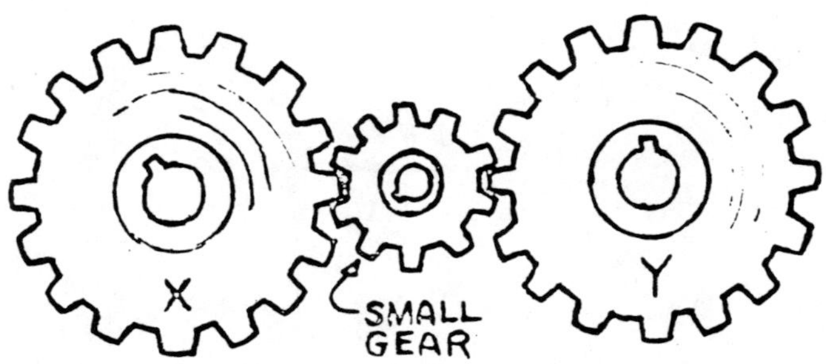

A. increase the speed of the larger gears
B. allow the larger gears to turn in different directions
C. decrease the speed of the larger gears
D. make the larger gears turn in the same direction

3. Each of these three-foot-high water cans have a bottom with an area of one square foot. The pressure on the bottom of the cans is 3. ____

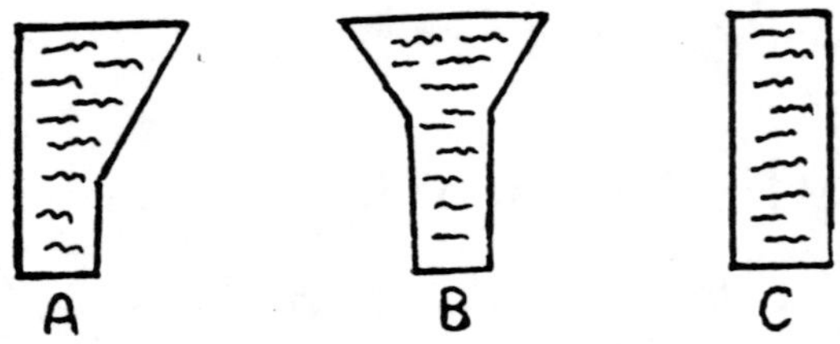

A. least in A
B. least in B
C. least in C
D. the same in all

4. The reading on the scale should be 4. ____

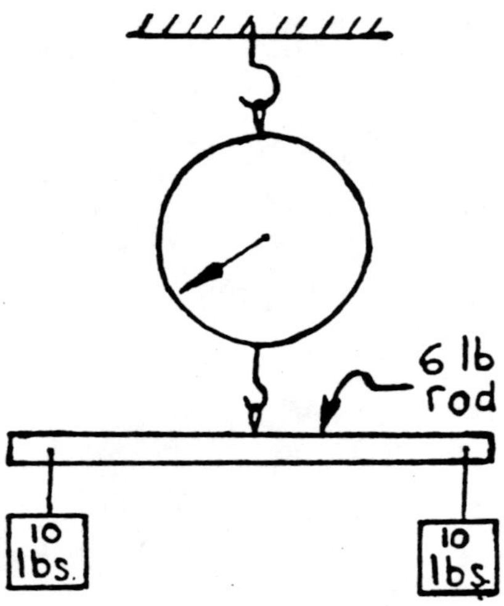

A. zero
B. 10 pounds
C. 13 pounds
D. 26 pounds

KEY (CORRECT ANSWERS)

1. A
2. D
3. D
4. D

TEST 2

TOOLS AND THEIR USE

DIRECTIONS: Questions 1 to 6 test knowledge of tools and how to use them. For each question, decide which one of the four things shown in the boxes labeled A,B,C,or D normally is used with or goes best with the thing in the picture on the left. Then *PRINT THE LETTER OF THE CORRECT ANSWER IN THE SPACE AT THE RIGHT*.

NOTE: All tools are NOT drawn to the same scale.

1. 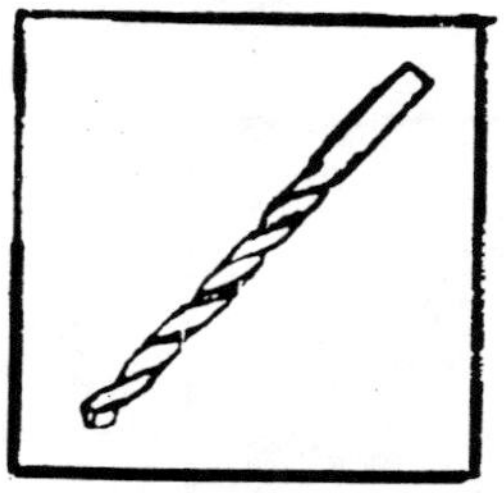

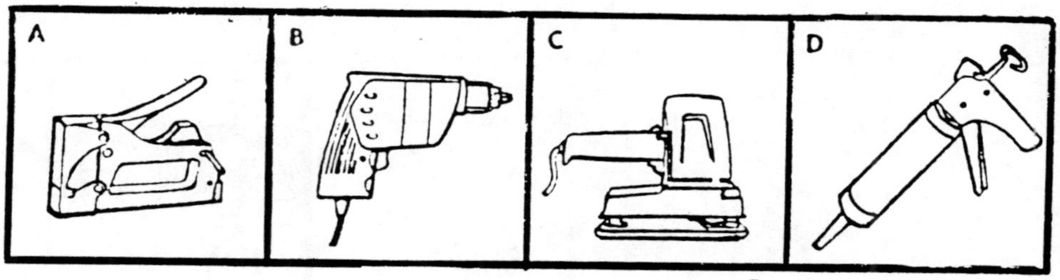

1. ____

2. 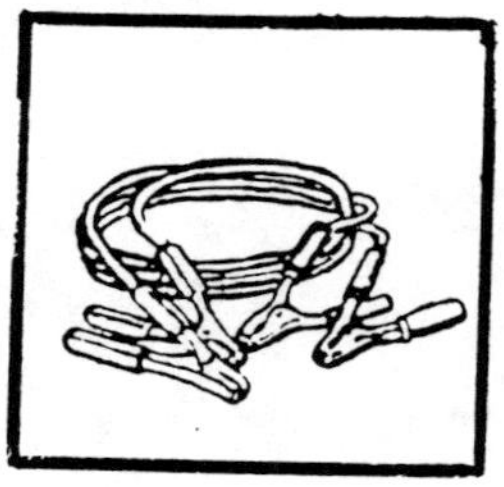

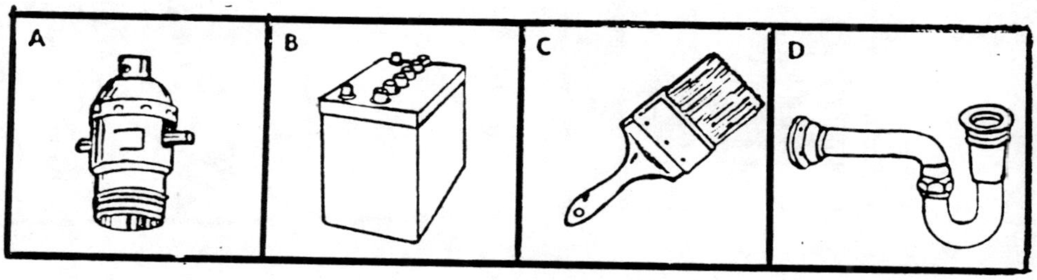

2. ____

3. 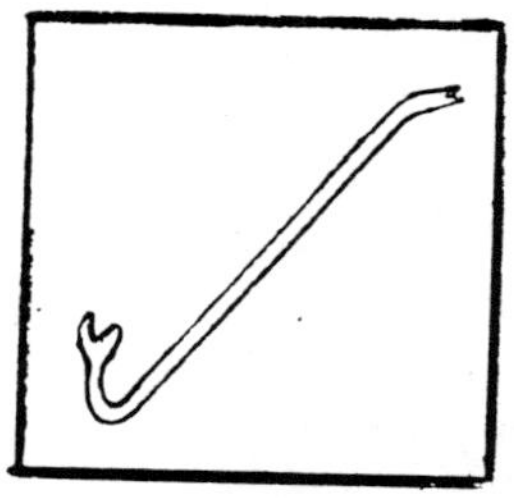

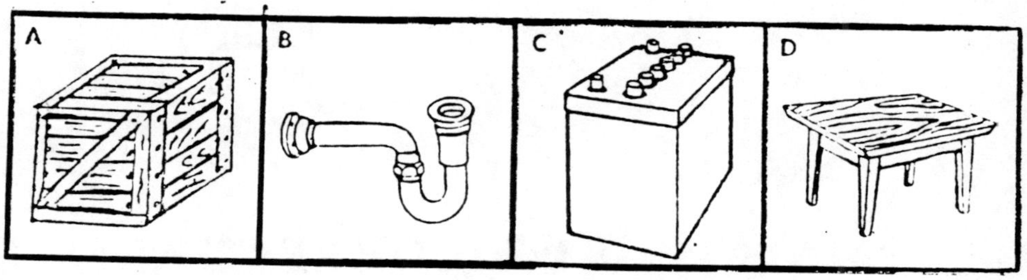

3. ____

4.

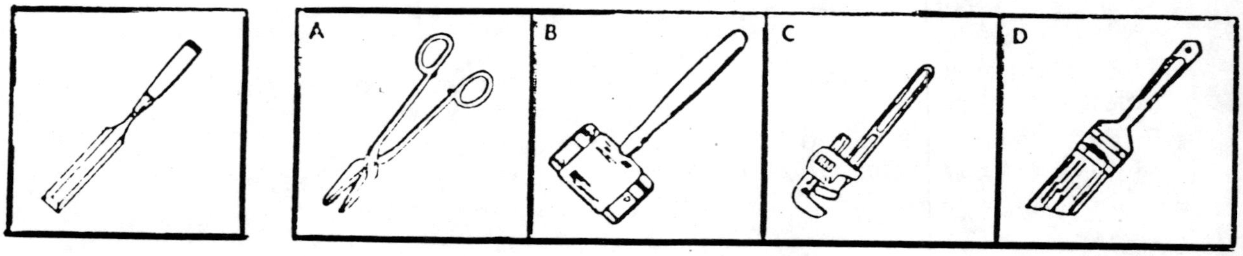

4. ___

5.

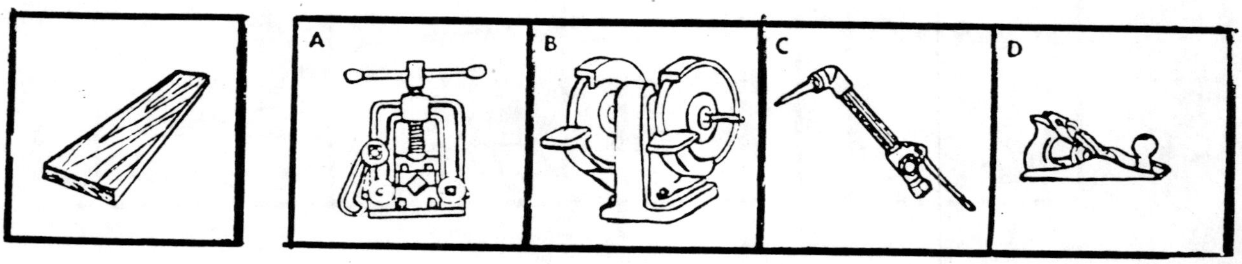

5. ___

6.

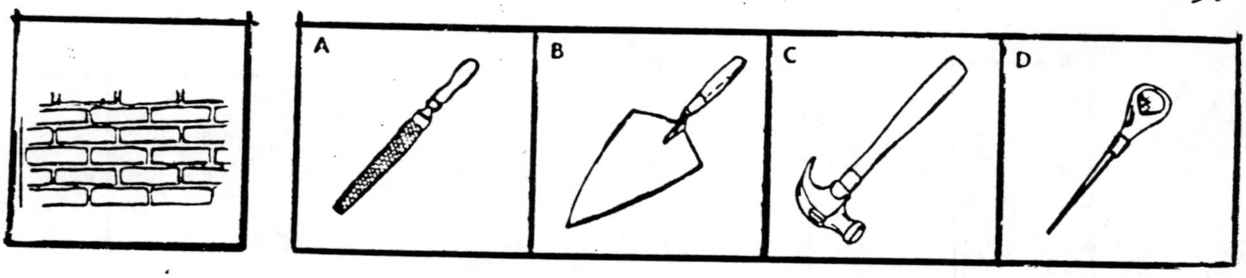

6. ___

KEY (CORRECT ANSWERS)

1. B
2. B
3. A
4. B
5. D
6. B

MECHANICAL APTITUDE

EXAMINATION SECTION

QUESTIONS 1-6.

Questions 1 through 6 are questions designed to test your ability to distinguish identical forms from unlike forms.

In each question, there are five drawings, lettered A, B, C, D, and E. Four of the drawings are alike. You are to find the one drawing that is different from the other four in the question. Then, on the Answer Sheet, blacken the space lettered the same as the figure that you have selected.

1. 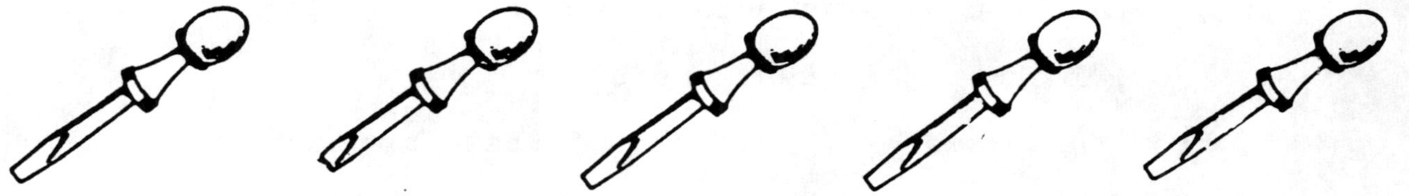

A B C D E

2. 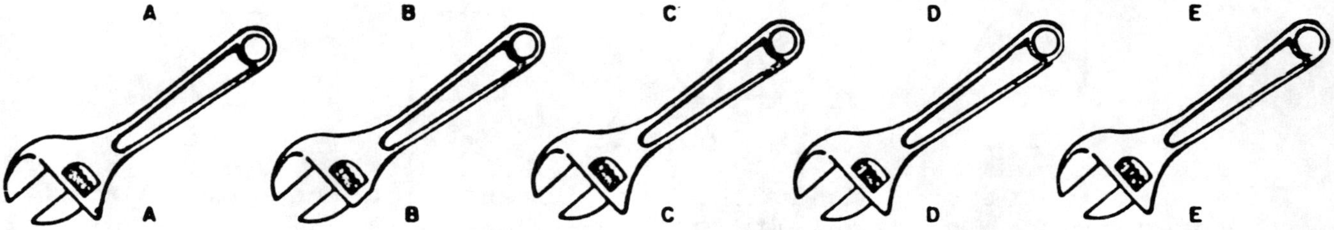

A B C D E

3. 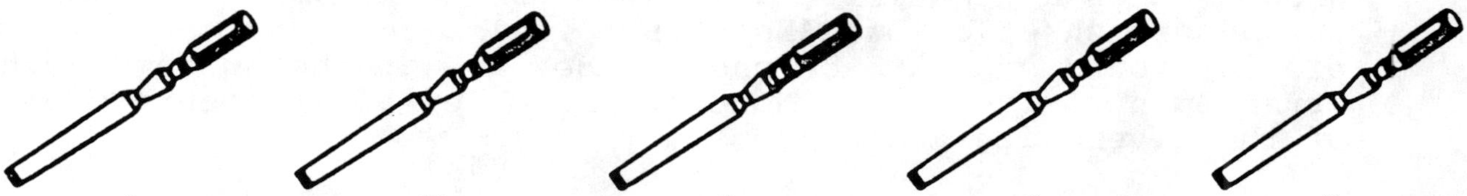

A B C D E

4. 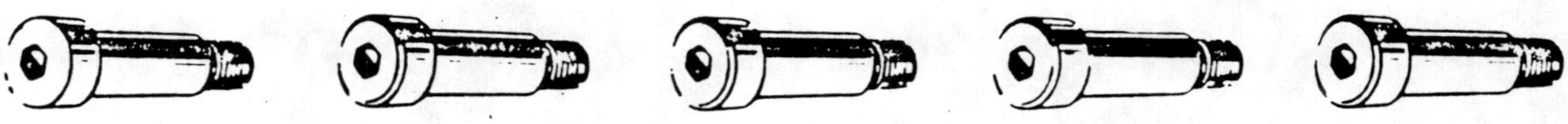

A B C D E

5. 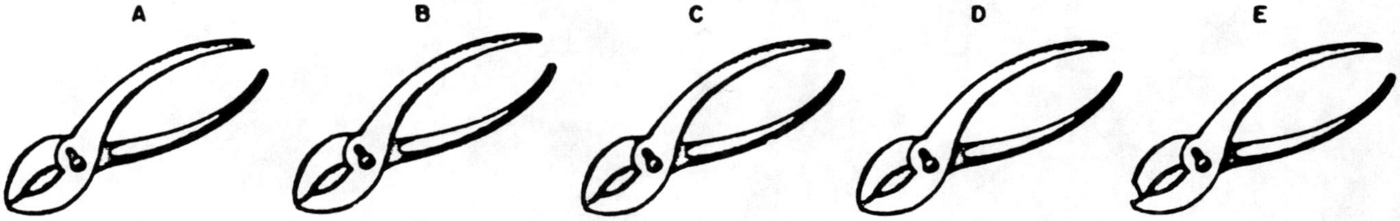

A B C D E

6. 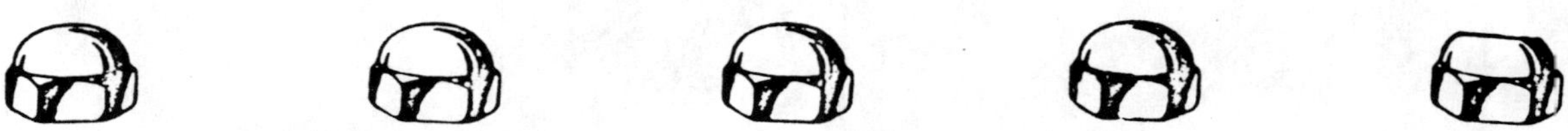

A B C D E

ANSWER SHEET

1 Ⓐ Ⓑ Ⓒ Ⓓ Ⓔ   4 Ⓐ Ⓑ Ⓒ Ⓓ Ⓔ

2 Ⓐ Ⓑ Ⓒ Ⓓ Ⓔ   5 Ⓐ Ⓑ Ⓒ Ⓓ Ⓔ

3 Ⓐ Ⓑ Ⓒ Ⓓ Ⓔ   6 Ⓐ Ⓑ Ⓒ Ⓓ Ⓔ

QUESTIONS 7-8.

Questions 7 and 8 are questions designed to test your knowledge of pattern matching.

Questions 7 and 8 present problems found in making patterns. Each shows, at the left side, two or more separate flat pieces. In each question , select the arrangement lettered A, B, C, or D that shows how these pieces at the left can be fitted together without gaps or overlapping. The pieces may be turned around or turned over in any way to make them fit together.

On the Answer Sheet blacken the space lettered the same as the figure that you have selected.

Now, look at the questions below.

7. From these pieces, *WHICH ONE* of these arrangements can you make?

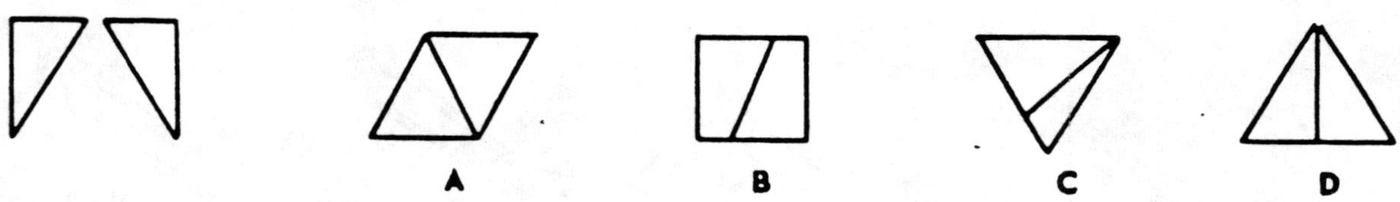

In question 7, only the arrangement D can be made from the pieces shown at the left, so space D is marked for Question 7 on the answer sheet below. (Note that it is necessary to turn the pieces around so that the short sides are at the bottom in the arrangement lettered D. None of the other arrangements show pieces of the given size and shape.)

8. From these pieces, *WHICH ONE* of these arrangements can you make?

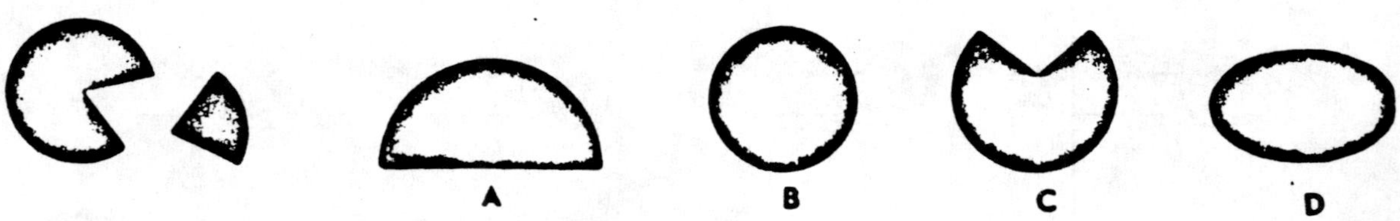

ANSWER SHEET

7 Ⓐ Ⓑ Ⓒ Ⓓ

8 Ⓐ Ⓑ Ⓒ Ⓓ

QUESTIONS 9-10.

Questions 9 and 10. are questions designed to test your ability to identify forms of *LIKE* and *UNLIKE* proportions.

In each of the questions, select from the drawings of objects labeled A, B, C, and D, the one that would have the Top, Front, and Right views shown in the drawing at the left. Then on your Answer Sheet blacken the space that has the same letter as your answer.

9.

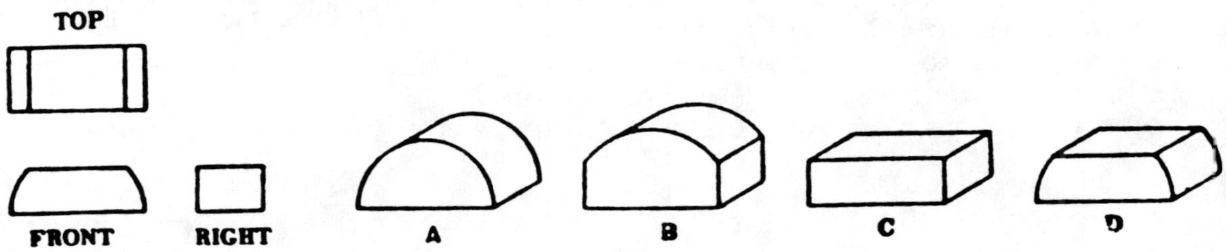

10.

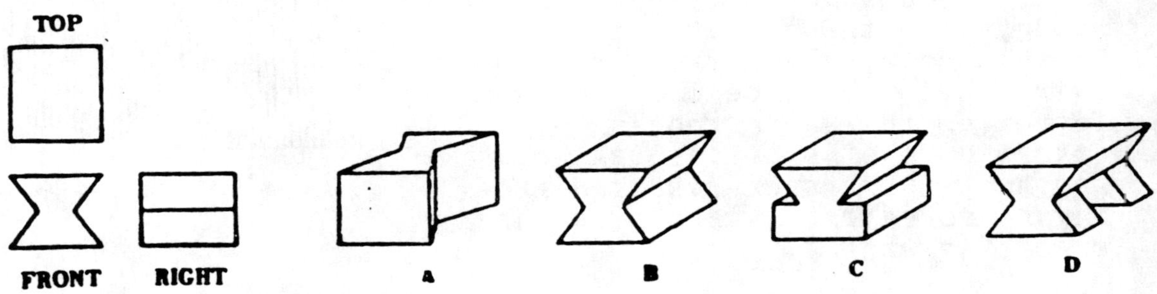

ANSWER SHEET

9 (A) (B) (C) (D)

10 (A) (B) (C) (D)

QUESTIONS 11-14.
Explanation and Commentary:

In each question, *ONE* rectangle is clearly *WRONG*. For each question, use the measuirng gage to check each of the rectangles and to find the *WRONG* one. Do this by putting the measuring gage rectangle on the question rectangle with the same letter so that the rectangles slightly overlap and the thin lines are parallel, like the one at the right. In this case, the height of the question rectangle exactly matches the height of the measuring gage rectangle, so the question rectangle is the right height. In this case, you do *NOT* mark your answer sheet.

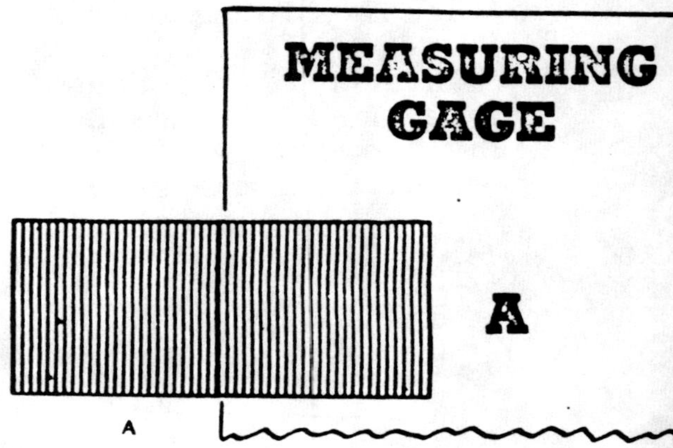

Once in every question, when you put a measuring gage rectangle on a question rectangle, you will find that the heights do *NOT* match and that the question rectangle is clearly wrong, like the one at the right. In this case, you mark on the answer sheet the space with the same letter as the *WRONG* rectangle. *REMEMBER TO LINE UP THE MEASURING RECTANGLE WITH EACH QUESTION RECTANGLE SO THAT THE THIN LINES ARE EXACTLY PARALLEL.*

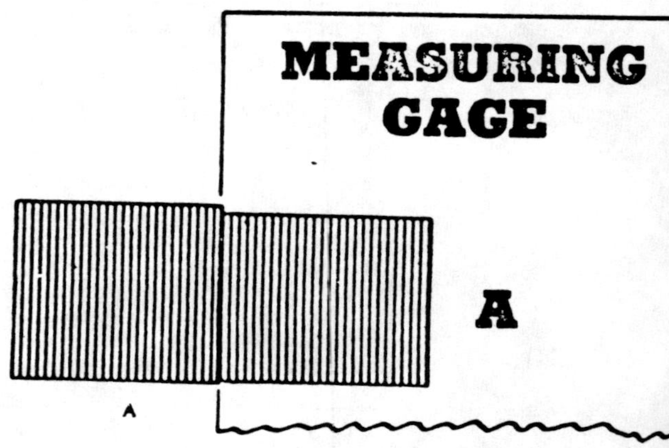

Now, cut out the measuring gage on the last page and practice on the questions. The test will be timed, so practice doing them rapidly and accurately.

Questions 11 through 14 test how quickly and accurately you can check the heights of rectangles with a measuring gage. Each question has five rectangles of different heights. The height is the dimension that runs the same way as the thin lines.

11.

12.

13.

14.

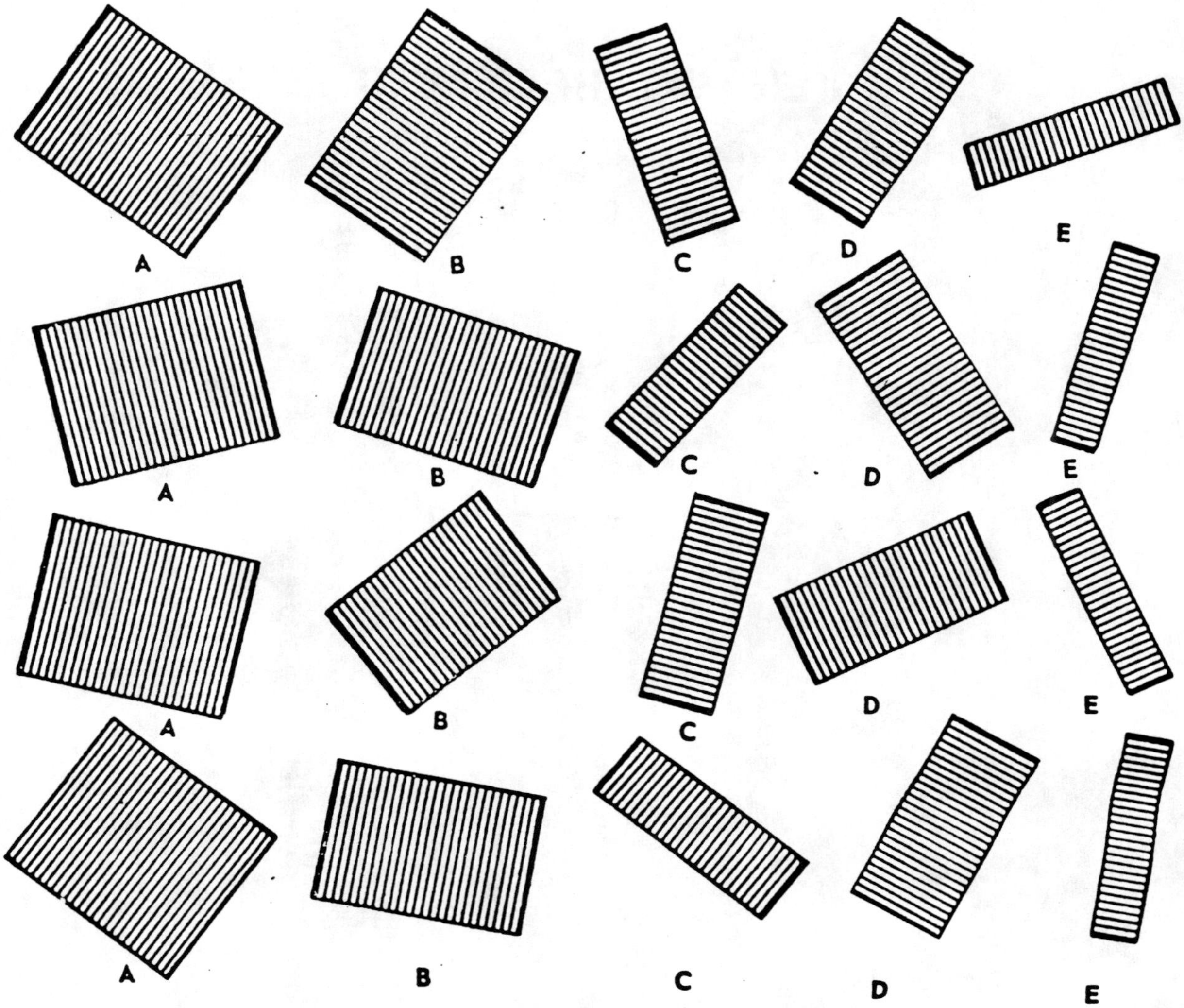

ANSWER SHEET

11 Ⓐ Ⓑ Ⓒ Ⓓ Ⓔ

12 Ⓐ Ⓑ Ⓒ Ⓓ Ⓔ

13 Ⓐ Ⓑ Ⓒ Ⓓ Ⓔ

14 Ⓐ Ⓑ Ⓒ Ⓓ Ⓔ

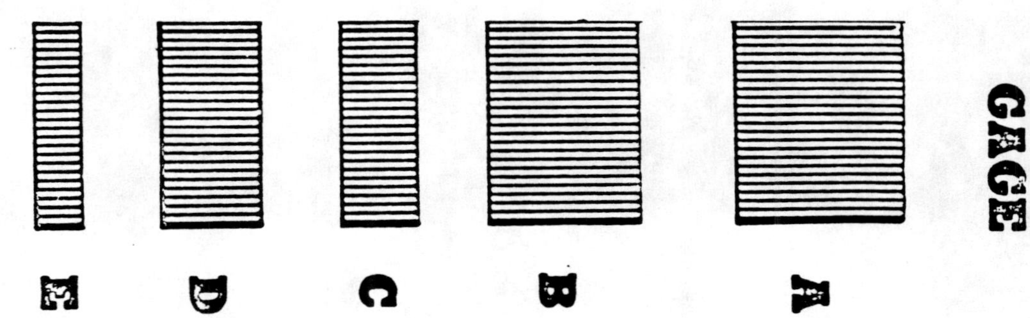

KEY (CORRECT ANSWERS)

1. B
2. B
3. C
4. A
5. E
6. E
7. D
8. B
9. D
10. B
11. D
12. C
13. B
14. A

EXAMINATION SECTION

DIRECTIONS: Each question or incomplete statement is followed by two suggested answers or completions. Select A or B, or C if the two figures have the same value, as the BEST answer that completes the statement or completes the statement. *PRINT THE LETTER OF THE CORRECT ANSWER IN THE SPACE AT THE RIGHT.*

1. 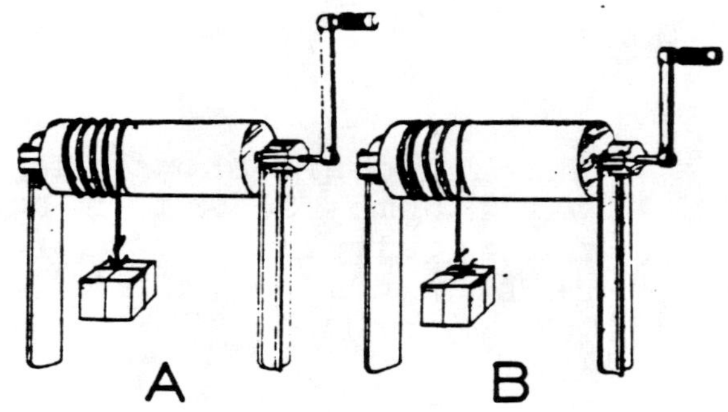

With which windlass can a man raise the heavier weight? 1.___

2. 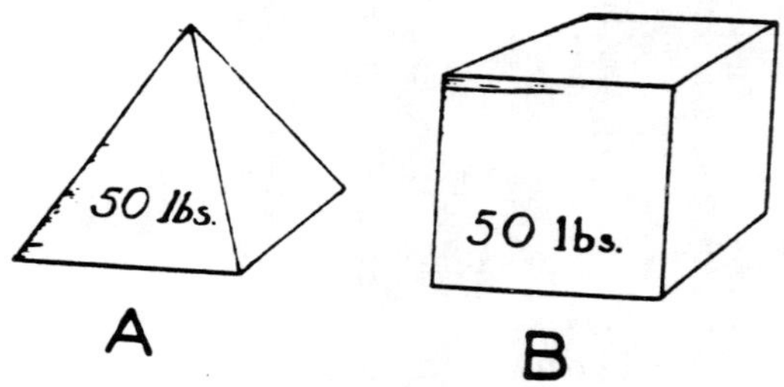

Which of these solid blocks will be the harder to tip over? 2.___

3. 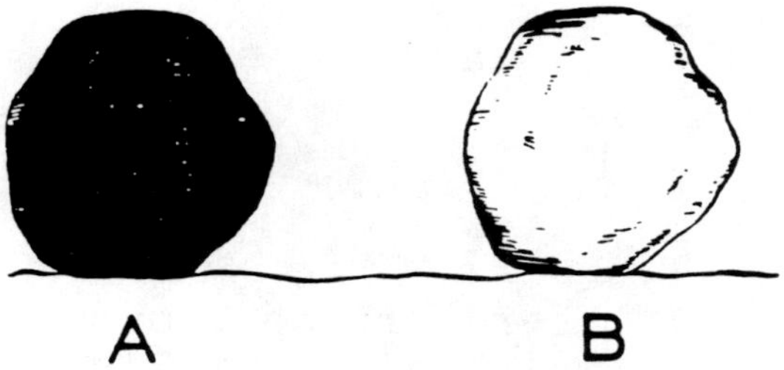

Which rock will get hotter in the sun? 3.___

4. 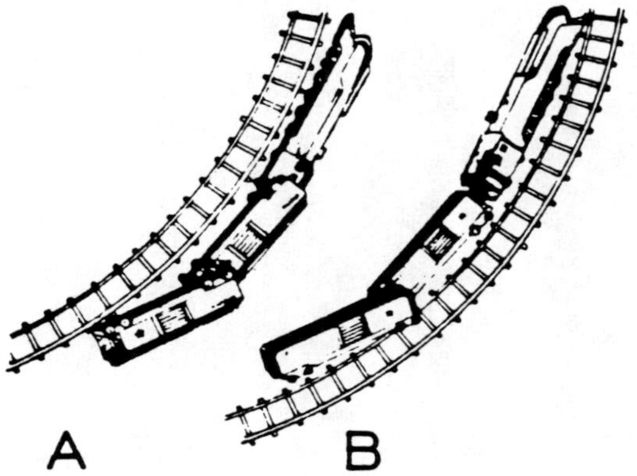

Which of these is the more likely picture of a train wreck? 4.___

5.

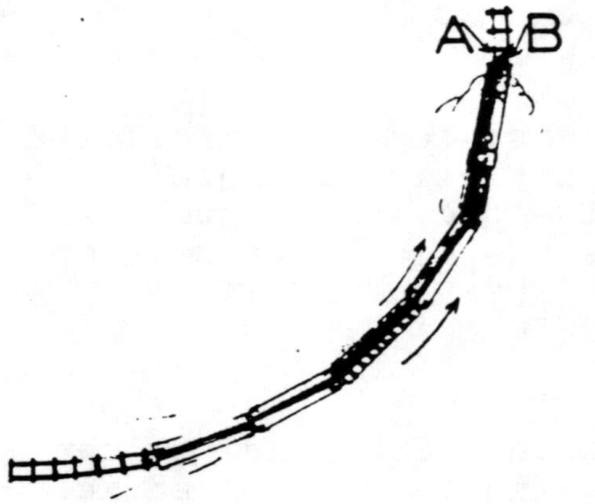

If the track is exactly level, on which rail does more pressure come?

5.____

6.

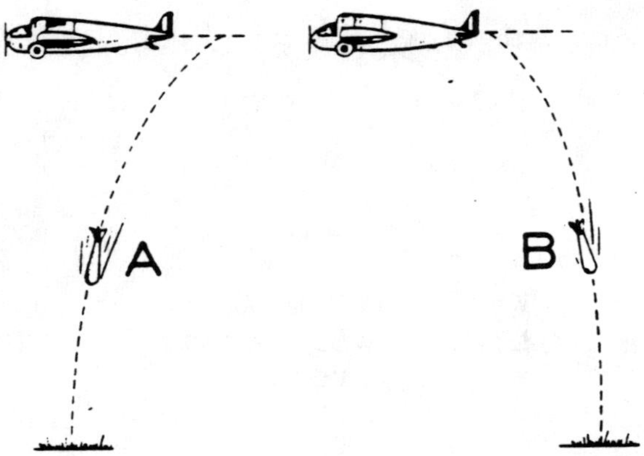

Which picture shows the way a bomb falls from a moving airplane if there is no wind?

6.____

7.

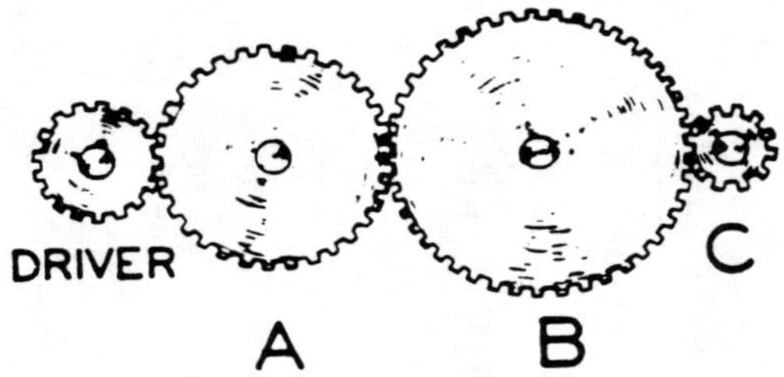

Indicate a gear which turn the same direction as the driver.

7.____

8.

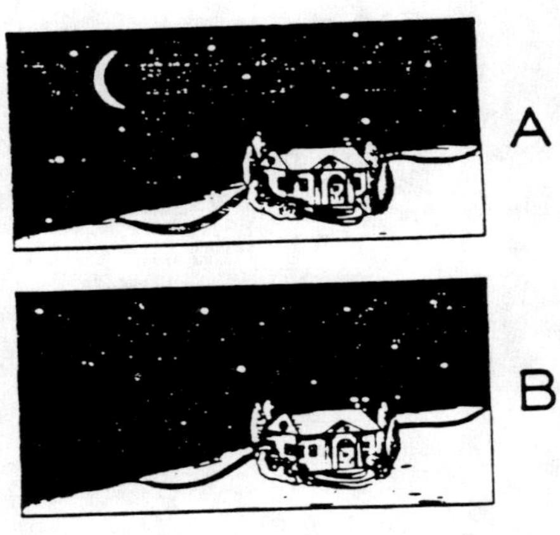

If there are no clouds, on which night will you be able to see more stars?

8.____

9. 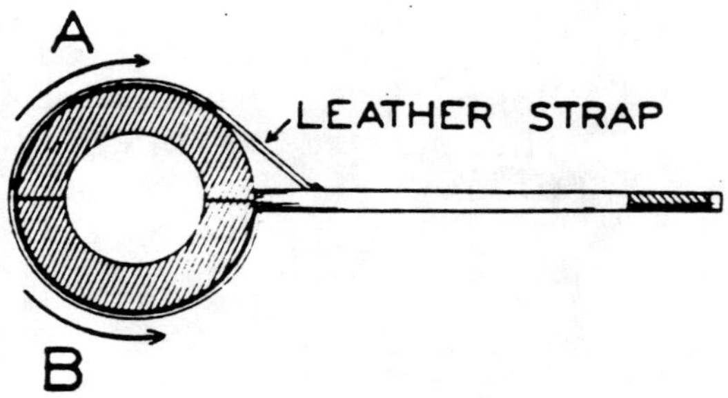

This wrench can be used to turn the pipe in direction: 9.___

10. 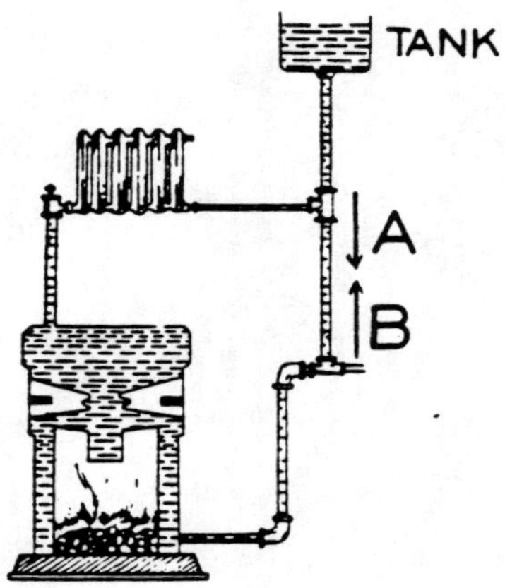

In which direction does the water in the right-hand pipe go? 10.___

11. 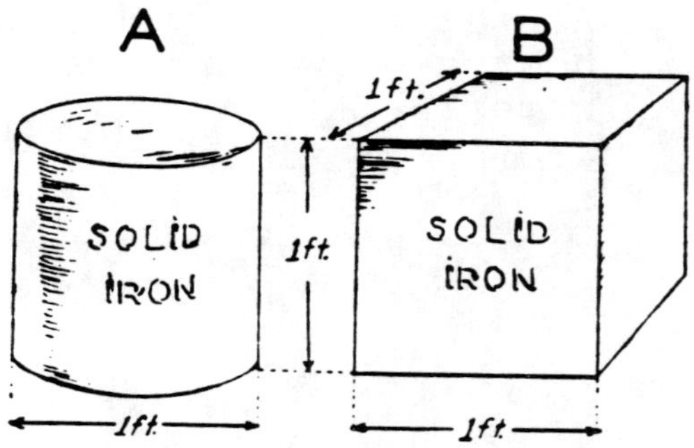

Which weighs more? 11.___

12. 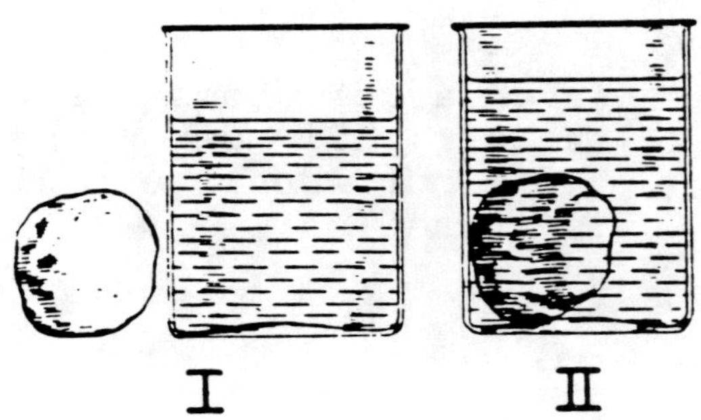

If the rock and tank of water together in picture I weigh 100 pounds, what will they weigh in picture II? 12.___

13. 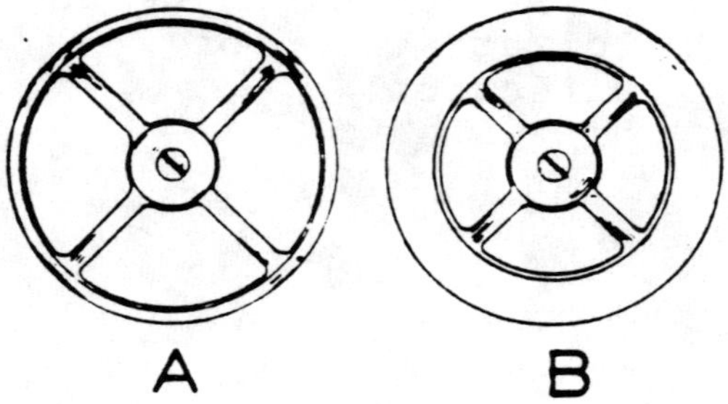

Which steel wheel will keep going longer after the power has been shut off? 13.___

14. 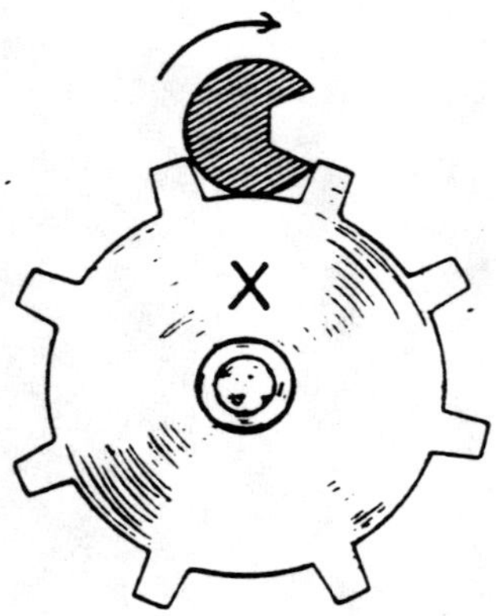

The top of the wheel *X* will go 14.___
  A. steadily to the right
  B. steadily to the left
  C. by jerks to the left

15. 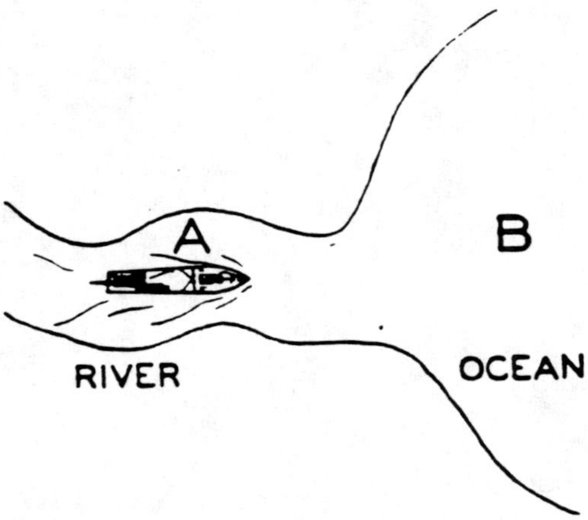

At which point will the boat be lower in the water? 15.___

16. 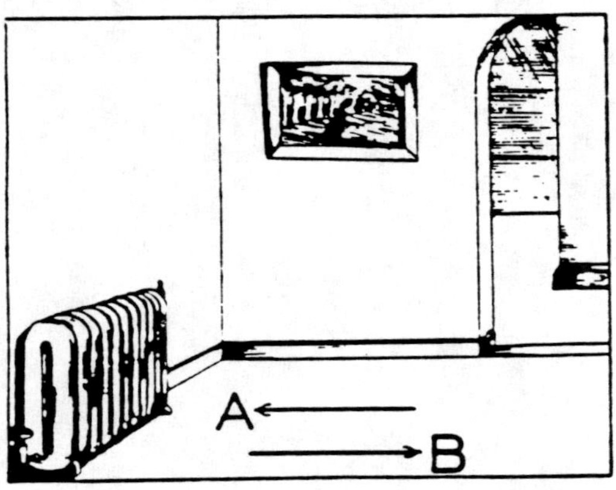

Which arrow shows the way the air will move along the floor when the radiator is turned on? 16.___

17. 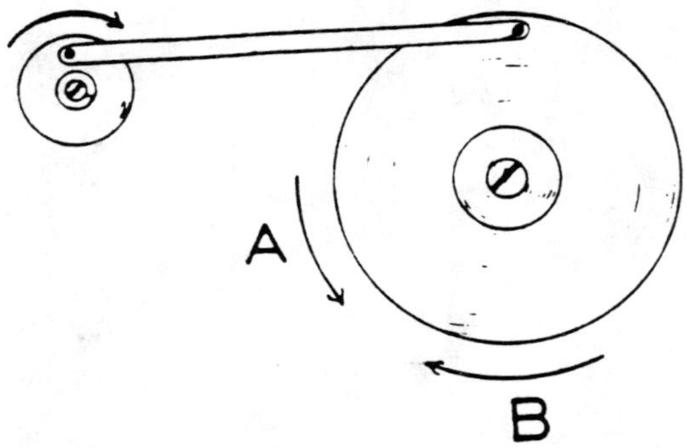

When the little wheel turns around, the big wheel will
- A. turn in direction A
- B. turn in direction B
- C. move back and forth

17.___

18. 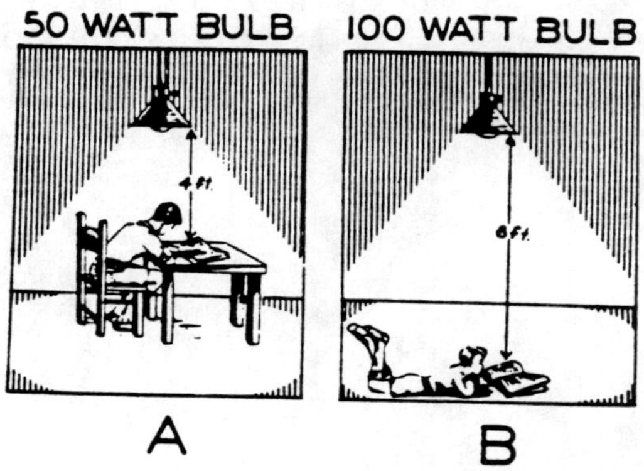

Which boy gets more light on the pages of his book?

18.___

19. 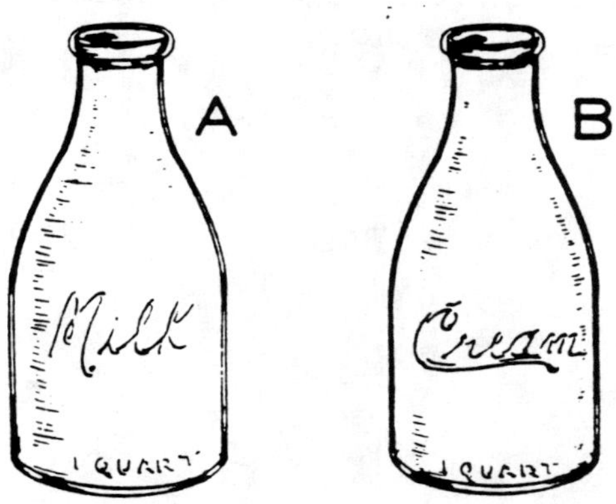

Which weighs more?

19.___

20. 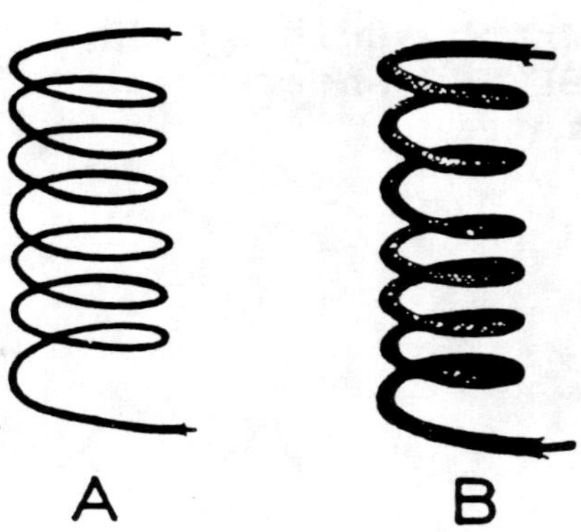

Which of these wires offers more resistance to the passage of an electric current?

20.___

21. 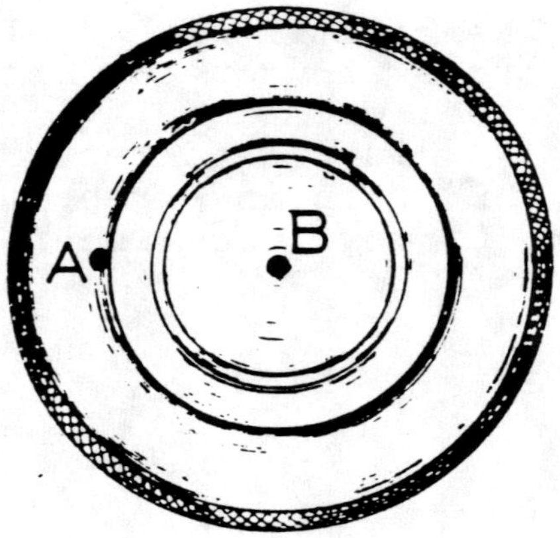

Which spot on the wheel travels faster? 21.___

22. 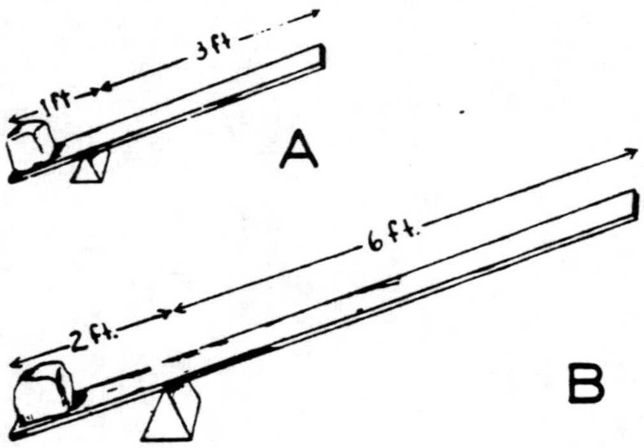

With which arrangement can a man lift the heavier weight? 22.___

23. 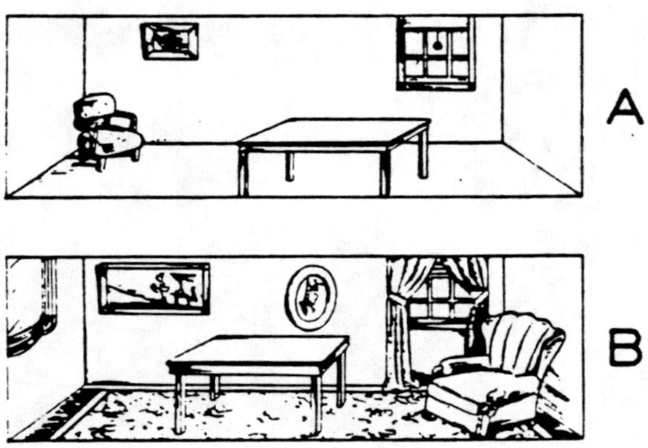

Which room has more of an echo? 23.___

24. 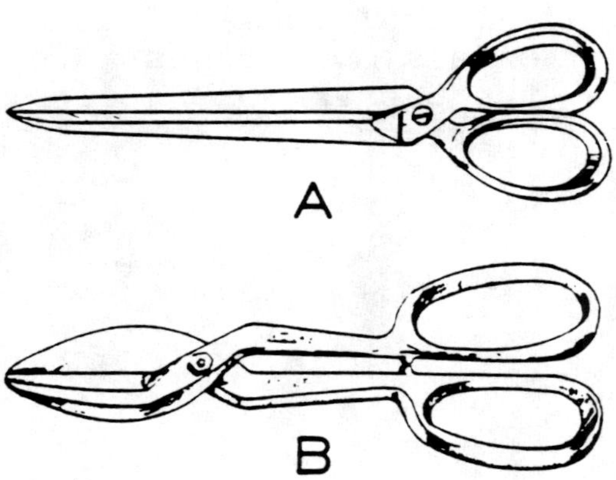

Which would be the BETTER shears for cutting metal? 24.___

KEY (CORRECT ANSWERS)

1. B
2. A
3. A
4. A
5. B

6. A
7. B
8. B
9. A
10. A

11. B
12. C
13. A
14. C
15. A

16. B
17. C
18. B
19. B
20. B

21. B
22. A
23. A
24. B

MECHANICAL APTITUDE

MECHANICAL COMPREHENSION

EXAMINATION SECTION

DIRECTIONS FOR THIS SECTION:
Each question or incomplete statement below is followed by several suggested answers or completions. Select the *one* that *BEST* answers the question or completes the statement. *PRINT THE LETTER OF THE CORRECT ANSWER IN THE SPACE AT THE RIGHT.*

TEST 1

Questions 1-3.

DIRECTIONS: Questions 1 to 3 inclusive are based upon the following paragraph.

The only openings permitted in fire partitions except openings for ventilating ducts shall be those required for doors. There shall be but one such door opening unless the provision of additional openings would not exceed, in total width of all doorways, 25 percent of the length of the wall. The minimum distance between openings shall be three feet. The maximum area for such a door opening shall be 80 square feet, except that such openings for the passage of motor trucks may be a maximum of 140 square feet.

1. According to the above paragraph, openings in fire partitions are permitted *only* for 1. ...
   A. doors B. doors and windows
   C. doors and ventilation ducts
   D. doors, windows, and ventilation ducts

2. In a fire partition, 22 feet long and 10 feet high, the *MAXIMUM* number of doors, 3 feet wide and 7 feet high, is 2. ...
   A. 1 B. 2 C. 3 D. 4

3. 3. ...

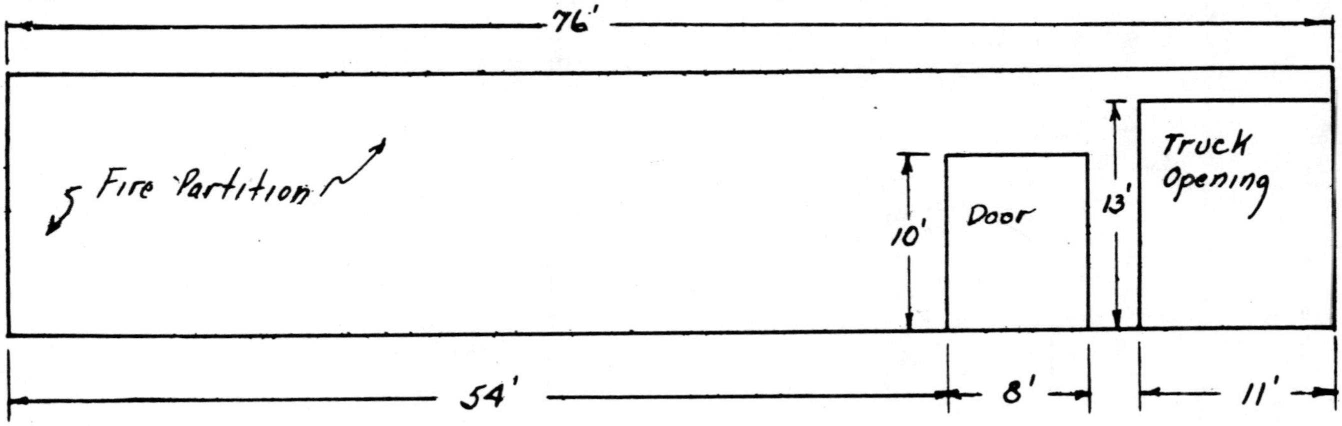

The *one* of the following statements about the layout shown above that is *MOST* accurate is that the
   A. total width of the openings is too large
   B. truck opening is too large
   C. truck and door openings are too close together
   D. layout is acceptable

4. At a given temperature, a wet hand will freeze to a bar of metal, but *NOT* to a piece of wood, *because* the 4. ...
   A. metal expands and contracts more than the wood
   B. wood is softer than the metal
   C. wood will burn at a lower temperature than the metal
   D. metal is a better conductor of heat than the wood

5. Of the following items commonly found in a household, the *one* that uses the *MOST* electric current is a(n) 5. ...
A. 150-watt light bulb B. toaster
C. door buzzer D. 8" electric fan

6. Sand and ashes are frequently placed on icy pavements to prevent skidding. The effect of the sand and ashes is to increase 6. ...
A. inertia B. gravity C. momentum D. friction

7. The air near the ceiling of a room usually is warmer than the air near the floor because 7. ...
A. there is better air circulation at the floor level
B. warm air is lighter than cold air
C. windows usually are nearer the floor than the ceiling
D. heating pipes usually run along the ceiling

8. 8. ...

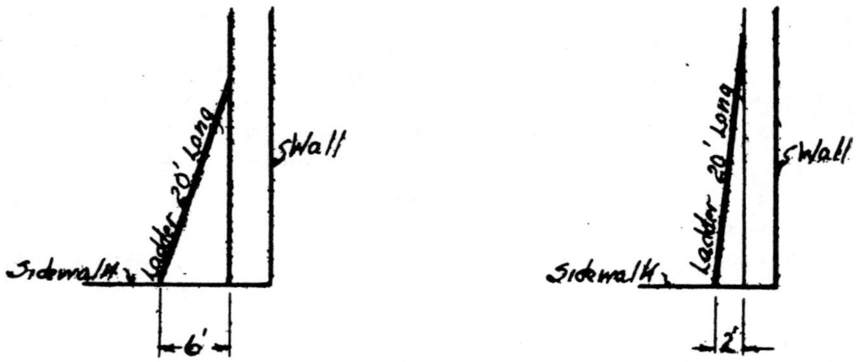

DIA. 1 DIA. 2

It is safer to use the ladder positioned as shown in diagram 1 than as shown in diagram 2 because, in diagram 1,
A. less strain is placed upon the center rungs of the ladder
B. it is easier to grip and stand on the ladder
C. the ladder reaches a lower height
D. the latter is less likely to tip over backwards

9. 9. ...

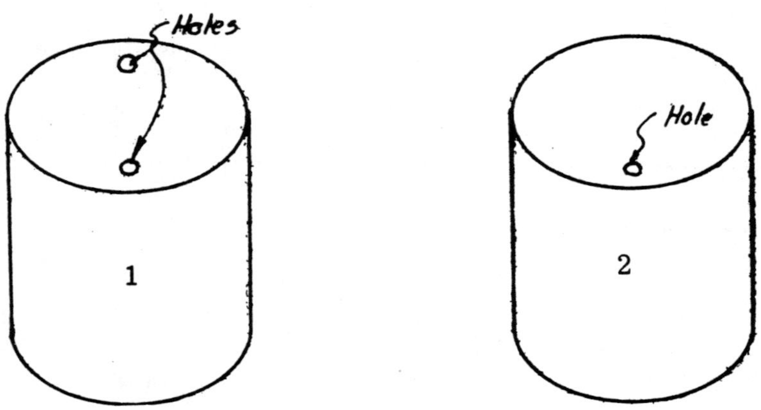

It is *easier* to pour a liquid from:
A. Can 1 because there are two holes from which the liquid can flow
B. Can 1 because air can enter through one hole while the liquid comes out the other hole

C. Can 2 because the liquid comes out under greater pressure
D. Can 2 because it is easier to direct the flow of the liquid when there is only one hole

10. A substance which is subject to "spontaneous combustion" is one that 10. ...
A. is explosive when heated
B. is capable of catching fire without an external source of heat
C. acts to speed up the burning of material
D. liberates oxygen when heated

11. The sudden shutting down of a nozzle on a hose discharging water under high pressure is a *bad* practice *CHIEFLY* because the 11. ...
A. hose is likely to whip about violently
B. hose is likely to burst
C. valve handle is likely to snap
D. valve handle is likely to jam

12. Fire can continue where there are present fuel, oxygen from the air or other source, and a sufficiently high temperature to maintain combustion. The method of extinguishment of fire *MOST* commonly used is to 12. ...
A. remove the fuel
B. exclude the oxygen from the burning material
C. reduce the temperature of the burning material
D. smother the flames of the burning material

13. 13. ...

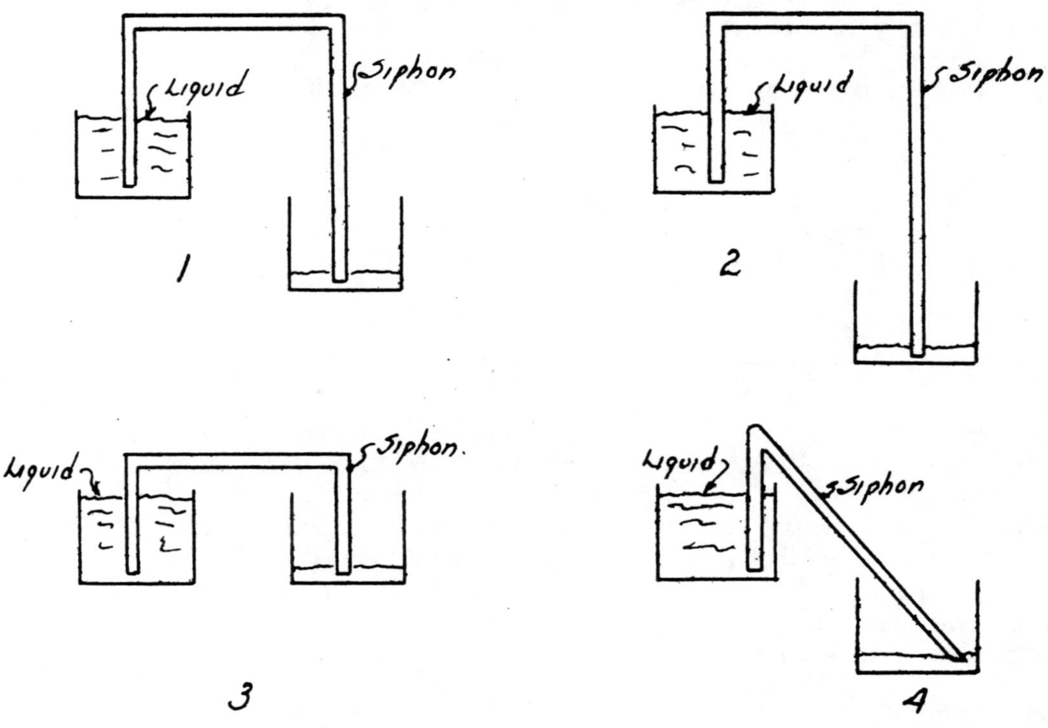

The *one* of the siphon arrangements shown above which would *MOST* quickly transfer a solution from the container on the left side to the one on the right side is numbered
A. 1 B. 2 C. 3 D. 4

14. Static electricity is a hazard in industry *CHIEFLY* because it may cause 14. ...
A. dangerous or painful burns
B. chemical decomposition of toxic elements

C. sparks which can start an explosion
D. overheating of electrical equipment

15. 15. ...

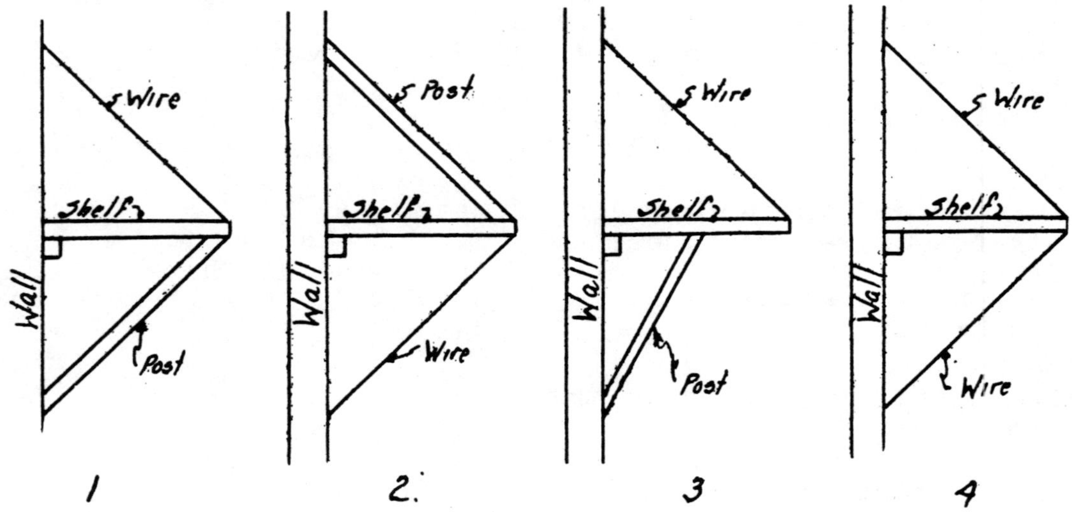

The *STRONGEST* method of supporting the shelf is shown in diagram
A. 1 B. 2 C. 3 D. 4

16. A row boat will float *deeper* in fresh water than in salt water *because* 16. ...
A. in the salt water the salt will occupy part of the space
B. fresh water is heavier than salt water
C. salt water is heavier than fresh water
D salt water offers less resistance than fresh water

17. 17. ...

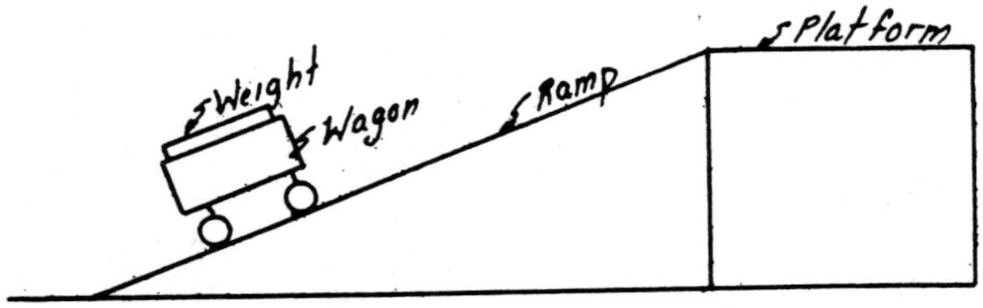

It is easier to get the load onto the platform by using the ramp than it is to lift it directly onto the platform.
This is *true* because the effect of the ramp is to
A. reduce the amount of friction so that less force is required
B. distribute the weight over a larger area
C. support part of the load so that less force is needed to move the wagon
D. increase the effect of the moving weight

18. 18. ...

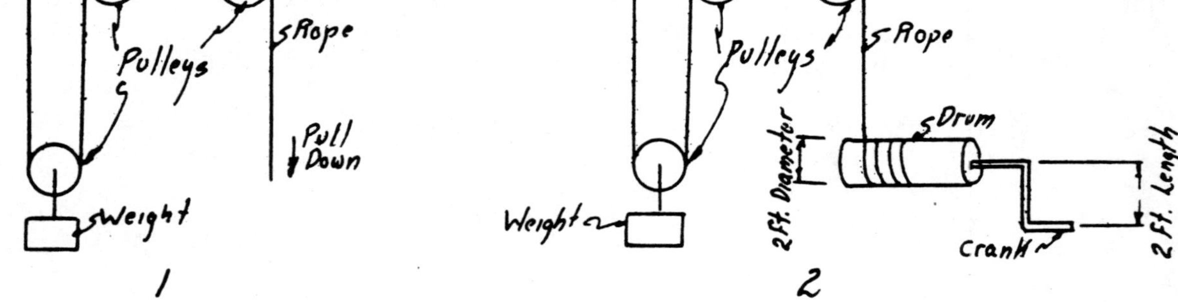

More weight can be lifted by the method shown in diagram 2 than as shown in diagram 1 *because*

A. it takes less force to turn a crank than it does to pull in a straight line
B. the drum will prevent the weight from falling by itself
C. the length of the crank is larger than the radius of the drum
D. the drum has more rope on it easing the pull

19. 19. ...

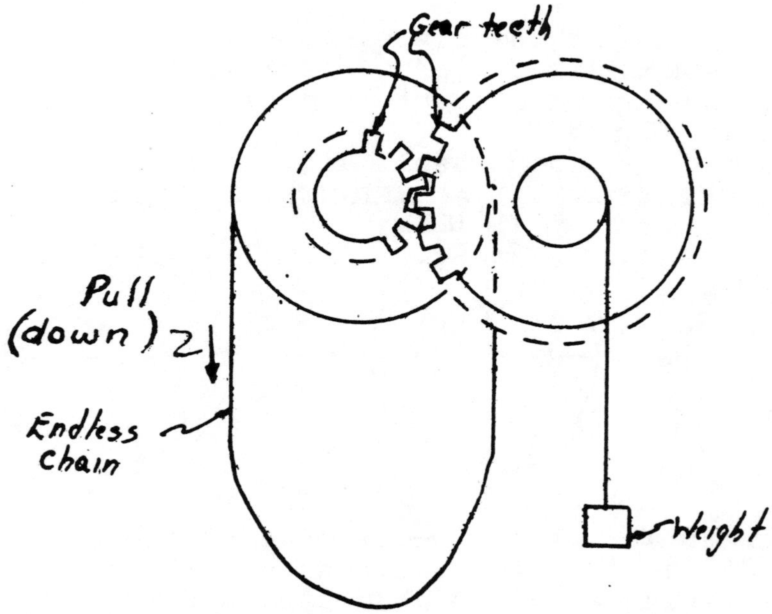

As the endless chain is pulled down in the direction shown, the weight will move

A. *up* faster than the endless chain is pulled down
B. *up* slower than the endless chain is pulled down
C. *down* faster than the endless chain is pulled down
D. *down* slower than the endless chain is pulled down

20. Two balls of the same size, but different weights, are both dropped from a 10-ft. height. The *one* of the following statements that is *MOST* accurate is that 20. ...

A. both balls will reach the ground at the same time because they are the same size
B. both balls will reach the ground at the same time because the effect of gravity is the same on both balls
C. the heavier ball will reach the ground first because it weighs more
D. the lighter ball will reach the ground first because air resistance is greater on the heavier ball

21. It is considered poor practice to increase the leverage of a wrench by placing a pipe over the handle of the wrench. This is *true PRINCIPALLY* because 21. ...

A. the wrench may break
B. the wrench may slip off the nut
C. it is harder to place the wrench on the nut
D. the wrench is more difficult to handle

22. 22. ...

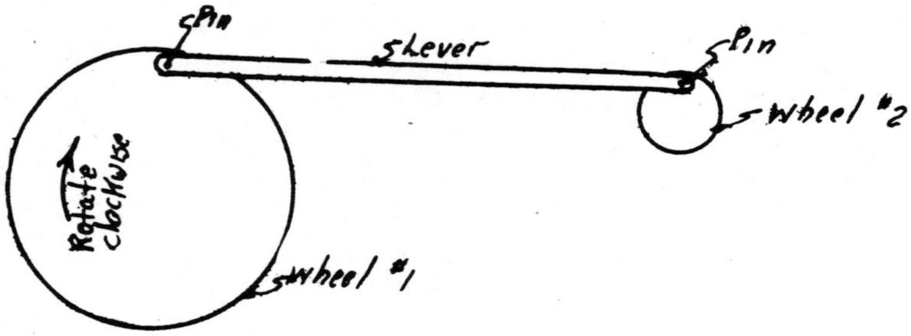

If wheel #1 is turned in the direction shown, wheel #2 will
   A. turn continuously in a clockwise direction
   B. turn continuously in a counterclockwise direction
   C. move back and forth
   D. become jammed and both wheels will stop

23. ALL SOLID AREAS REPRESENT EQUAL WEIGHTS ATTACHED TO THE FLYWHEEL 23. ...

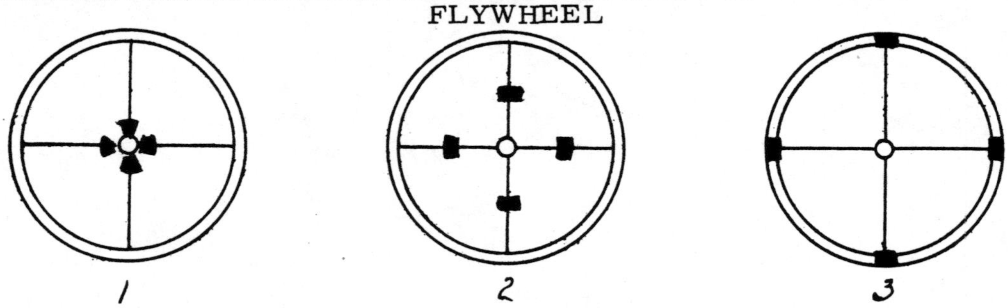

The above diagrams are of flywheels made of the same material with the same dimensions and attached to similar engines. The solid areas represent equal weights attached to the flywheel. If all three engines are running at the *same* speed for the *same* length of time, and the power to the engines is shut off *simultaneously*,
   A. wheel 1 will continue turning longest
   B. wheel 2 will continue turning longest
   C. wheel 3 will continue turning longest
   D. all three wheels will continue turning for the same time

24. The *one* of the following substances which *expands* when freezing is 24. ...
   A. alcohol   B. ammonia   C. mercury   D. water

25. When drilling a hole through a piece of wood with an auger bit, it is considered good practice to clamp a piece of scrap wood to the underside of the piece through which the hole is being drilled. 25. ...
The *MAIN* reason for this is to
   A. direct the auger bit B. speed up the drilling operation
   C. prevent the drill from wobbling
   D. prevent splintering of the wood

TEST 2

Questions 1-2.

DIRECTIONS: Questions 1 and 2 are to be answered in accordance with the information in the following statement:

The electrical resistance of copper wires varies directly with their lengths and inversely with their cross section areas.

1. A piece of copper wire 30 feet long is cut into two pieces, 20 feet and 10 feet. The resistance of the *longer* piece, compared to the shorter, is 1. ...
   A. one-half as much B. two-thirds as much
   C. one and one-half as much D. twice as much
2. Two pieces of copper wire are each 10 feet long but the cross section area of one is 2/3 that of the other. The resistance of the piece with the *larger* cross-section area is 2. ...
   A. one-half the resistance of the smaller
   B. two-thirds the resistance of the smaller
   C. one and one-half times the resistance of the smaller
   D. twice the resistance of the smaller
3. 3. ...

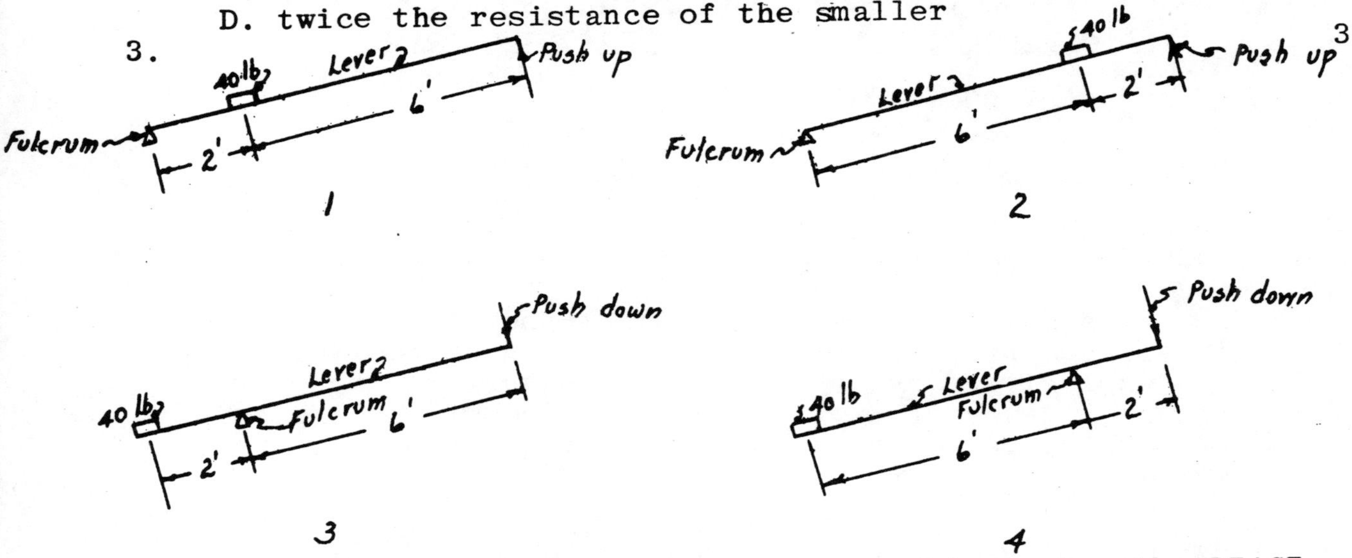

   The arrangement of the lever which would require the *LEAST* amount of force to move the weight is shown in the diagram numbered
   A. 1 B. 2 C. 3 D. 4
4. Steel supporting beams in buildings often are surrounded by a thin layer of concrete to keep the beams from becoming hot and collapsing during a fire. 4. ...
   The *one* of the following statements which *BEST* explains how collapse is prevented by this arrangement is that concrete
   A. becomes stronger as its temperature is increased
   B. acts as an insulating material
   C. protects the beam from rust and corrosion
   D. reacts chemically with steel at high temperatures
5. If boiling water is poured into a drinking glass, the glass is likely to crack. If, however, a metal spoon first is placed in the glass, it is much less likely to crack. 5. ...
   The reason that the glass with the spoon is *less likely* to crack is that the spoon
   A. distributes the water over a larger surface of the glass
   B. quickly absorbs heat from the water
   C. reinforces the glass
   D. reduces the amount of water which can be poured into the glass
6. It takes *more* energy to force water through a *long* pipe than through a *short* pipe of the same diameter. The *PRINCIPAL* reason for this is 6. ...
   A. gravity B. friction C. inertia D. cohesion
7. A pump, discharging at 300 lbs.-per-sq.-inch pressure, de- 7. ...

livers water through 100 feet of pipe laid horizontally. If the valve at the end of the pipe is shut so that no water can flow, then the pressure at the valve is, for practical purposes,

A. *greater* than the pressure at the pump
B. *equal to* the pressure at the pump
C. *less* than the pressure at the pump
D. *greater or less* than the pressure at the pump, depending on the type of pump used

8. The explosive force of a gas when stored under various pressures is given in the following table: 8. ...

Storage Pressure	Explosive Force
10	1
20	8
30	27
40	64
50	125

The *one* of the following statements which *BEST* expresses the relationship between the storage pressure and explosive force is that

A. there is no systematic relationship between an increase in storage pressure and an increase in explosive force
B. the explosive force varies as the square of the pressure
C. the explosive force varies as the cube of the pressure
D. the explosive force varies as the fourth power of the pressure

9. 9. ...

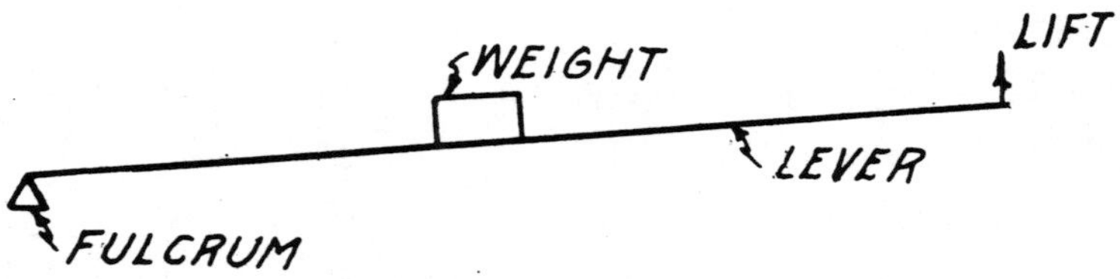

The leverage system in the sketch above is used to raise a weight. In order to *reduce* the amount of force required to raise the weight, it is necessary to

A. decrease the length of the lever
B. place the weight closer to the fulcrum
C. move the weight closer to the person applying the force
D. move the fulcrum further from the weight

10. In the accompanying sketch of a block and fall, if the end of the rope P is pulled so that it moves one foot, the distance the weight will be *raised* is 10. ...

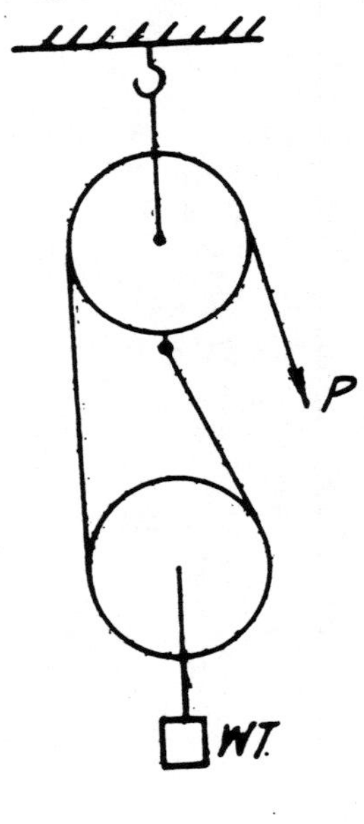

A. 1/2 ft.
B. 1 ft.
C. 1 1/2 ft.
D. 2 ft.

11. 11. ...

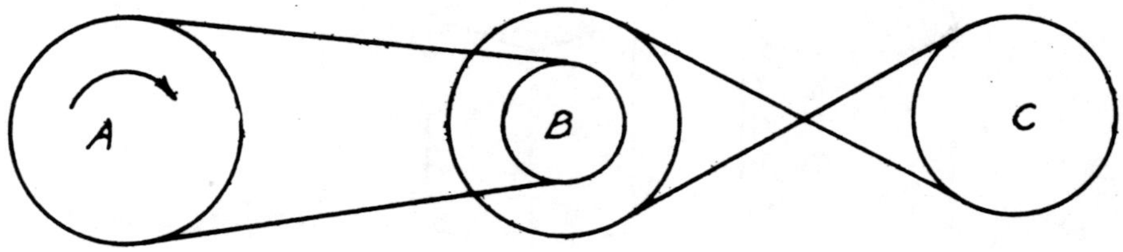

The above sketch diagrammatically shows a pulley and belt system.
If pulley A is made to rotate in a clockwise direction, *then* pulley C will rotate

A. faster than pulley A and in a clockwise direction
B. slower than pulley A and in a clockwise direction
C. faster than pulley A and in a counter-clockwise direction
D. slower than pulley A and in a counter-clockwise direction

12. 12. ...

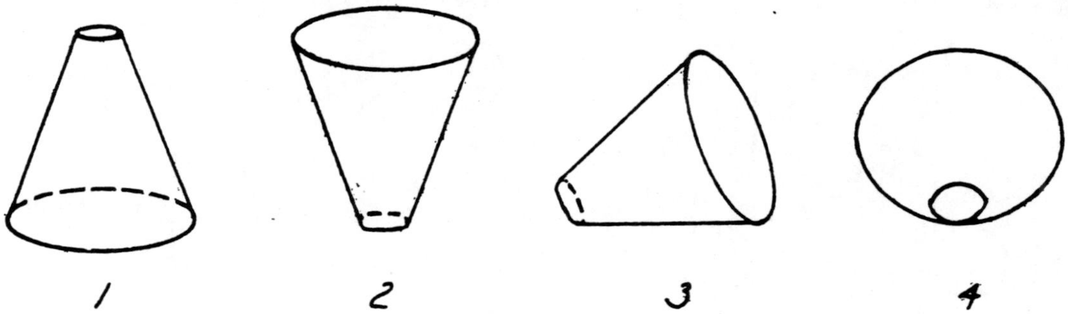

The above diagrams show four positions of the same object.
The position in which this object is *MOST* stable is

A. 1 B. 2 C. 3 D. 4

13. The accompanying sketch diagrammatically shows a system of meshing gears with relative diameters as drawn. 13. ...
If gear 1 is made to rotate in the direction of the arrow, *then* the gear that will turn *FASTEST* is numbered

A. 1 B. 2 C. 3 D. 4

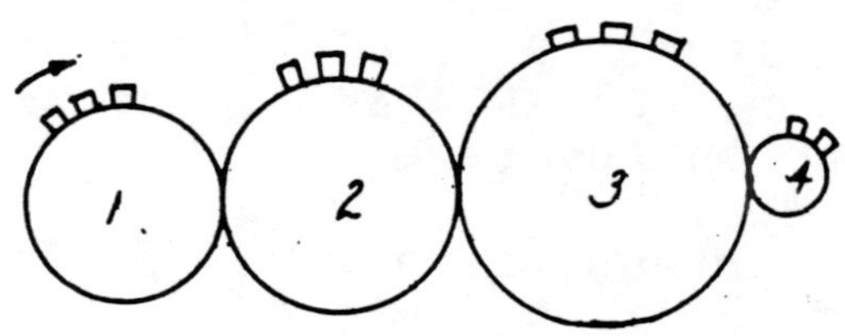

14. 14. ...

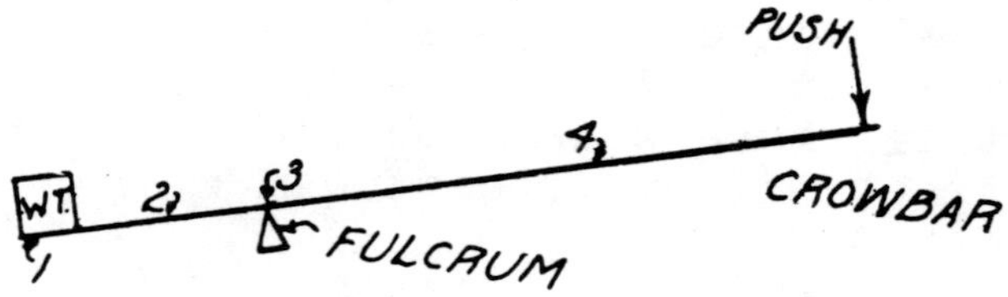

The above sketch shows a weight being lifted by means of a crowbar.
The point at which the tendency for the bar to break is *GREATEST* is

A. 1 B. 2 C. 3 D. 4

15. 15. ...

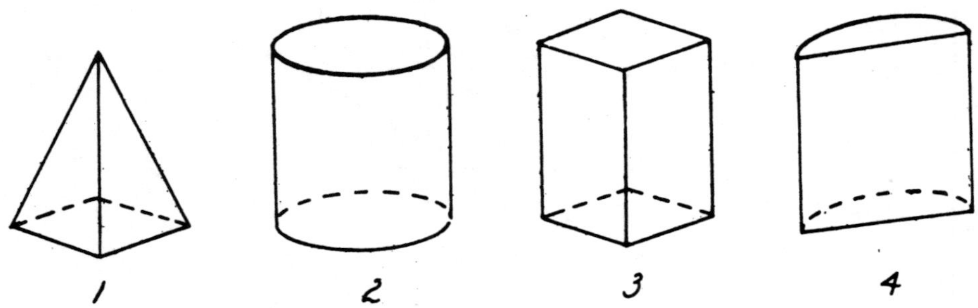

The above sketches show four objects which weigh the same but have different shapes.
The object which is *MOST* difficult to tip over is numbered

A. 1 B. 2 C. 3 D. 4

16. 16. ...

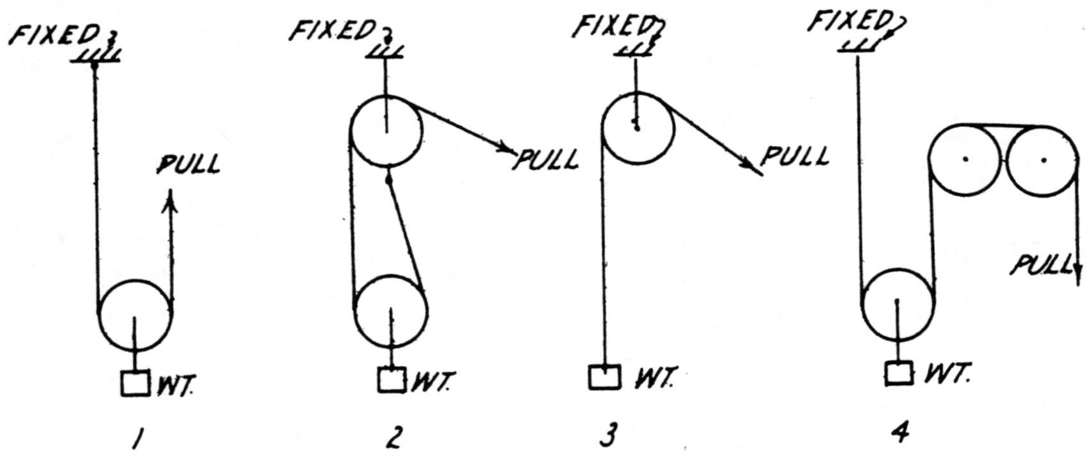

An object is to be lifted by means of a system of lines and pulleys. Of the systems shown above, the *one* which would require the *GREATEST* force to be used in lifting the weight is the one numbered

A. 1 B. 2 C. 3 D. 4

17. An intense fire develops in a room in which carbon dioxide cylinders are stored. The *PRINCIPAL* hazard in this situation is that 17. ...

A. the CO_2 may catch fire B. toxic fumes may be released
C. the cylinders may explode
D. released CO_2 may intensify the fire

18. At a fire involving the roof of a 5-story building, the firemen trained their hose stream on the fire from a vacant lot across the street, aiming the stream at a point about 15 feet above the roof. 18. ...
In this situation, water in the stream would be traveling at the *GREATEST* speed

A. as it leaves the hose nozzle
B. at a point midway between the ground and the roof
C. at the maximum height of the stream
D. as it drops on the roof

19. A principle of lighting is that the intensity of illumination at a point is inversely proportional to the square of the distance from the source of illumination. 19. ...
Assume that a pulley lamp is lowered from a position of 6

feet to one of three feet above a desk. According to the above principle, we would expect that the amount of illumination reaching the desk from the lamp in the lower position, as compared to the higher position, will be

A. half as much　　B. twice as much
C. four times as much　　D. nine times as much

20. 20. ...

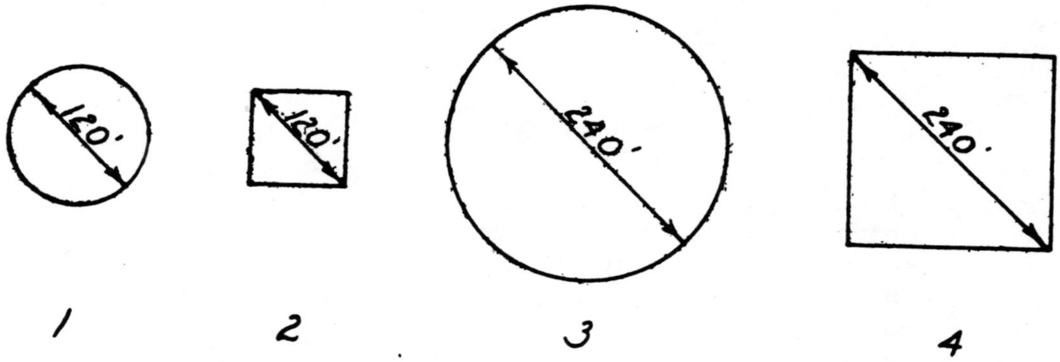

When standpipes are required in a structure, sufficient risers must be installed so that no point on the floor is more than 120 feet from a riser.
The *one* of the above diagrams which gives the *MAXIMUM* area which can be covered by *one* riser is

A. 1　　B. 2　　C. 3　　D. 4

21. Spontaneous combustion may be the reason for a pile of oily rags catching fire. 21. ...
In general, spontaneous combustion is the *DIRECT* result of

A. application of flame　　B. falling sparks
C. intense sunlight　　D. chemical action
E. radioactivity

22. In general, firemen are advised not to direct a solid stream of water on fires burning in electrical equipment. 22. ...
Of the following, the *MOST* logical reason for this instruction is that

A. water is a conductor of electricity
B. water will do more damage to the electrical equipment than the fire
C. hydrogen in water may explode when it comes in contact with electric current
D. water will not effectively extinguish fires in electrical equipment
E. water may spread the fire to other circuits

23. The height at which a fireboat will float in still water is determined *CHIEFLY* by the 23. ...

A. weight of the water displaced by the boat
B. horsepower of the boat's engines
C. number of propellers on the boat
D. curve the bow has above the water line
E. skill with which the boat is maneuvered

24. When firemen are working at the nozzle of a hose they usually lean forward on the hose. 24. ...
The *most likely* reason for taking this position is that

A. the surrounding air is cooled, making the firemen more comfortable
B. a backward force is developed which must be counteracted
C. the firemen can better see where the stream strikes

D. the fireman are better protected from injury by falling debris
E. the stream is projected further

25. In general, the color and odor of smoke will *BEST* indicate 25. ...
A. the cause of the fire B. the extent of the fire
C. how long the fire has been burning
D. the kind of material on fire
E. the exact seat of the fire

TEST 3

1. As a demonstration, firemen set up two hose lines identical in every respect except that one was longer than the other. Water was then delivered through these lines from one pump and it was seen that the stream from the longer hose line had a shorter "throw." 1. ...
Of the following, the *MOST* valid explanation of this difference in "throw" is that the
A. air resistance to the water stream is proportional to the length of hose
B. time required for water to travel through the longer hose is greater than for the shorter one
C. loss due to friction is greater in the longer hose than in the shorter one
D. rise of temperature is greater in the longer hose than in the shorter one
E. longer hose line probably developed a leak at one of the coupling joints

2. Of the following toxic gases, the *one* which is *MOST* dangerous because it cannot be seen and has no odor, is 2. ...
A. ether B. carbon monoxide C. chlorine
D. ammonia E. cooking gas

3. You are visiting with some friends when their young son rushes into the room with his clothes on fire. You immediately wrap him in a rug and roll him on the floor. 3. ...
The *MOST* important reason for your action is that the
A. flames are confined within the rug
B. air supply to the fire is reduced
C. burns sustained will be third degree, rather than first degree
D. whirling action will put out the fire
E. boy will not suffer from shock

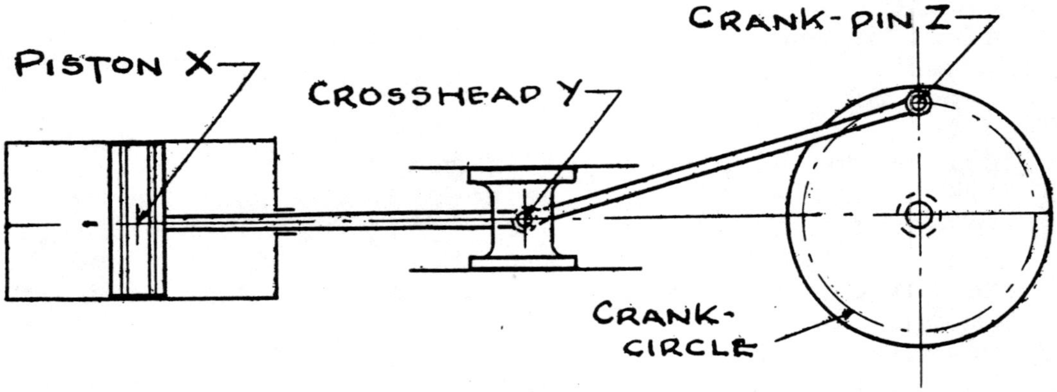

FIGURE I

Questions 4-6.

DIRECTIONS: The device shown in Figure I above represents schematically a mechanism commonly used to change reciprocating (back and forth) motion to rotation (circular) motion.

The following questions, numbered 4 to 6 inclusive, are to be answered with reference to this device.

4. Assume that piston X is placed in its extreme left position so that X, Y, and Z are in a horizontal line. If a horizontal force to the right is applied to the piston X, we may then expect that 4. ...
   A. the crank-pin Z will revolve clockwise
   B. the crosshead Y will move in a direction opposite to that of X
   C. the crank-pin Z will revolve counterclockwise
   D. no movement will take place
   E. the crank-pin Z will oscillate back and forth
5. If we start from the position shown in the above diagram, and move piston X to the right, the result will be that 5. ...
   A. the crank-pin Z will revolve counterclockwise and crosshead Y will move to the left
   B. the crank-pin Z will revolve clockwise and crosshead Y will move to the left
   C. the crank-pin Z will revolve clockwise and crosshead Y will move to the right
   D. the crank-pin Z will revolve clockwise and crosshead Y will move to the right
   E. crosshead Y will move to the left as piston X moves to the right
6. If crank-pin Z is moved closer to the center of the crank circle, then the length of the 6. ...
   A. stroke of piston X is increased
   B. stroke of piston X is decreased
   C. stroke of piston X is unchanged
   D. rod between the piston X and crosshead Y is increased
   E. rod between the piston X and crosshead Y is decreased

Questions 7-8.

DIRECTIONS: Figure II represents schematically a block-and-fall tackle. The advantage derived from this machine is that the effect of the applied force is multiplied by the number of lines of rope directly supporting the load. The following two questions, numbered 7 and 8, are to be answered with reference to this figure.

7. Pull P is exerted on line T to raise the load L. The line in which the *LARGEST* strain is finally induced is line 7. ...
   A. T B. U C. V D. X E. Y
8. If the largest pull P that two men can apply to line T is 280 lbs., the *MAXIMUM* load L that they can raise without regard to frictional losses is, *most nearly*, ______ lbs. 8. ...
   A. 1960 B. 1680 C. 1400
   D. 1260 E. 1120

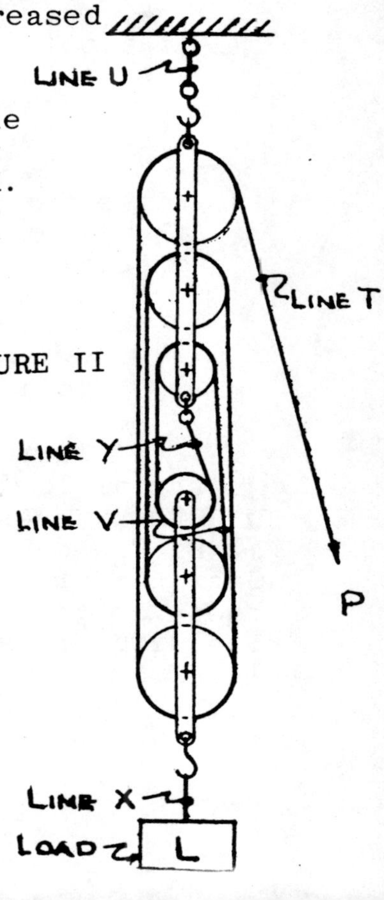

FIGURE II

Questions 9-13.

DIRECTIONS: Answer Questions 9 to 13 on the basis of Figure III.
The diagram schematically illustrates part of a water tank.
1 and 5 are outlet and inlet pipes, respectively.
2 is a valve which can be used to open and close the outlet pipe by hand.
3 is a float which is rigidly connected to valve 4 by an iron bar, thus causing that valve to open or shut as the float rises or falls.
4 is a hinged valve which controls the flow of water into the tank.

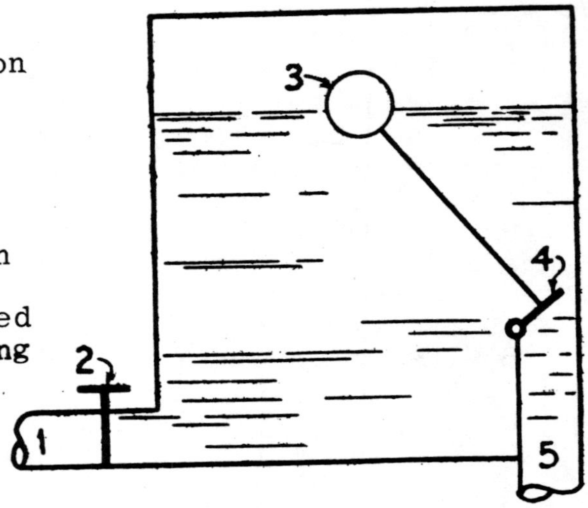

FIGURE III

9. If the tank is half filled and water is going out of pipe 1 more rapidly than it is coming in through pipe 5, *then* 9. ...
   A. valve 2 is closed B. float 3 is rising in the tank
   C. valve 4 is opening wider D. valve 4 is closed
   E. float 3 is stationary
10. If the tank is half filled with water and water is coming in through inlet pipe 5 more rapidly than it is going out through outlet pipe 1, *then* 10. ...
   A. valve 2 is closed B. float 3 is rising in the tank
   B. valve 4 is opening wider D. valve 4 is closed
   E. float 3 is stationary
11. If the tank is empty, then it can *normally* be expected that 11. ...
   A. float 3 is at its highest position
   B. float 3 is at its lowest position
   C. valve 2 is closed D. valve 4 is closed
   E. water will not come into the tank
12. If float 3 develops a leak, *then* 12. ...
   A. the tank will tend to empty
   B. water will tend to stop coming into the tank
   C. valve 4 will tend to close D. valve 2 will tend to close
   E. valve 4 will tend to remain open
13. Without any other changes being made, if the bar joining the float to valve 4 is removed and a slightly shorter bar substituted, *then* 13. ...
   A. a smaller quantity of water in the tank will be required before the float closes valve 4
   B. valve 4 will not open C. valve 4 will not close
   D. it is not possible to determine what will happen
   E. a greater quantity of water in the tank will be required before the float closes valve 4

Questions 14-18.

DIRECTIONS: Answer Questions 14 to 18 on the basis of Figure IV.
A, B, C and D are four meshed gears forming a gear train.
Gear A is the driver. Gears A and D each have twice as many teeth as gear B, and gear C has four times as many teeth as gear B.
The diagram is schematic: the teeth go all around each gear.

14. *Two* gears which turn in the *same* direction are: 14. ...
   A. A and B B. B and C C. C and D
   D. B and D E. D and C

15. The *two* gears which revolve at the *same* speed are gears 15. ...
   A. A and C B. A and D
   C. B and C D. B and D
   E. D and C
16. If all the teeth on gear C are stripped without affecting the teeth on gears A, B, and D, then rotation would occur *only* in gear(s) 16. ...
   A. C B. D C. A and B
   D. A, B, and D E. B and D
17. If gear D is rotating at the rate of 100 R.P.M., then gear B is rotating at the rate of ______ R.P.M. 17. ...
   A. 25 B. 50 C. 100 D. 200 E. 400

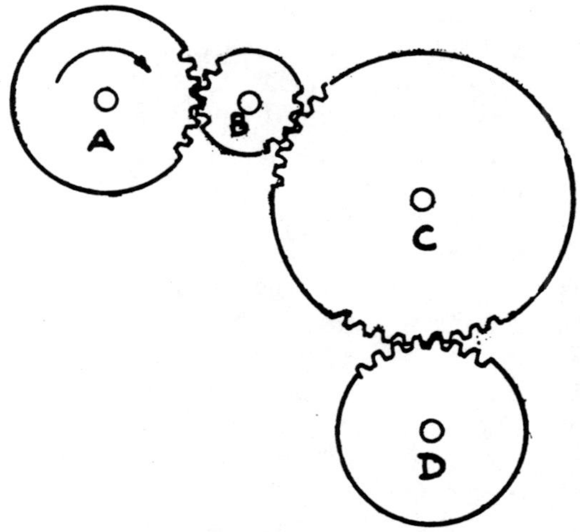

FIGURE IV

18. If gear A turns at the rate of two revolutions per second, then the number of revolutions per second that gear C turns is 18. ...
   A. 1 B. 2 C. 3 D. 4 E. 8

Questions 19-23.
DIRECTIONS: Answer Questions 19 to 23 on the basis of Figure V.
The diagram shows a water pump in cross section.
1 is a check valve, 2 and 3 are the spring and diaphragm ,respectively, of the discharge valve; 4 is the pump piston; 5 is the inlet valve, and 6 is the pump cylinder.
All valves permit the flow of water in one direction only.

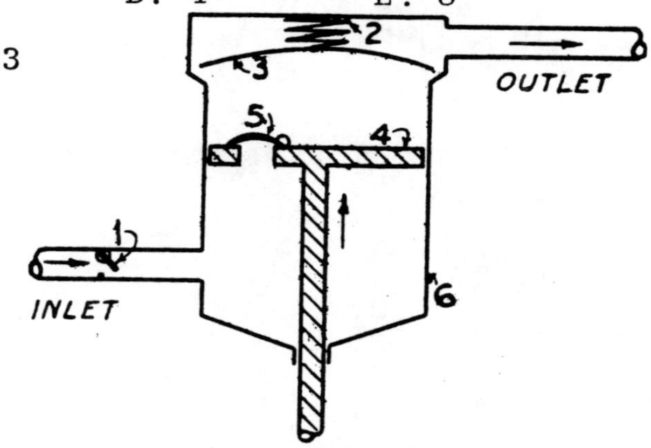

FIGURE V

19. When water is flowing through the outlet pipe, 19. ...
   A. check valve 1 is closed B. diaphragm 3 is closed
   C. valve 5 is closed D. spring 2 is fully extended
   E. the piston is on the downstroke
20. If valve 5 does not work properly and stays closed, *then* 20. ...
   A. the piston cannot move down B. the piston cannot move up
   C. diaphragm 3 cannot open D. check valve 1 cannot close
   E. the flow of water will be reversed
21. If diaphragm 3 does not work properly and stays in the open position, *then* 21. ...
   A. check valve 1 will not open B. valve 5 will not open
   C. spring 2 will be compressed D. spring 2 will be extended
   E. water will not flow through the inlet pipe
22. When valve 5 is open during normal operation of the pump, *then* 22. ...
   A. spring 2 is fully compressed
   B. the piston is on the upstroke
   C. water is flowing through check valve 1
   D. a vacuum is formed between the piston and the bottom of the cylinder
   E. diaphragm 3 is closed
23. If check valve 1 jams and stays closed, *then* 23. ...
   A. valve 5 will be open on both the upstroke and down-

stroke of the piston

B. a vacuum will tend to form in the inlet pipe between the source of the water supply and check valve 1

C. pressure on the cylinder side of check valve 1 will increase

D. less force will be required to move the piston down

E. more force will be required to move the piston down

24. The one of the following which *BEST* explains why smoke usually rises from a fire is that 24. ...

A. cooler, heavier air displaces lighter, warm air

B. heat energy of the fire propels the smoke upward

C. suction from the upper air pulls the smoke upward

D. burning matter is chemically changed into heat energy

25. The practice of racing a car engine to warm it up in cold weather, generally, is 25. ...

A. *good, MAINLY* because repeated stalling of the engine and drain on the battery is avoided

B. *bad, MAINLY* because too much gas is used to get the engine heated

C. *good, MAINLY* because the engine becomes operational in the shortest period of time

D. *bad, MAINLY* because proper lubrication is not established rapidly enough

---

KEYS (CORRECT ANSWERS)

TEST 1

1.	C	11.	B
2.	A	12.	C
3.	B	13.	B
4.	D	14.	C
5.	B	15.	A
6.	D	16.	C
7.	B	17.	C
8.	D	18.	C
9.	B	19.	D
10.	B	20.	B
		21.	A
		22.	D
		23.	C
		24.	D
		25.	D

TEST 2

1.	D	11.	C
2.	B	12.	A
3.	A	13.	D
4.	B	14.	C
5.	B	15.	A
6.	B	16.	C
7.	B	17.	C
8.	C	18.	A
9.	B	19.	C
10.	A	20.	C
		21.	D
		22.	A
		23.	A
		24.	B
		25.	D

TEST 3

1.	C	11.	B
2.	B	12.	E
3.	B	13.	A
4.	D	14.	E
5.	D	15.	B
6.	B	16.	C
7.	B	17.	D
8.	B	18	A
9.	C	19.	C
10.	B	20.	A
		21.	C
		22.	E
		23.	D
		24.	A
		25.	D

MECHANICAL APTITUDE

TOOL RECOGNITION AND USE

TEST 1

DIRECTIONS: Each question or incomplete statement below is followed by several suggested answers or completions. Select the one that *BEST* answers the question or completes the statement.

KEY : CORRECT ANSWERS APPEAR AT THE END OF THIS TEST.

1. 1. ...

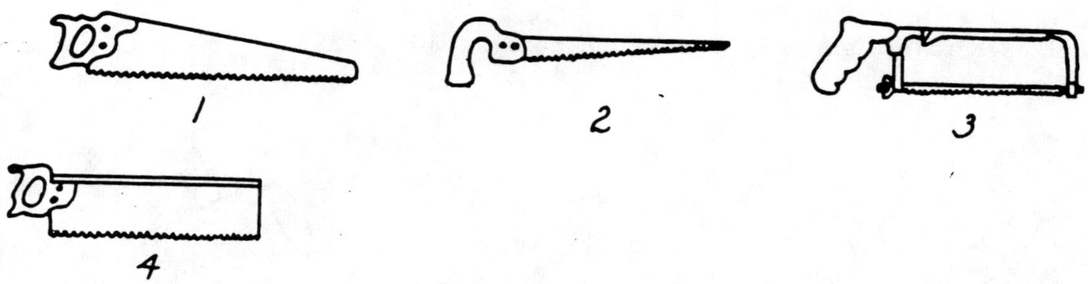

The saw that is used principally where curved cuts are to be made is numbered
1. 1   2. 2   3. 3   4. 4

2. 2. ...

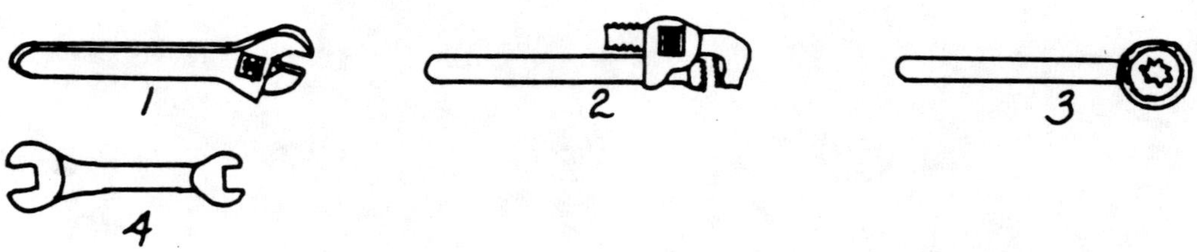

The wrench that is used principally for pipe work is numbered
1. 1   2. 2   3. 3   4. 4

3. 3. ...

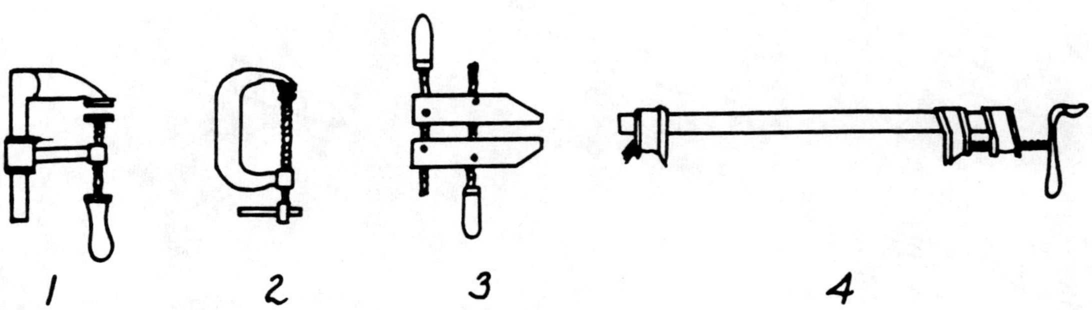

The carpenter's "hand screw" is numbered
1. 1   2. 2   3. 3   4. 4

4. 4. ...

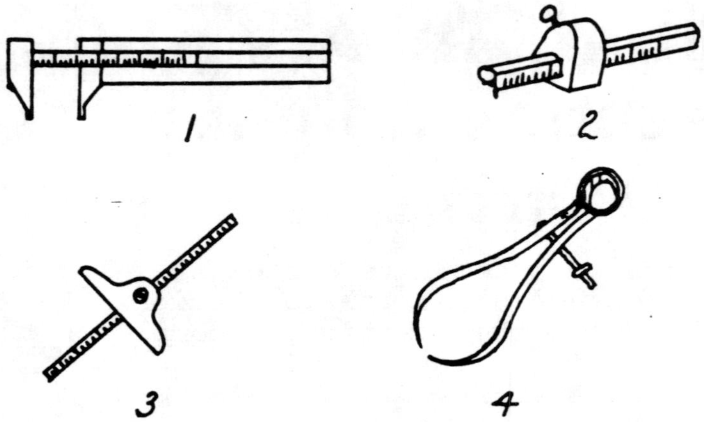

The tool used to measure the depth of a hole is numbered
1. 1 2. 2 3. 3 4. 4

5. 5. ...

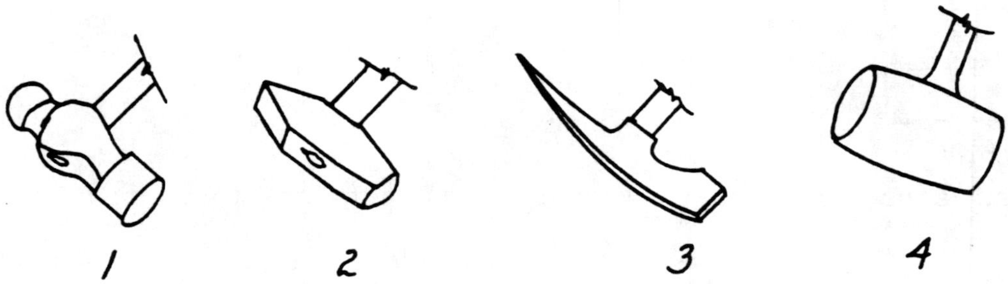

The tool that is best suited for use with a wood chisel is numbered
1. 1 2. 2 3. 3 4. 4

6. 6. ...

The screw head that would be tightened with an "Allen" wrench is numbered
1. 1 2. 2 3. 3 4. 4

7. 7. ...

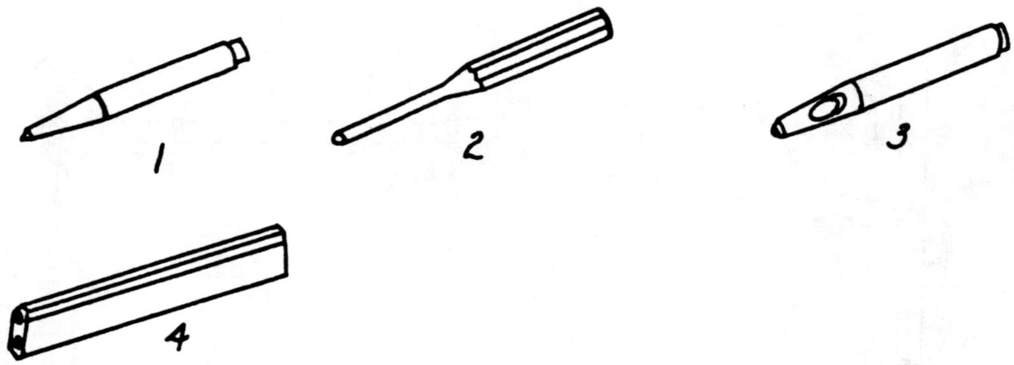

The center punch is numbered
1. 1 2. 2 3. 3 4. 4

8. 8. ...

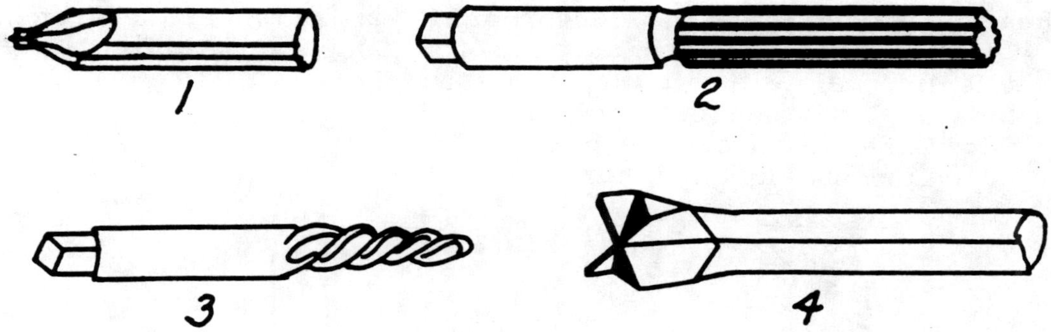

The tool used to drill a hole in concrete is numbered
1. 1 2. 2 3. 3 4. 4

9. 9. ...

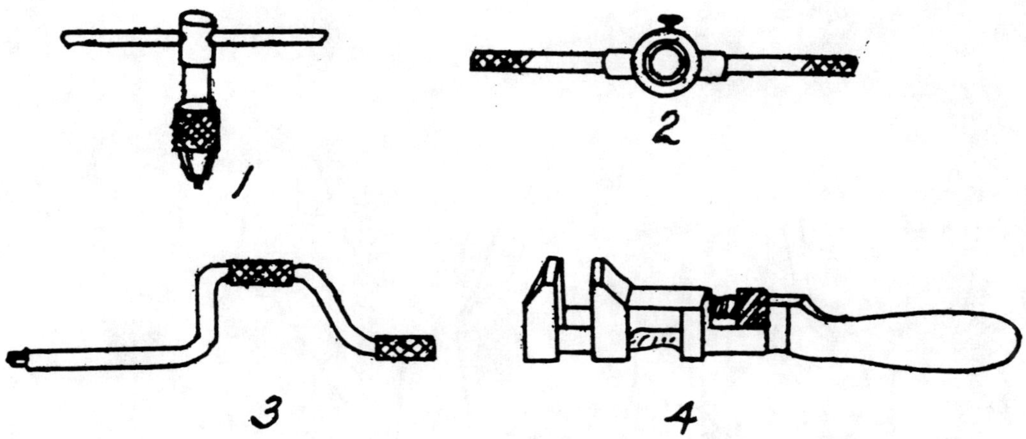

The wrench whose principal purpose is to hold taps for threading is numbered
1. 1 2. 2 3. 3 4. 4

10. 10. ...

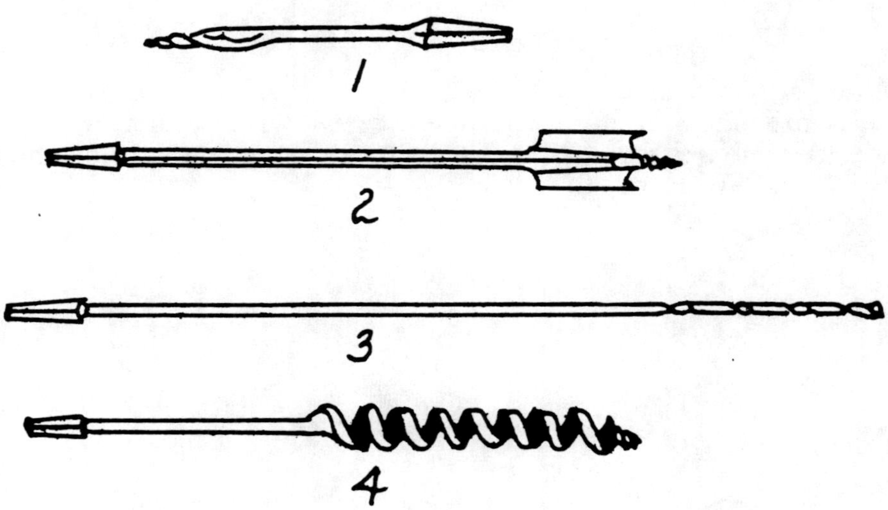

The electrician's bit is indicated by the number
1. 1 2. 2 3. 3 4. 4

11. The head of a cold chisel is "mushroomed" as shown in the sketch. The use of a chisel in this condition is poor practice because 11. ...
   1. it is impossible to hit the head squarely
   2. the chisel will not cut accurately
   3. chips might fly from the head
   4. the chisel has lost its "temper"

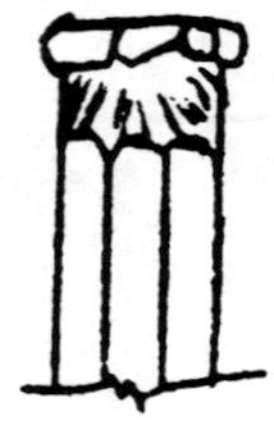

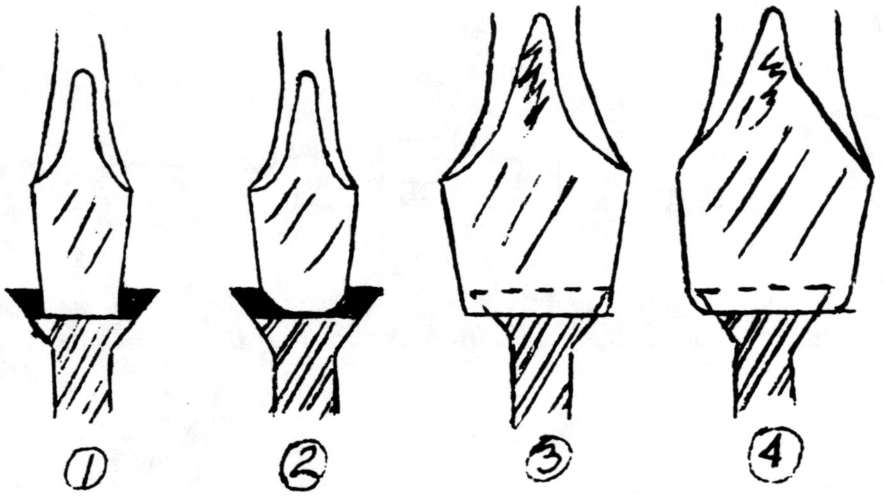

12. The above diagrams show a section of a screw with a screwdriver that is to be used with the screw. The one of the diagrams that shows the correct shape of screwdriver is 12. ..
   1. 1 2. 2 3. 3 4. 4

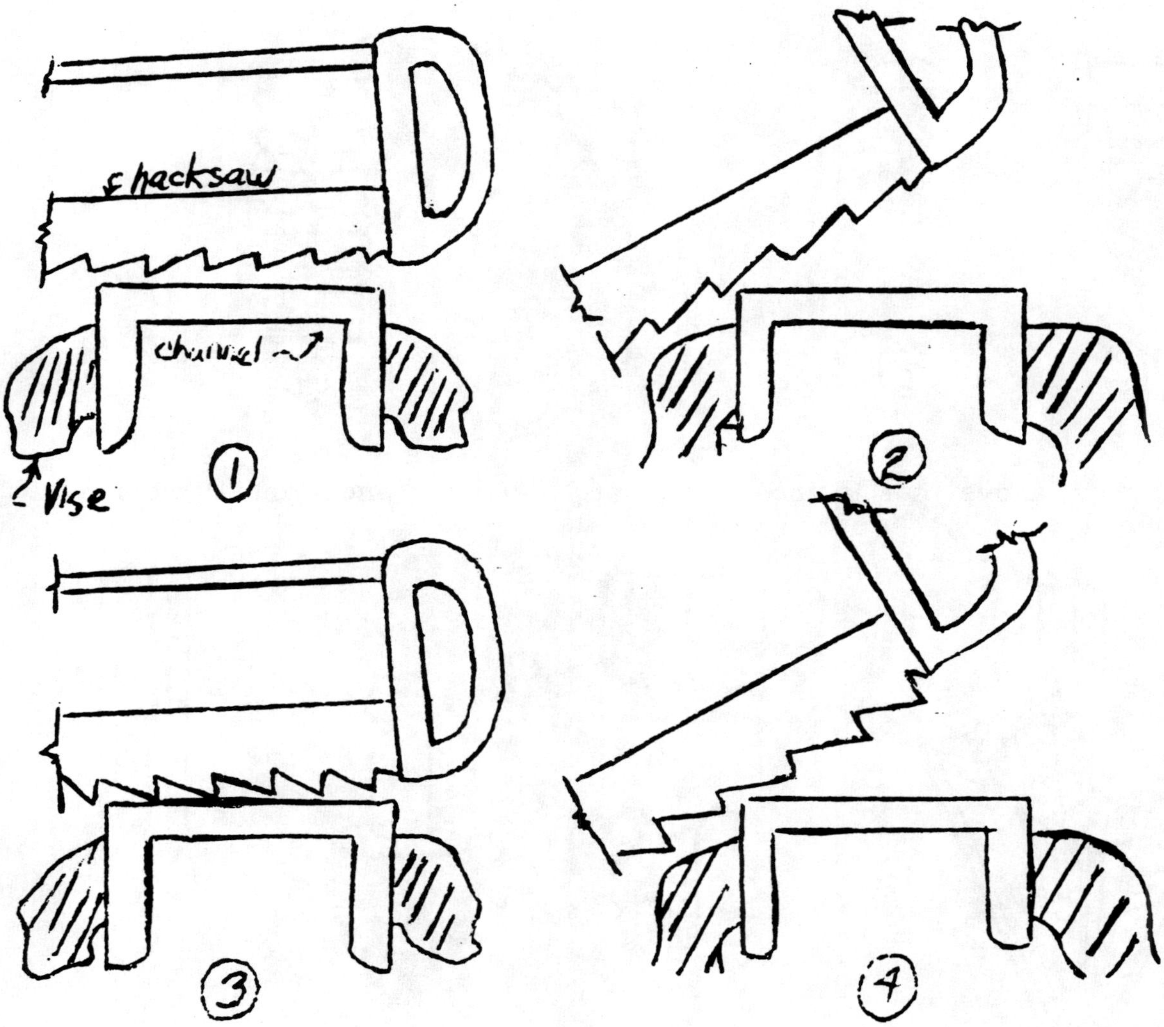

13. A steel channel is to be cut through with a hacksaw. The correct method for doing this is shown in the diagram numbered (diagrams above) 13. ...
    1. 1 2. 2 3. 3 4. 4

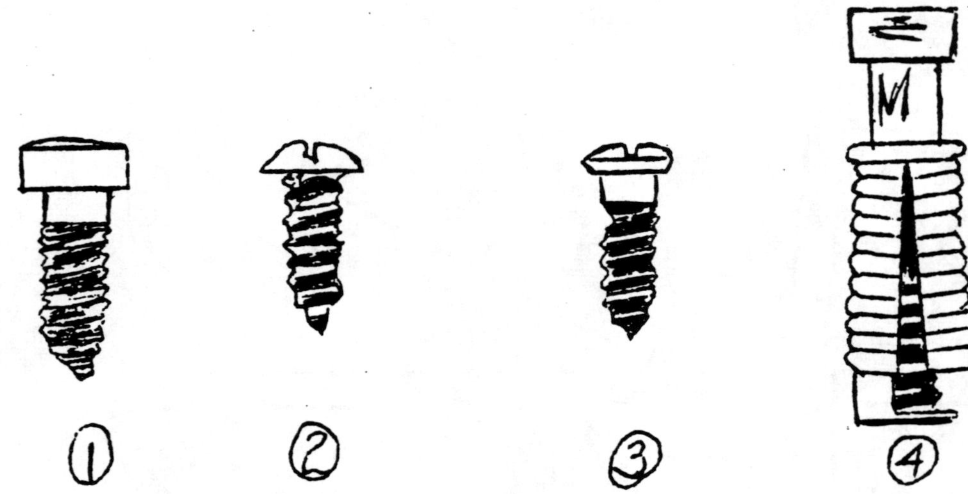

14. The screw above that is most frequently used for sheet metal work is numbered 14. ..
1. 1 2. 2 3. 3 4. 4

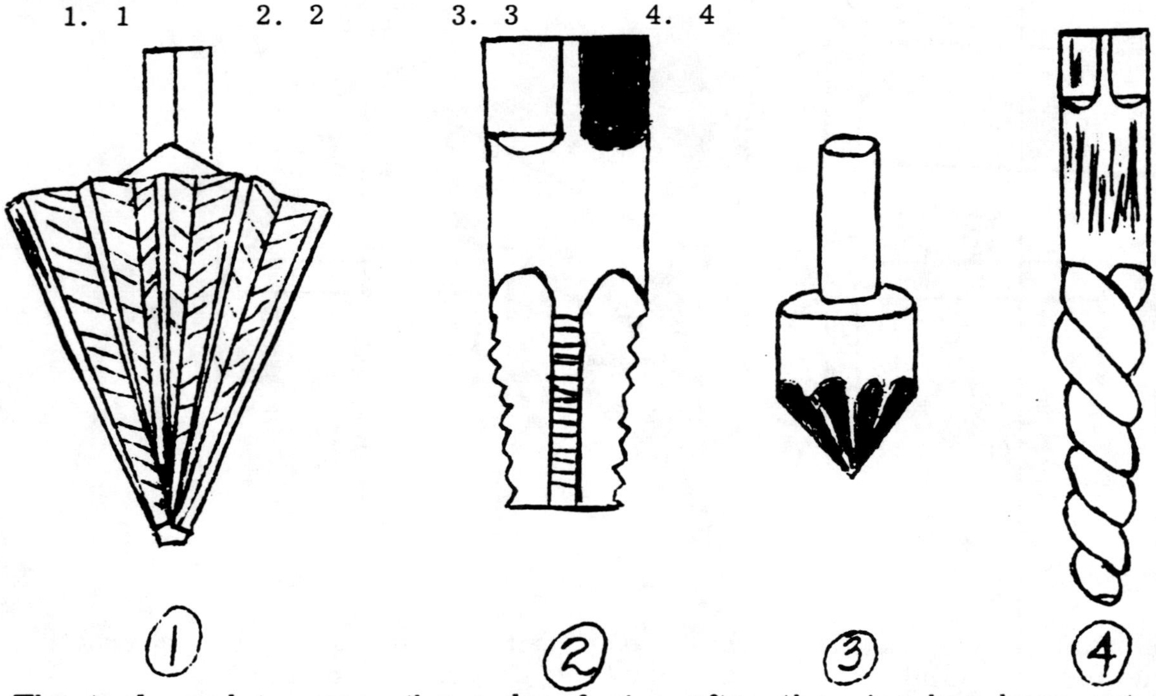

15. The tool used to ream the ends of pipe after the pipe has been cut is shown above in the diagram numbered 15. ..
1. 1 2. 2 3. 3 4. 4

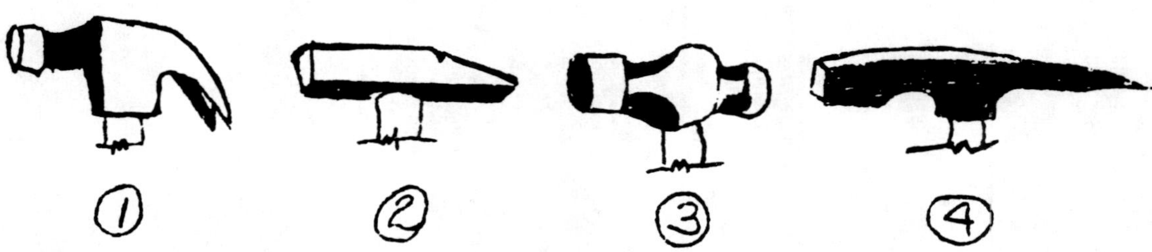

16. The hammer that would be used by a mason to trim brick is shown in the above diagram numbered 16. ..
1. 1 2. 2 3. 3 4. 4

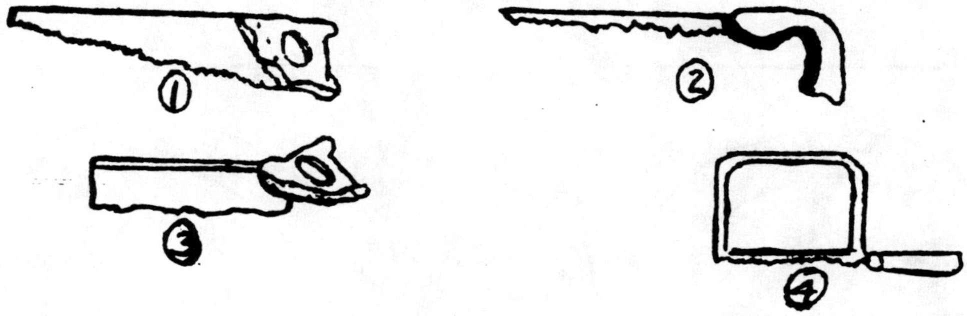

17. The saw intended especially to make accurate miter cuts is shown in the above diagram numbered 17. ...
   1. 1   2. 2   3. 3   4. 4

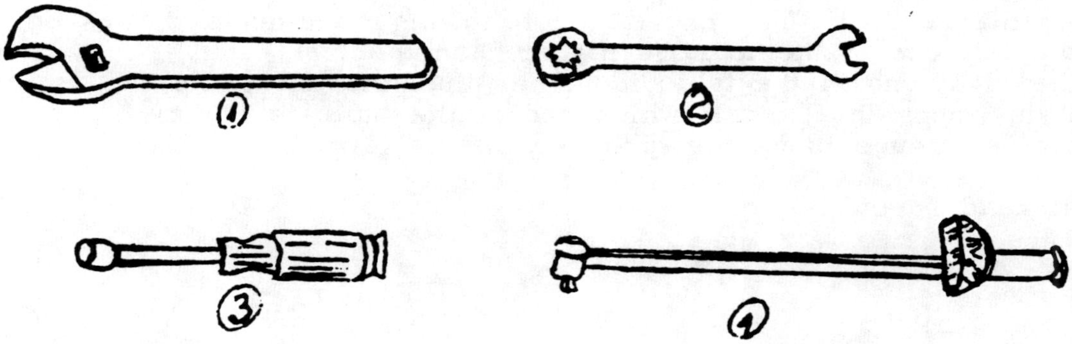

18. A wrench used to tighten cylinder head bolts to a specified torque is shown in the above diagram numbered 18. ..
   1. 1   2. 2   3. 3   4. 4

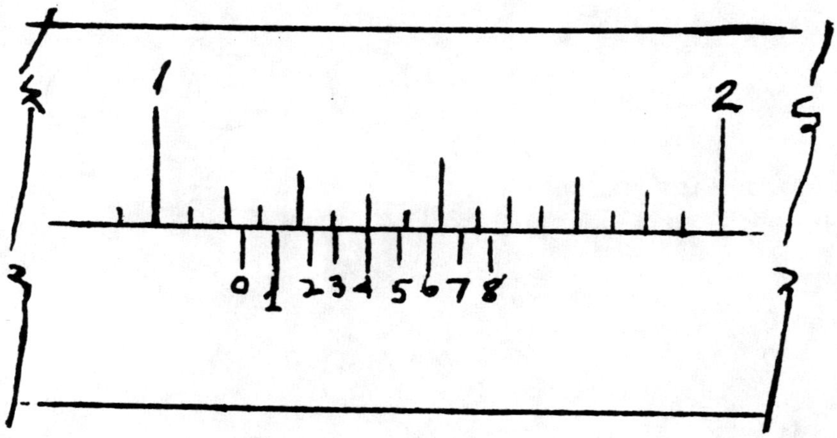

19. A section of the scale of a vernier caliper is shown above. The reading of this caliper setting is most nearly 19. ..
   1. 1 3/8   2. 1 5/64   3. 1 5/32   4. 1 7/64

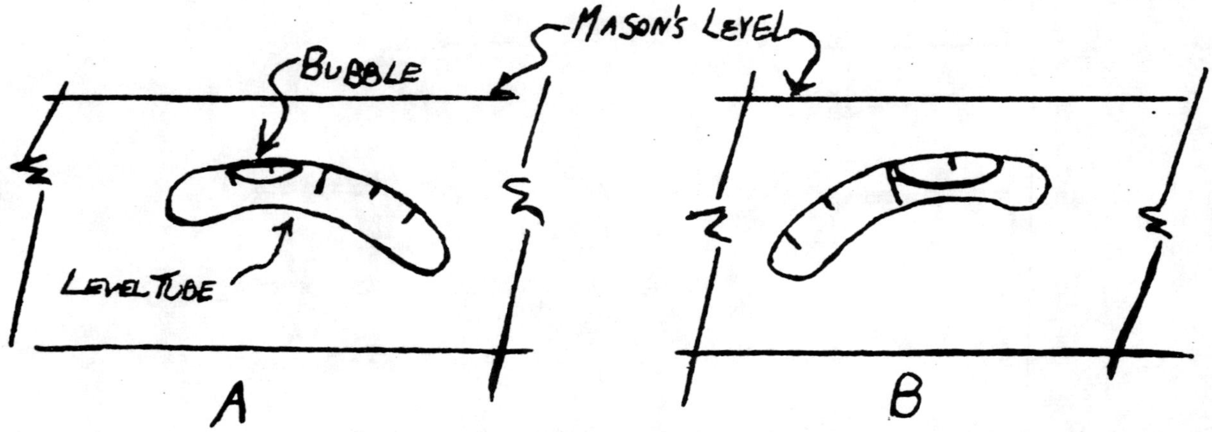

20. A level is placed on a table and the bubble moves to the position indicated in diagram A above. The level is then turned end for end and placed in the same location on the table as before. The bubble now appears as shown in diagram B. The one of the following statements that is correct is 20. ....
1. the left end of the table is higher than the right end
2, the right end of the table is higher than the left end
3. it is impossible to tell which end of the table is higher
4. the level tube is not set properly in the level

21. The flat-head screw is No. 21. ....
1. 1   2. 2   3. 3   4. 4

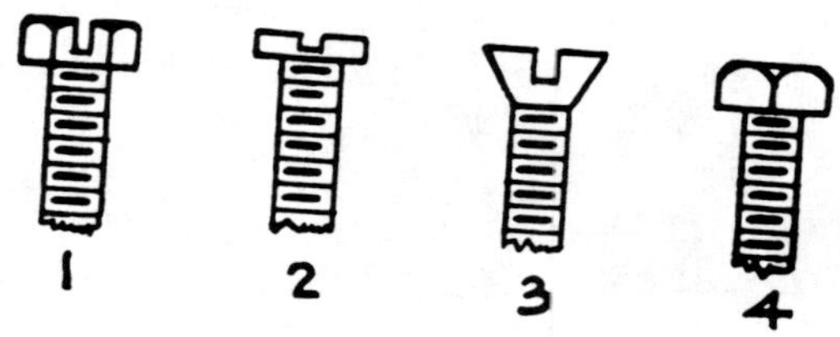

22. The "Phillips" head is No. 22. ....
1. 1   2. 2   3. 3   4. 4

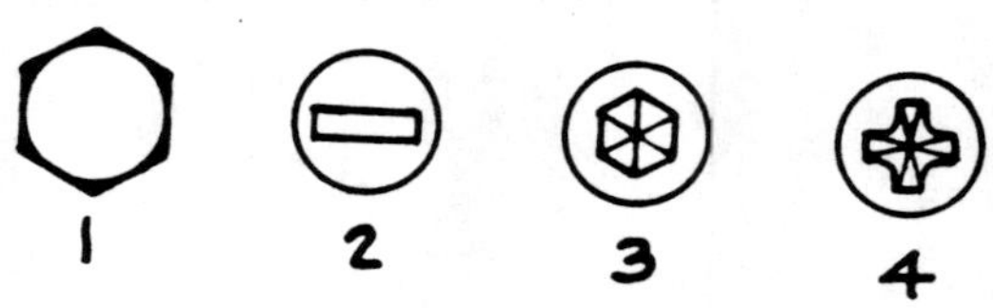

23. The standard coupling for rigid electrical conduit is 23. ....
1. 1   2. 2   3. 3   4. 4

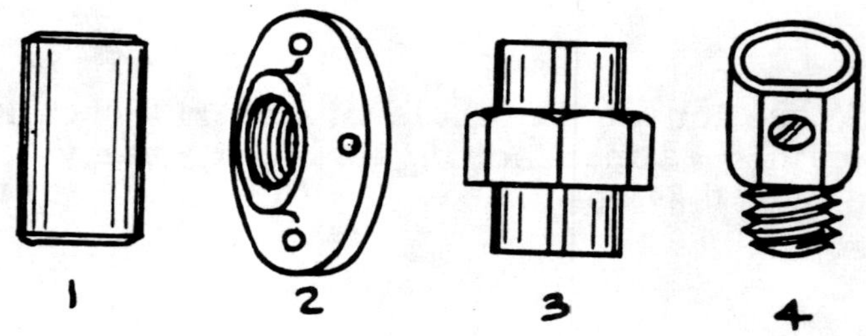

24. ...

24. The shape of nut most commonly used on electrical terminals is
1. 1 2. 2 3. 3 4. 4

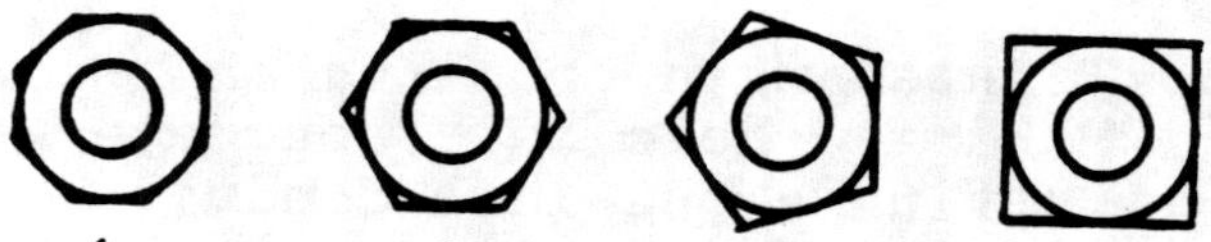

25. ...

25. The stove bolt is
1. 1 2. 2 3. 3 4. 4

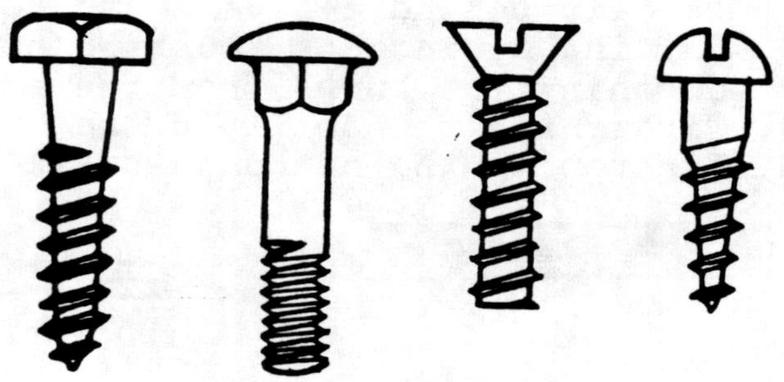

KEY (CORRECT ANSWERS)

1.	2	6.	3	11.	3	16.	4	21.	3
2.	2	7.	1	12.	1	17.	3	22.	4
3.	3	8.	4	13.	1	18.	4	23.	1
4.	3	9.	1	14.	2	19.	3	24.	2
5.	4	10.	3	15.	1	20.	4	25.	3

TEST 2

DIRECTIONS: The questions in this test refer to the use of tools shown below. Read the question, and for the operation given, select the proper tool to be used from those shown. *PRINT* on your answer sheet, in the correspondingly numbered item space, the letter given below your selected tool.

KEY: CORRECT ANSWERS APPEAR AT THE END OF THIS TEST.

1. Tightening a coupling on the end of a piece of conduit
2. Making a hole in a concrete wall for a lead anchor
3. Cutting a one-inch conduit
4. Loosening the wire connection on the terminal of a standard electric light socket
5. Cutting 3/0 insulated copper cable
6. Measuring the total length of several coupled pieces of straight conduit behind a live switchboard without an assistant
7. Cutting a piece of #10 bare copper wire
8. Cleaning the burrs from the end of a piece of conduit after cutting
9. Tightening the drill in the chuck of an electric drill
10. Tightening the nut on a small stud terminal

(A)

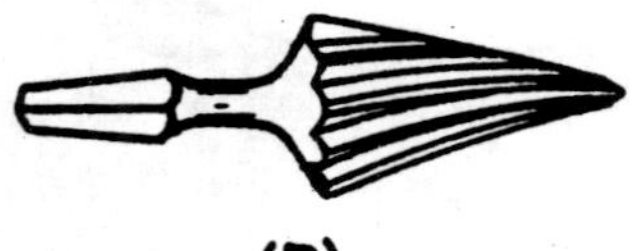

(B)

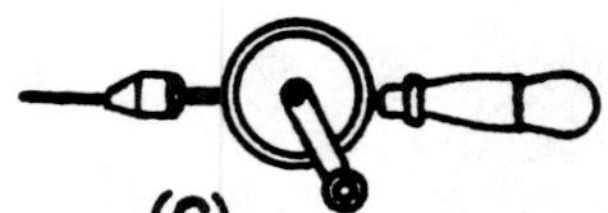

(C)

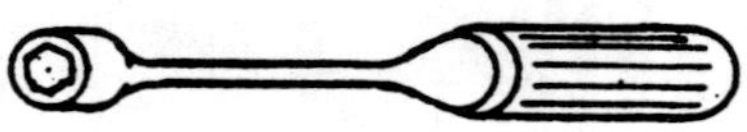

(D)

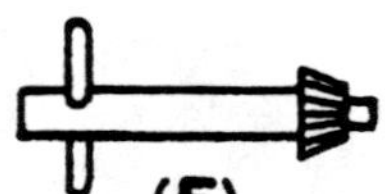

(E)

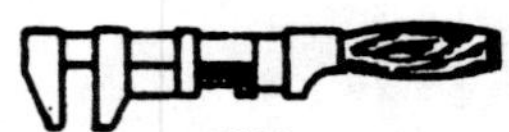

(H)

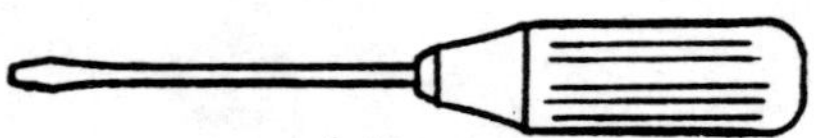

(J)

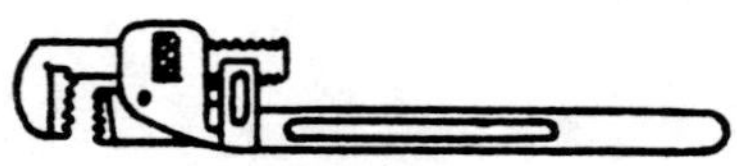

(K)

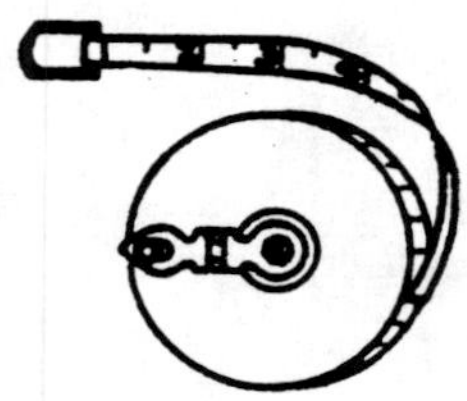

(L)

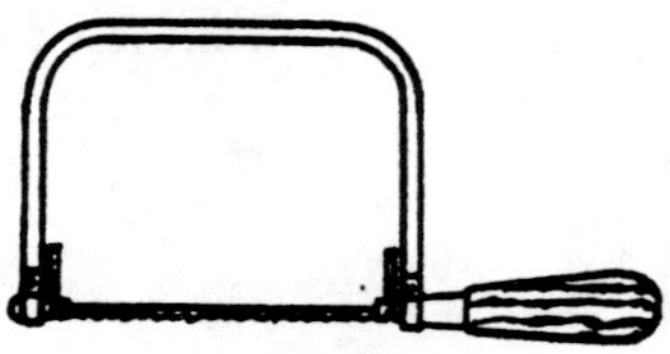

(M)

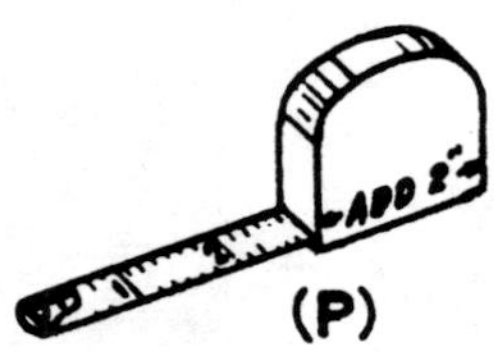

(P)

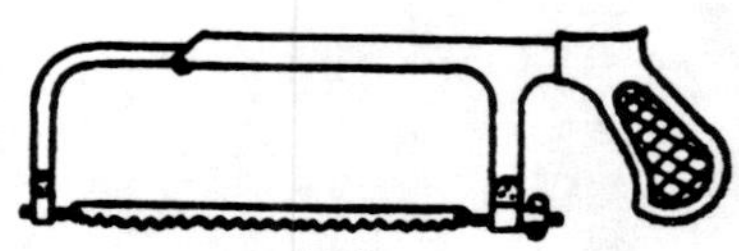

(S)

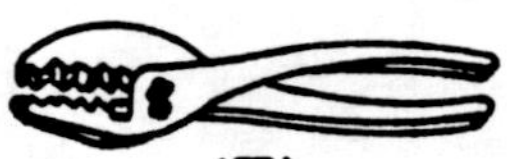

(T)

(V)

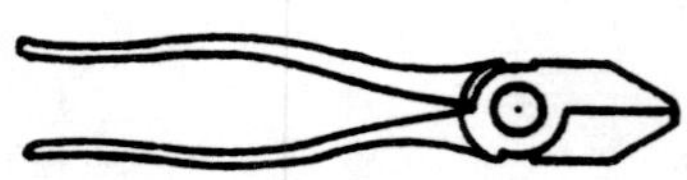

(W)

KEY (CORRECT ANSWERS)

1.	K	3.	S	5.	S	7.	W	9.	E
2.	V	4.	J	6.	A	8.	B	10.	D

TEST 3

DIRECTIONS: The questions in this test refer to the use of tools shown below. Read the question, and for the operation given, select the proper tool to be used from those shown. *PRINT* on your answer sheet, in the correspondingly numbered item space, the letter given below your selected tool.

KEY : CORRECT ANSWERS APPEAR AT THE END OF THIS TEST.

1. Tightening lag screws which hold a bracket to a wooden post
2. Making holes for sheet metal screws in 20-gauge sheet metal
3. Finishing the surface of a concrete sidewalk
4. Enlarging the hole in a steel strap to take a larger diameter machine screw
5. Installing an elbow fitting on the end of a pipe
6. Making a 3/4" hole in a wooden timber
7. Removing the rough edges from the outside of a pipe after cutting with a hacksaw
8. Cutting out a circular piece from a tin sheet
9. Removing the head from a bolt that is rusted in place
10. Making a hole through a brick wall for the installation of a 1" water pipe

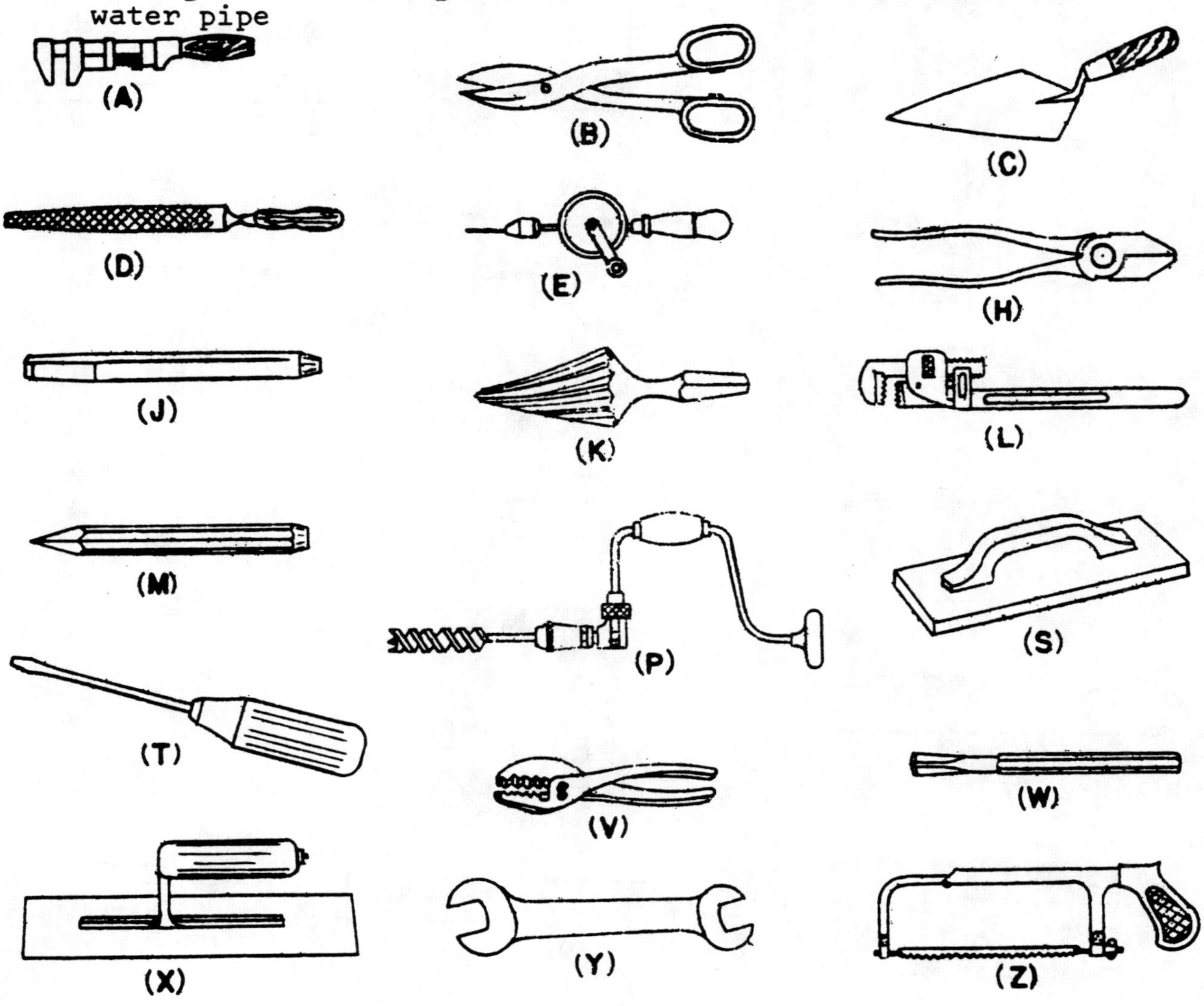

KEY (CORRECT ANSWERS)

1.	Y	3.	S or X	5.	L	7.	D	9.	J
2.	E	4.	E	6.	P	8.	B	10.	M or W

TEST 4

DIRECTIONS: The questions in this test refer to the use of tools shown below. Read the question, and for the operation given, select the proper tool to be used from those shown. *PRINT* on your answer sheet, in the correspondingly numbered item space, the letter given below your selected tool.

KEY: CORRECT ANSWERS APPEAR AT THE END OF THIS TEST.

1. Lifting a track rail to insert a steel plate between tie and rail
2. Drilling a shallow one-inch diameter hole in the concrete roadbed
3. Cutting a piece from a 2" diameter steel rod
4. Center-punching a steel plate before drilling a hole
5. Checking the two rails of a track for level
6. Tightening hexagon head screw spikes into a track tie
7. Lining up holes in two heavy metal plates before inserting a bolt
8. Making a half-twist in a 1/8"X3/4" iron strap held in a vise
9. Measuring the exact length of rail for a space approximately 30'long
10. Removing a bolt rusted in place by knocking off the nut or head
11. Cutting a shallow groove across a wooden tie

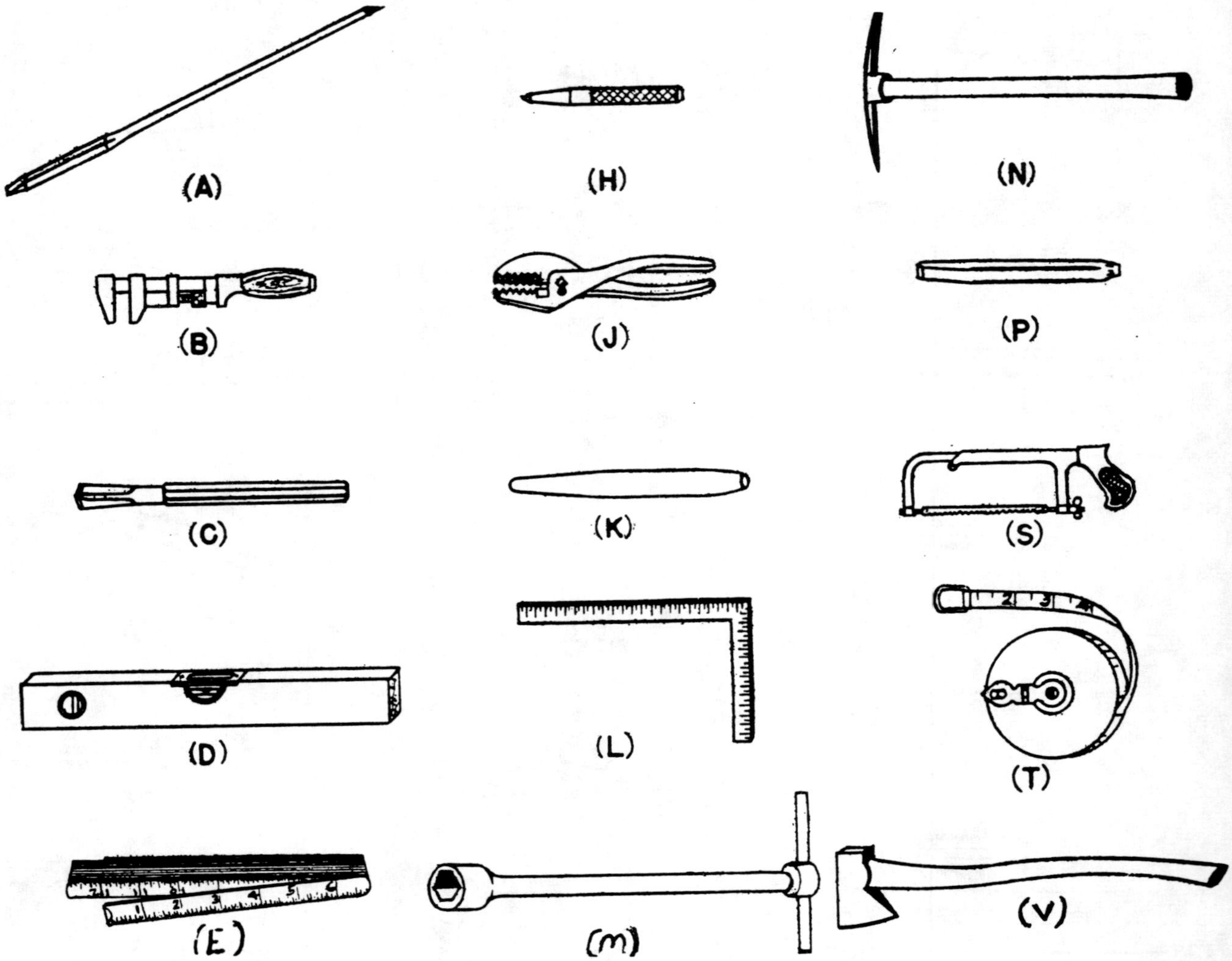

KEY (CORRECT ANSWERS)

1.	A	3.	S	5.	D	7.	K	9.	T
2.	C	4.	H	6.	M	8.	B	10.	P
								11.	V

TEST 5

DIRECTIONS: The questions in this test refer to the use of tools shown below. Read the question, and for the operation given, select the proper tool to be used from those shown. *PRINT* on your answer sheet, in the correspondingly numbered item space, the letter given below your selected tool.

KEY: CORRECT ANSWERS APPEAR AT THE END OF THIS TEST.

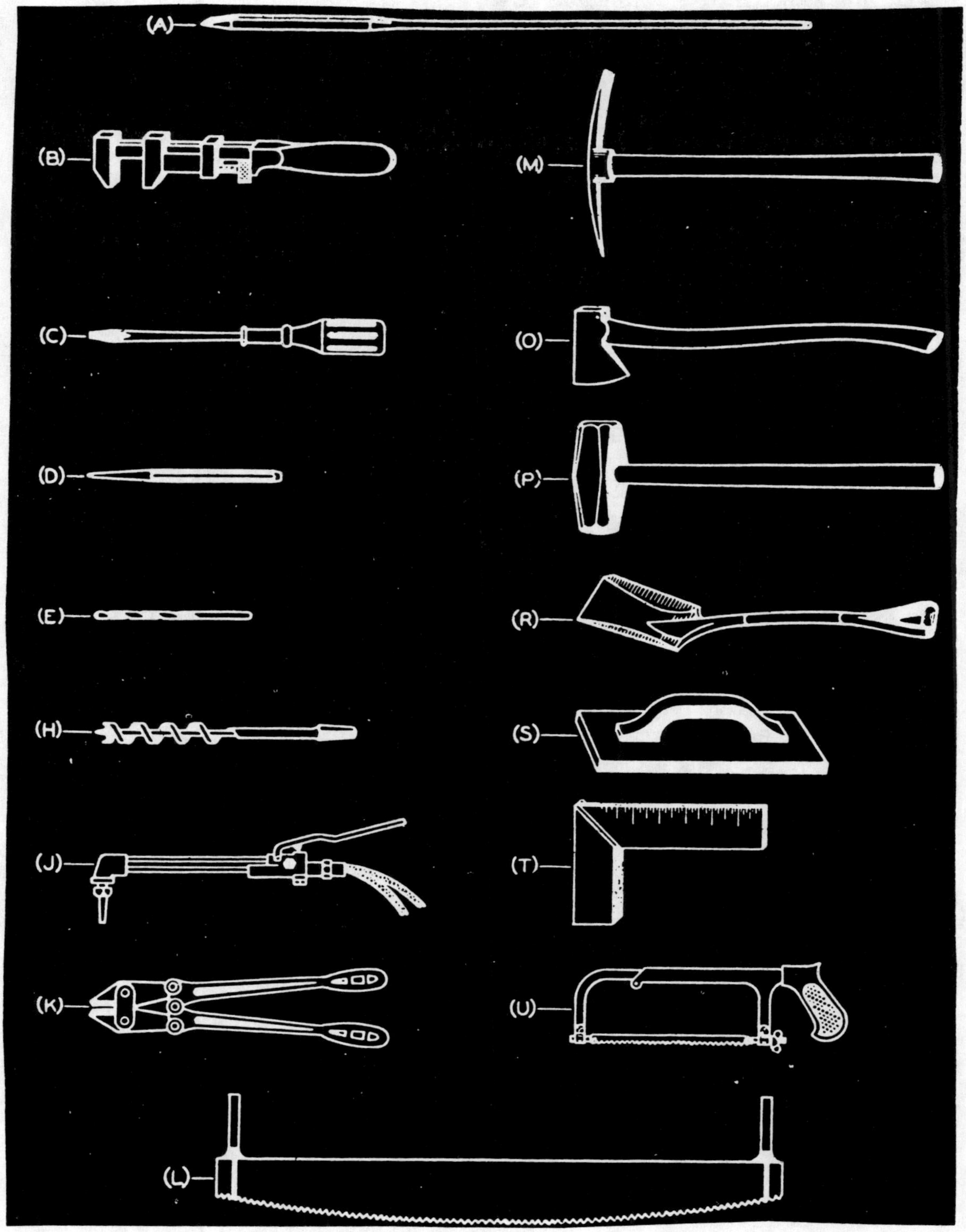

1. Sawing off the end of a bolt
2. Drilling a hole in a steel plate
3. Cutting scrap rail quickly into short lengths
4. Mixing concrete
5. Chopping off a piece of timber
6. Snipping off a piece of steel wire
7. Loading sand into a wheelbarrow
8. Loosening up a pile of solidly packed dirt and gravel
9. Drilling a large hole in a piece of timber
10. Breaking up a slab of concrete
11. Burning a hole in a piece of steel
12. Shifting a long piece of rail along the ground
13. Tightening a nut on a bolt
14. Making a straight cut through a heavy piece of timber
15. Inserting a round-head wood screw
16. Marking the center of a hole to be drilled in a steel plate
17. Determining if a piece of timber has been cut off squarely
18. Putting a smooth surface on concrete
19. Putting sharp points on the ends of wooden stakes
20. Measuring the thickness of a board

KEY (CORRECT ANSWERS)

1.	U	6.	K	11.	J	16.	D
2.	E	7.	R	12.	A	17.	T
3.	J	8.	M	13.	B	18.	S
4.	R	9.	H	14.	L	19.	O
5.	O	10.	P	15.	C	20.	T

TEST 6

TOOLS

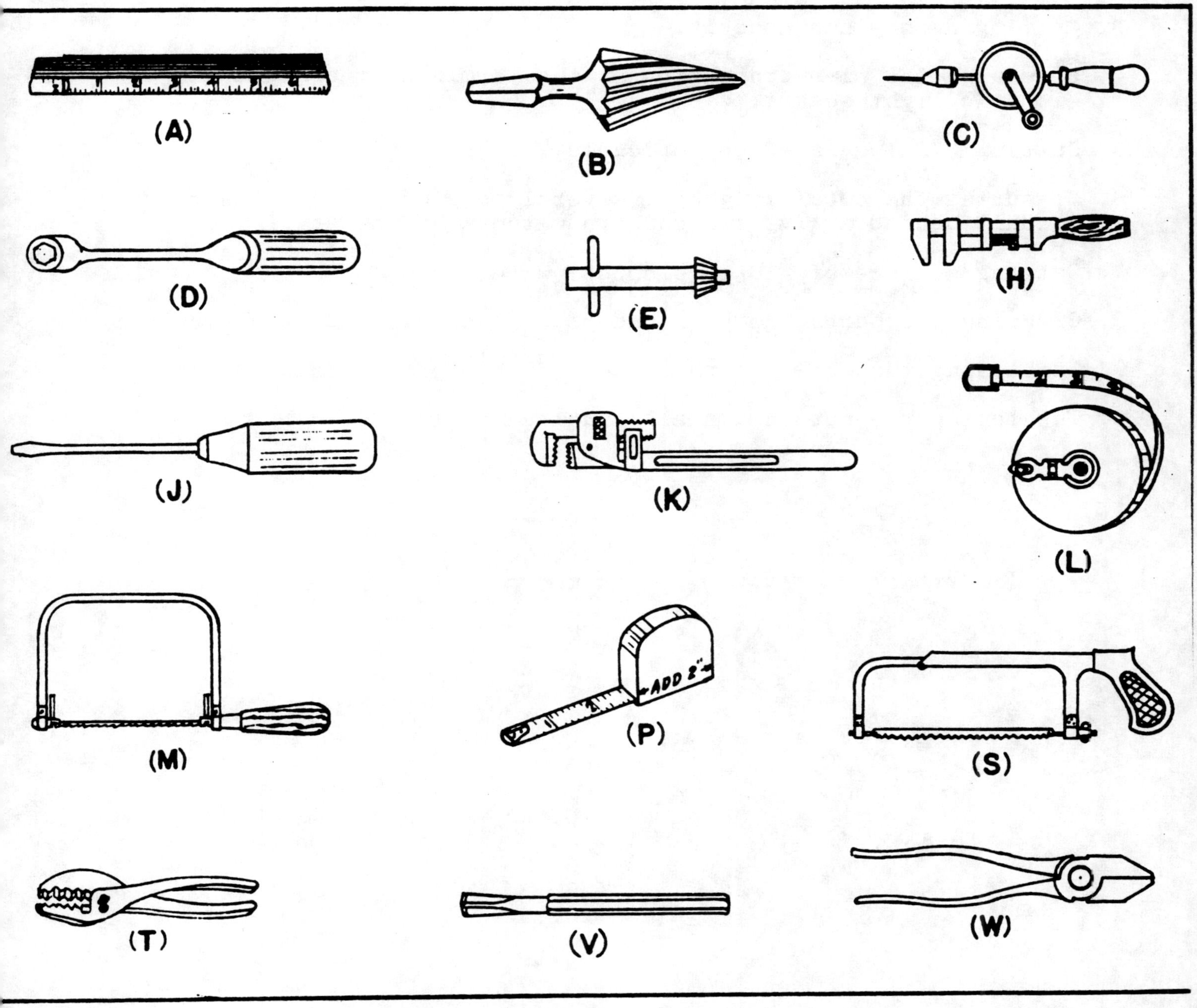

QUESTIONS

DIRECTIONS: 1 to 10 inclusive refer to the use of tools shown above. Read the item, and, for the operation given, select the proper tool to be used from those shown. *PRINT ON YOUR ANSWER SHEET, IN THE CORRESPONDINGLY NUMBERED ITEM SPACE, THE LETTER GIVEN BELOW YOUR SELECTED TOOL.*

1. Tightening a coupling on the end of a piece of conduit.

2. Making a hole in a concrete wall for a lead anchor.

3. Cutting a one-inch conduit.

4. Loosening the wire connection on the terminal of a standard electric light socket.

5. Cutting 3/0 insulated copper cable.

6. Measuring the total length of several coupled pieces of straight conduit behind a live switchboard without an assistant.

7. Cutting a piece of #10 bare copper wire.

8. Cleaning the burrs from the end of a piece of conduit after cutting.

9. Tightening the drill in the chuck of an electric drill.

10. Tightening the nut on a small stud terminal.

KEY (CORRECT ANSWERS)

1. K
2. V
3. S
4. J
5. S

6. A
7. W
8. B
9. E
10. D

TEST 7

TOOLS

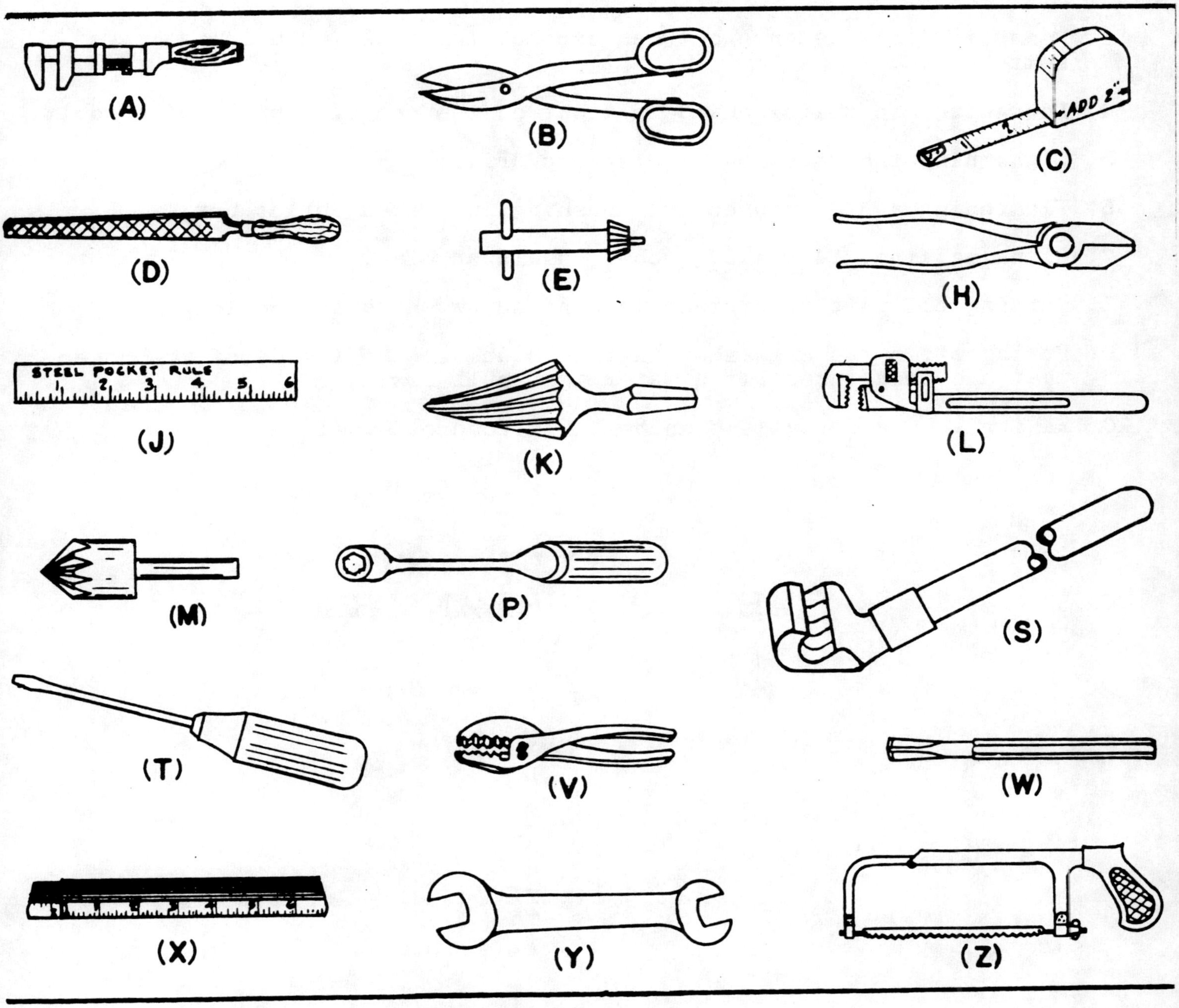

QUESTIONS

DIRECTIONS: 1 to 10 inclusive refer to the use of the tools shown above. Read the item, and, for the operation given, select the proper tool to be used from those shown. *PRINT ON YOUR ANSWER SHEET, IN THE CORRESPONDINGLY NUMBERED ITEM SPACE, THE LETTER GIVEN BELOW YOUR SELECTED TOOL.*

1. Loosening the nut holding a wire on a stud terminal.

2. Removing burrs from the inner edge of conduit after cutting it.

3. Measuring the distance between exposed terminals on a low-voltage switchboard.

4. Loosening a coupling which is tight on the end of a piece of conduit.

5. Tightening the chuck on an electric drill.

6. Tightening a 3/4 inch conduit bushing inside an outlet box.

7. Skinning a no. 14 A.W.G. rubber insulated wire.

8. Cutting off part of a brass machine screw which is too long.

9. Prying off a rubber gasket that is stuck to the inside of the cover that has been taken off a watertight pull box.

10. Making a hole for a lead anchor in a concrete wall.

KEY (CORRECT ANSWERS)

1. P
2. K
3. X
4. L
5. E

6. V
7. H
8. Z
9. T
10. W

TEST 8

TOOLS

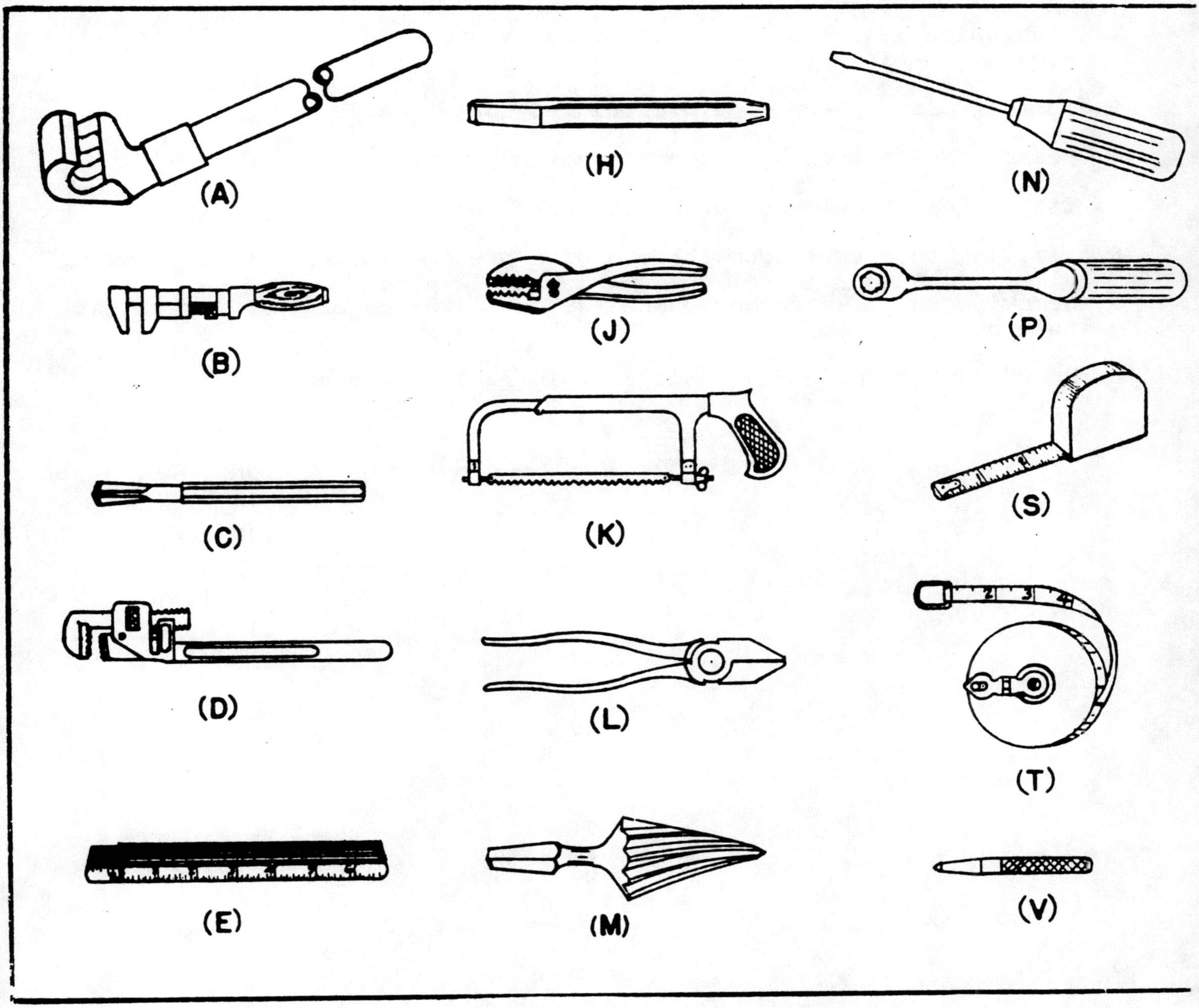

QUESTIONS

DIRECTIONS: 1 to 10 inclusive refer to the use of tools shown above. Read the item, and, for the operation given, select the proper tool to be used from those shown. *PRINT ON YOUR ANSWER SHEET, IN THE CORRESPONDINGLY NUMBERED ITEM SPACE, THE LETTER GIVEN BELOW YOUR SELECTED TOOL.*

1. Tightening a coupling on a piece of one-inch conduit.

2. Drilling a hole in a concrete wall for a lead anchor.

3. **Bending a piece of 3/4-inch conduit.**
4. **Tightening a wire on the terminal of a standard electric light socket.**
5. **Cutting off a piece of 4/0 insulated copper cable.**
6. **Measuring the length of a proposed long conduit run.**
7. **Tightening a small nut on a terminal board.**
8. **Removing the burrs from the end of a piece of conduit after cutting.**
9. **Removing the flat rubber gasket stuck to the cover of a watertight pull box.**
10. **Knocking the head off a bolt that is rusted in place.**

KEY (CORRECT ANSWERS)

1. D
2. C
3. A
4. N
5. K
6. T
7. P
8. M
9. N
10. H

ABSTRACT REASONING

SPATIAL RELATIONS/TWO DIMENSIONS

COMMENTARY

Since intelligence exists in many forms or phases and the theory of differential aptitudes is now firmly established in testing, other manifestations and measurements of intelligence than verbal or purely arithmetical must be identified and measured.

The spatial relations test, including that phase designated as spatial perception, involves and measures the ability to solve problems, drawn up in the form of outlines or pictures, which are concerned with the shapes of objects or the interrelationship of their parts. While, concededly, little is known about the nature and scope of this aptitude, it appears that this ability is required in science, mathematics, engineering, and drawing courses and curricula. Accordingly, tests of spatial perception involving the reconstruction of two-dimensional patterns, are presented in this section.

It is to be noted that the relationships expressed in spatial tests are geometric, definitive, and exact. Keeping these basic characteristics in mind, the applicant is to proceed to solve the spatial perception problems in his own way. There is no set method of solving these problems. The examinee may find that there are different methods for different types of spatial problems. Therefore, the BEST way to prepare for this type of test is to *TAKE* and study the work-practice problems in two-dimensional patterns provided in this section.

ABSTRACT REASONING

SPATIAL RELATIONS/TWO DIMENSIONS

·The tests of spatial relations that follow consist of items which involve the visualization of two dimensions.

Each of the items of these tests consists of a line of figures -- a complete figure on the left and four lettered alternatives of component parts on the right, only one of which can be fitted together exactly to form the complete figure on the left.

The candidate is then required to select that choice of component parts which could be fitted together to form the complete figure given at the left.

SAMPLE QUESTIONS AND EXPLANATIONS

DIRECTIONS: The items in this part constitute a test of spatial relations involving two dimensions. Each item consists of a line of figures. The first figure is the complete figure. This is followed by four lettered choices of component parts, only one of which can be fitted together exactly to form the first (complete) figure.

Rules to be followed:

1. The lettered choice of component parts selected as the answer must have the same number of parts as the first (complete) figure.
2. The parts must fit exactly.
3. The parts may be turned around but may not be turned over.

1.

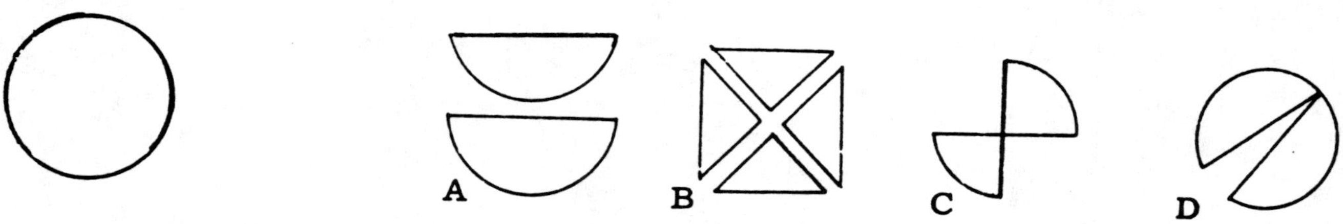

The correct answer is D. When the two parts of D are completely closed, they form the complete figure on the left.

2.

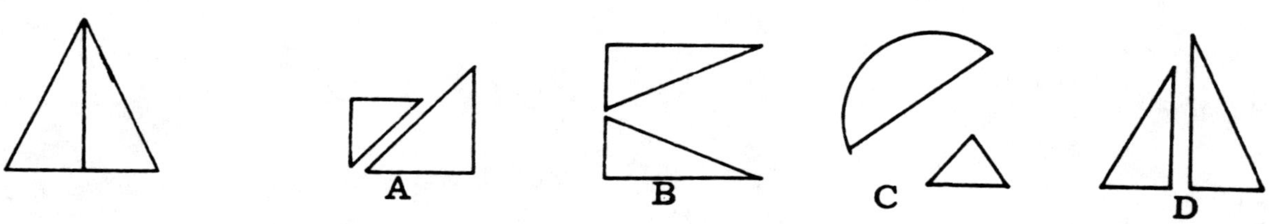

The correct answer is B. When the two parts of B are reversed in position, they form the complete figure on the left.

TEST 1

1.

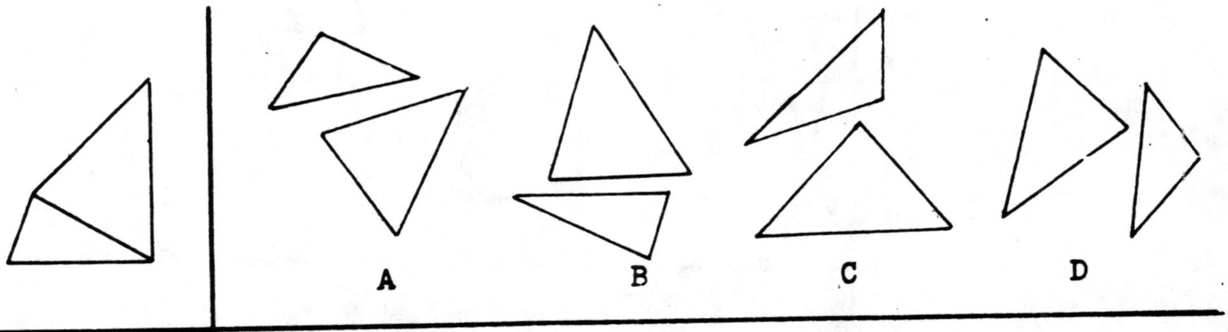

2.

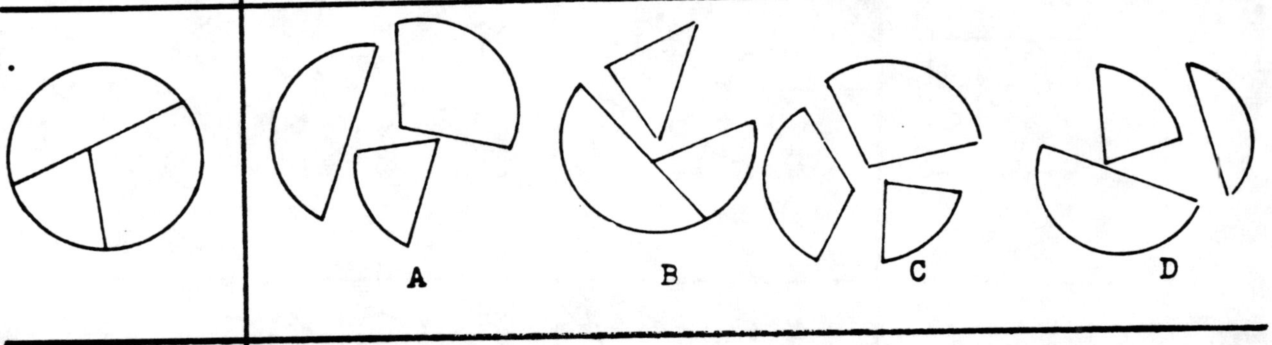

3.

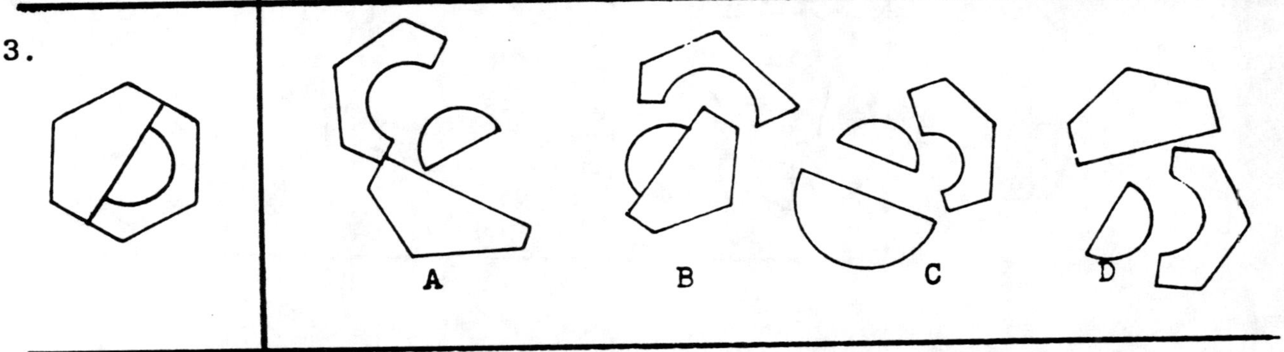

4.

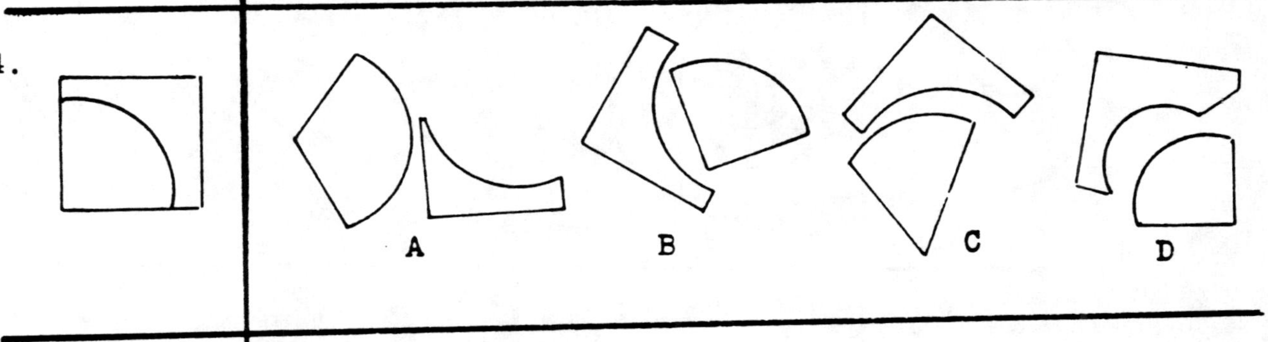

5.

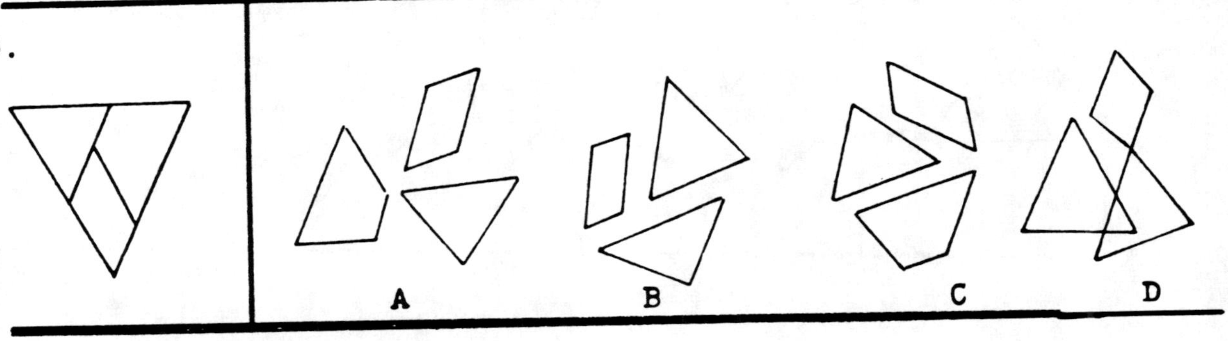

TEST 2

6. 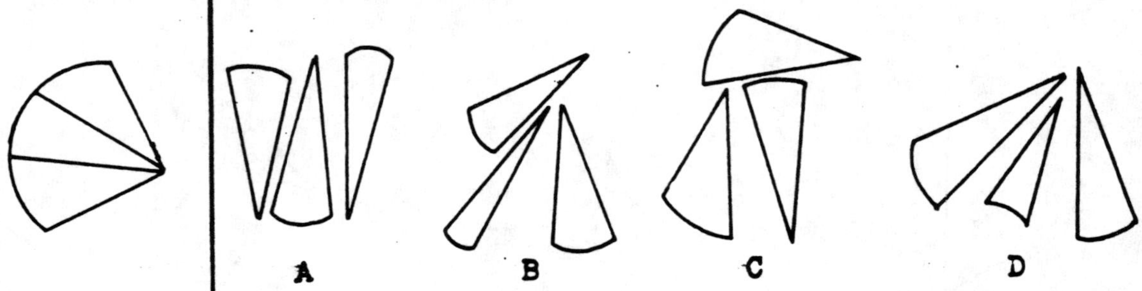

7. 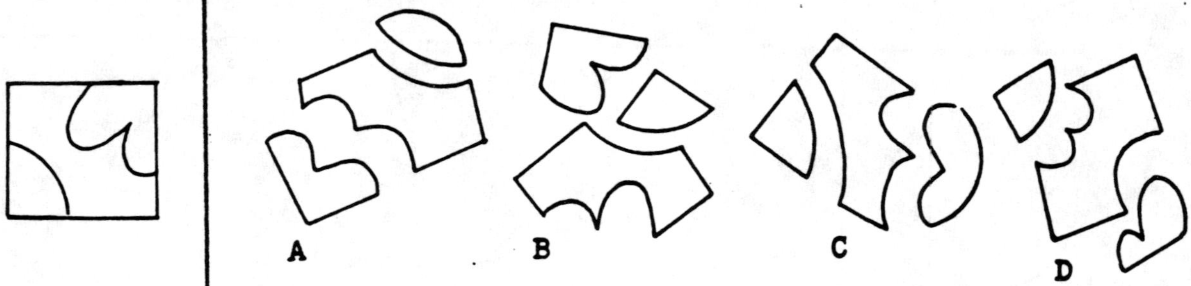

8. 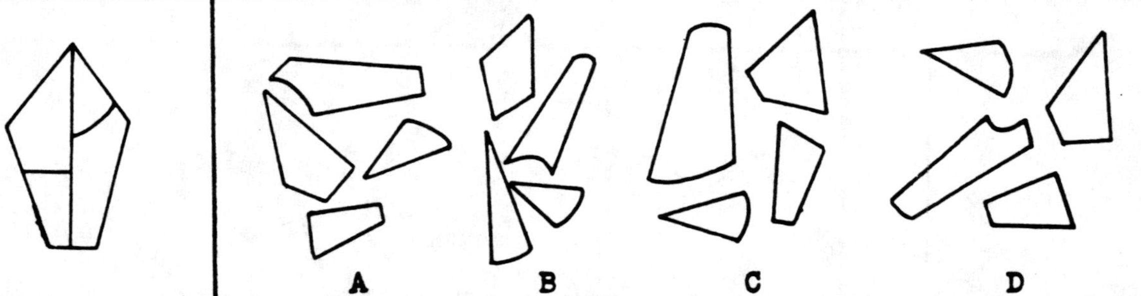

9. 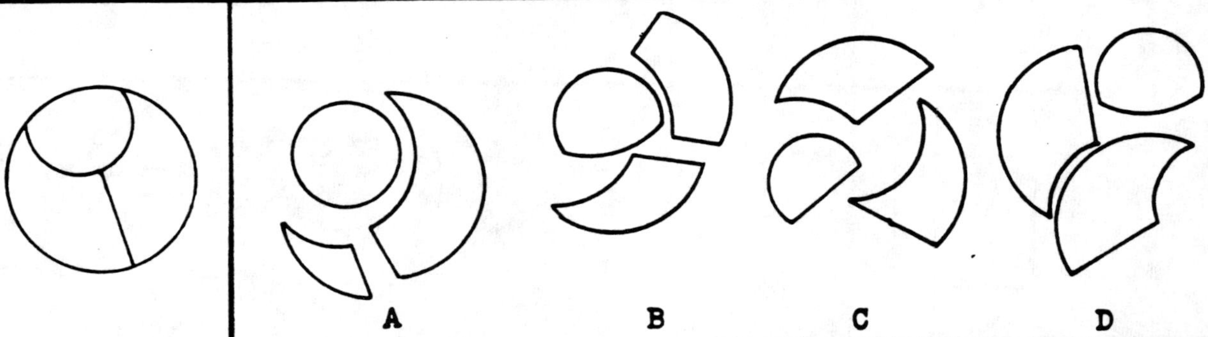

10. 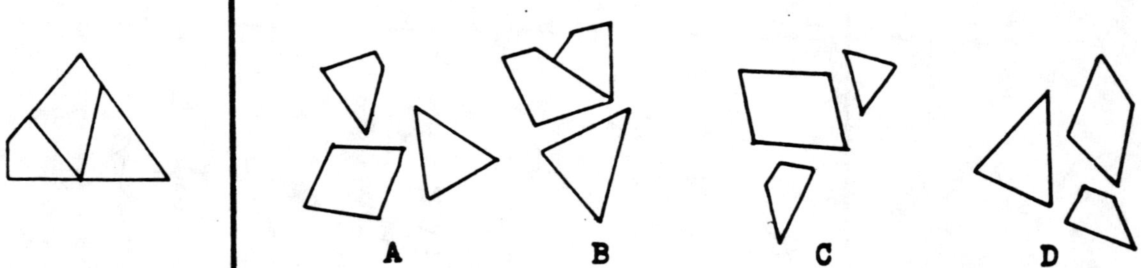

TEST 3

11.

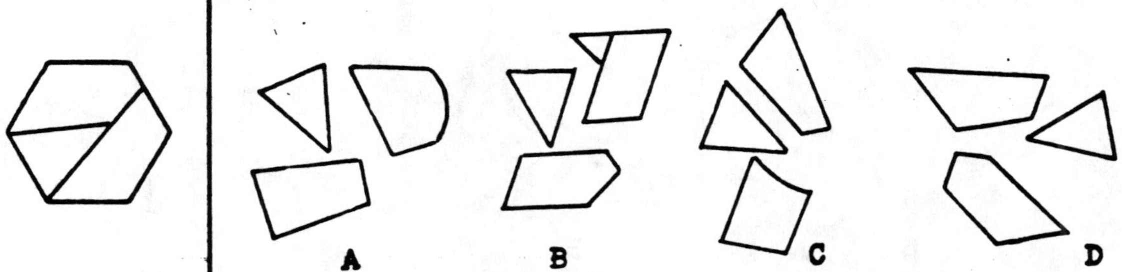

12.

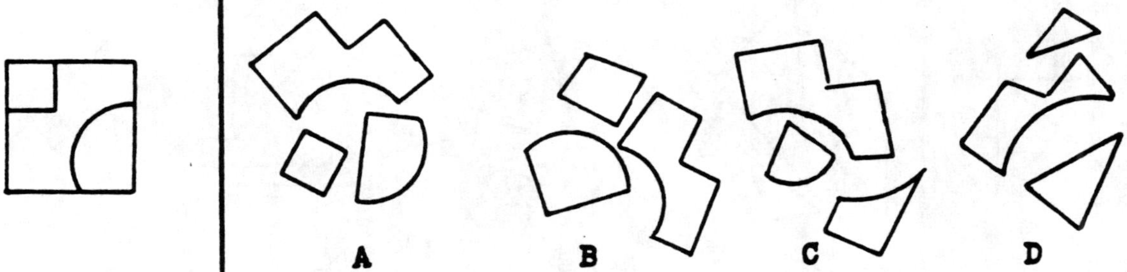

13.

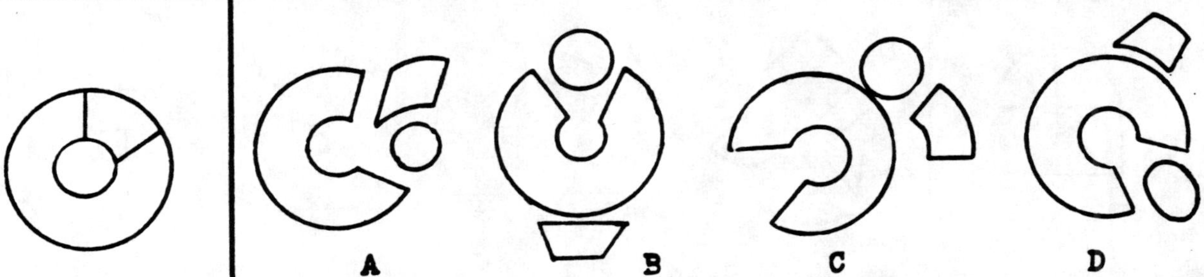

14.

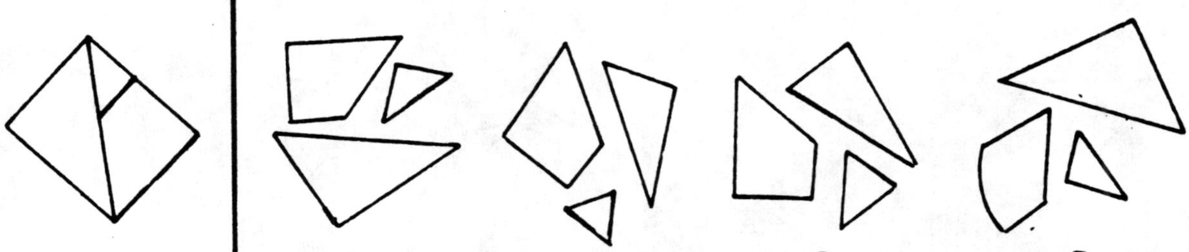

15.

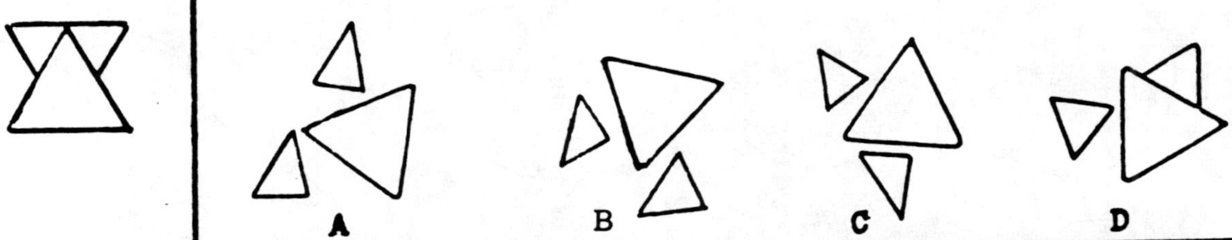

TEST 4

16. 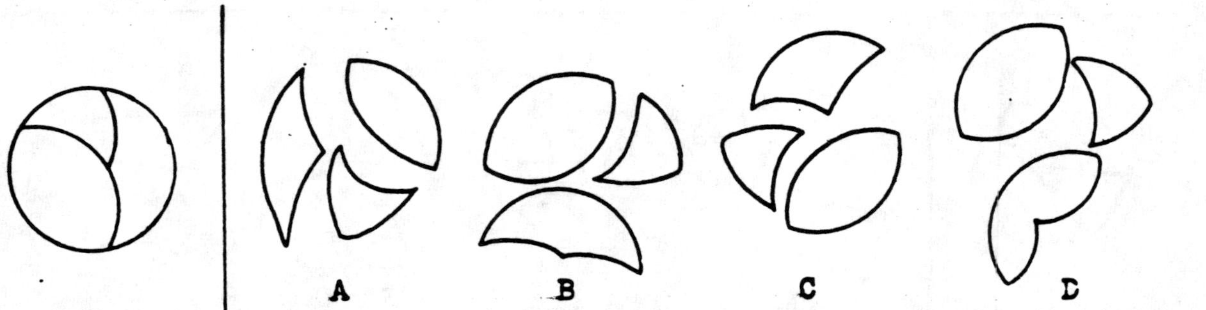

17. 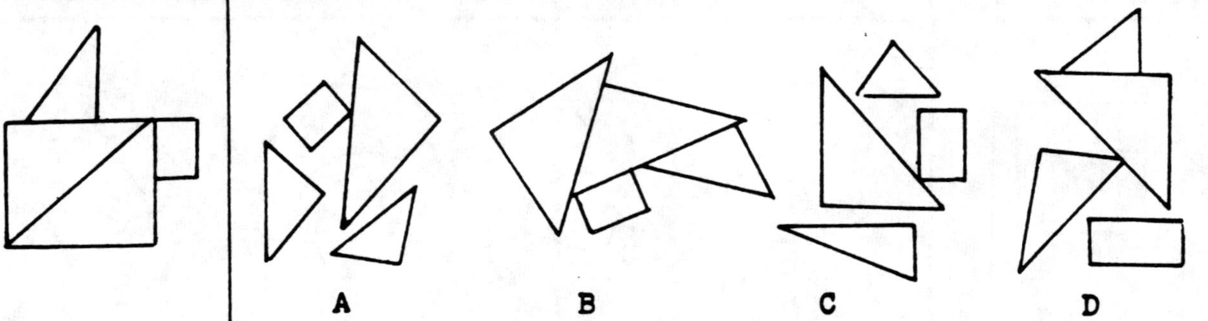

18. 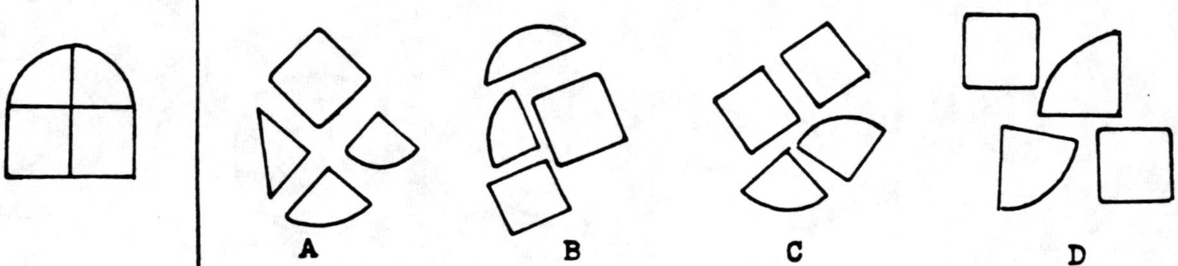

19. 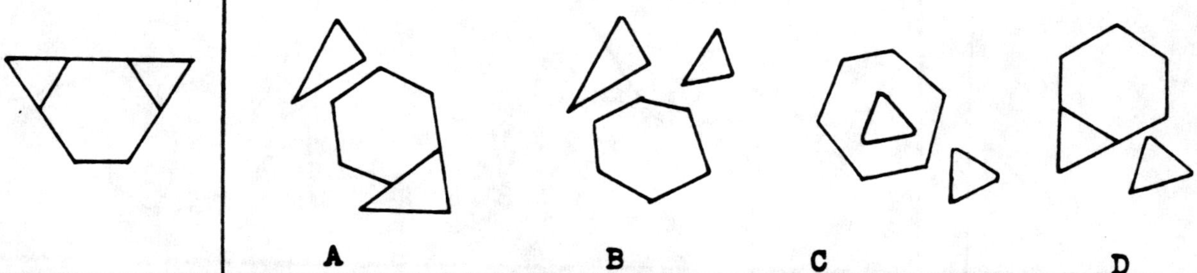

20. 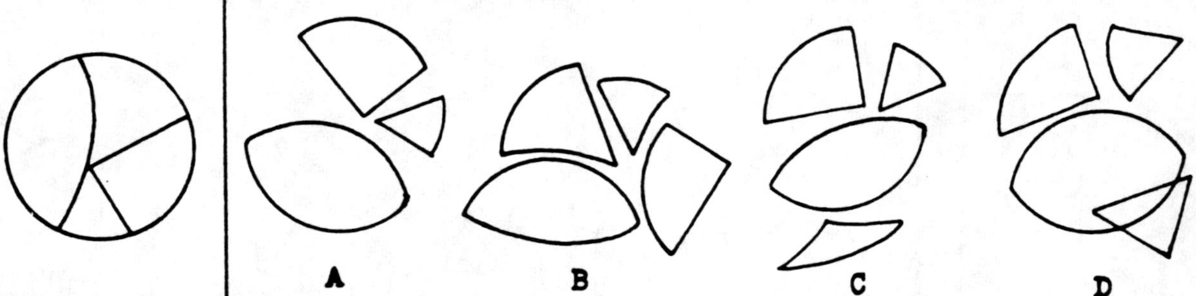

TEST 5

21.

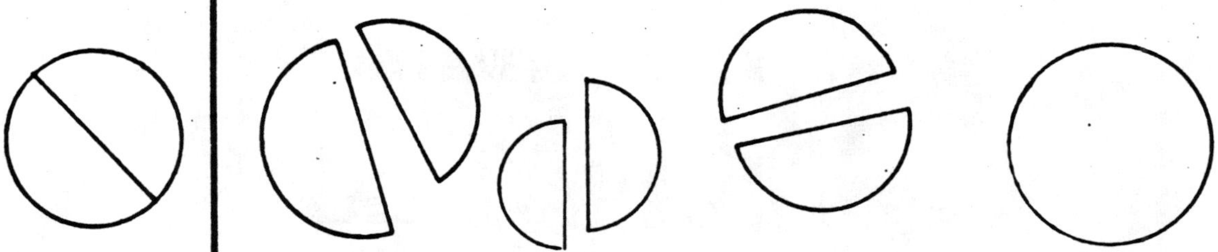

A B C D

22.

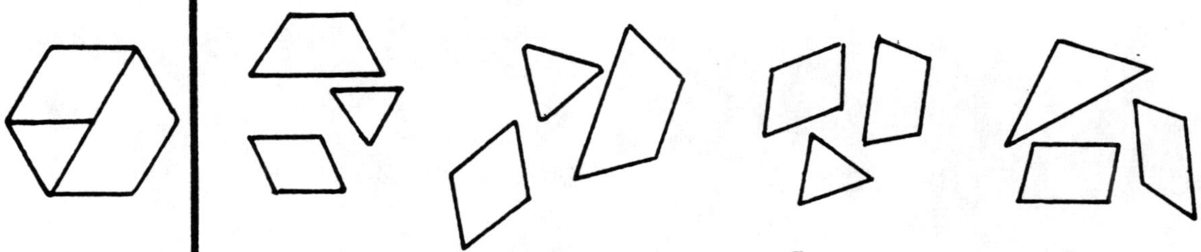

A B C D

23.

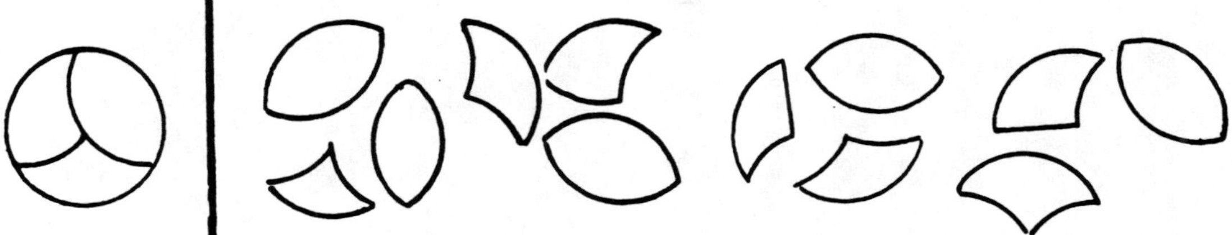

A B C D

24.

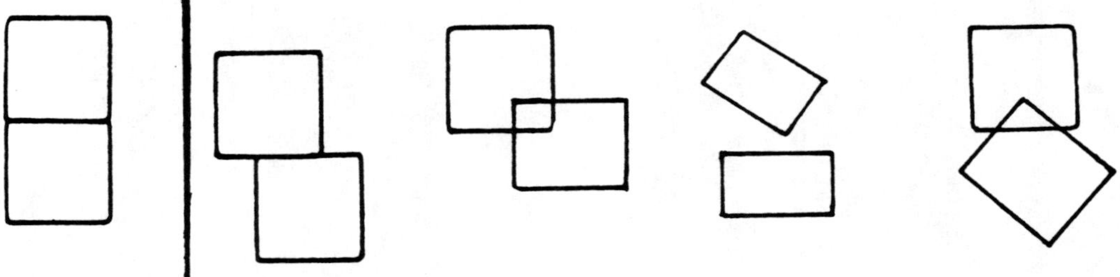

A B C D

25.

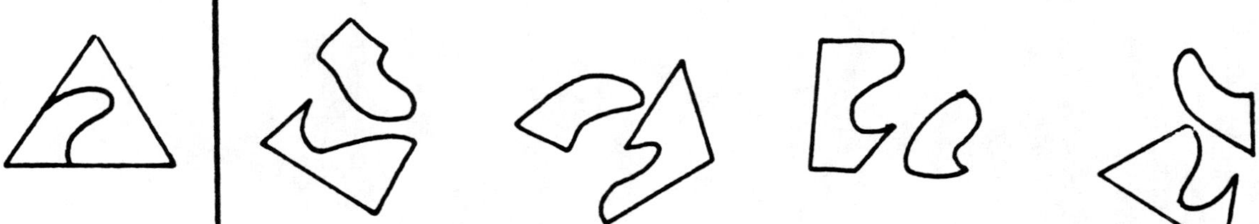

A B C D

KEYS (CORRECT ANSWERS)

TEST 1	TEST 2	TEST 3	TEST 4	TEST 5
1. B	6. C	11. D	16. B	21. C
2. A	7. B	12. A	17. B	22. B
3. D	8. A	13. C	18. C	23. B
4. B	9. D	14. A	19. D	24. A
5. C	10. B	15. D	20. B	25. D

ABSTRACT REASONING

COMMENTARY

The mathematical or quantitative ability of the candidate is generally measured through the form of questions and/or problems involving arithmetical reasoning, algebraic problem solving, and the interpretation of visual materials -- graphs, charts, tables, diagrams, maps, cartoons, and pictures.

A more recent development, which attempts to assay facets of quantitative ability not ordinarily discernible or measurable, is the nonverbal test of reasoning of the type commonly designated as the figure analogy. Figure analogies are novel and differentiated measures of non-numerical mathematics reasoning.

Since intelligence exists in many forms or phases and the theory of differential aptitudes is now firmly established in testing, other manifestations and measurements of intelligence than verbal or purely arithmetical must be identified and measured.

Classification inventory, or figure classification, involves the aptitude of form perception, i.e., the ability to perceive pertinent detail in objects or in pictorial or graphic material. It involves making visual comparisons and discriminations and discerning slight differences in shapes and shading figures and widths and lengths of lines.

—

One aspect of this type of nonverbal question takes the form of a *positive* requirement to find the *COMPATIBLE PATTERN* (i.e., the one that *does* belong) from among two (2) sets of figure groups. The prescription for this question-type is as follows:

> A group of three drawings lettered A,B,and C, respectively, is presented, followed on the same line by five (5) numbered alternative drawings labeled 1,2,3,4, and 5, respectively.
>
> The first two (2) drawings (A,B) in each question are related in some way.
>
> The candidate is then to decide what characteristic *each* of the figures labeled A and B has that causes them to be related, and is then to select the one alternative from the five (5) numbered figures that is related to figure C in the same way that drawing B is related to drawing A.

Leading examples of presentation are the figure analogy and the figure classification. The Section that follows presents progressive and varied samplings of this type of question.

—

FIGURE ANALOGIES

Figure analogies are a novel and differentiated measure of non-numerical mathematics reasoning.

This question takes the form of, and, indeed, is similar to, the one-blank verbal analogy. However, pictures or drawings are used instead of words.

SAMPLE QUESTIONS AND EXPLANATIONS

DIRECTIONS: Each question in this part consists of 3 drawings lettered A,B,C, followed by 5 alternative drawings, numbered 1 to 5. The first 2 drawings in each question are related in some way. Choose the number of the alternative that is related to the third drawing in the same way that the second drawing is related to the first, and mark the appropriate space on your answer sheet.

1.

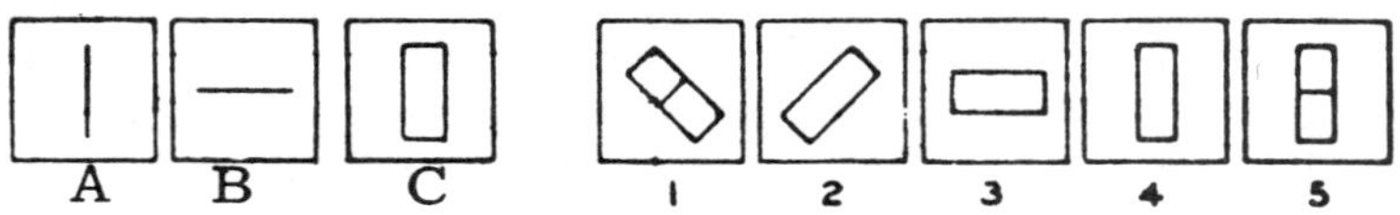

The CORRECT answer is 3. A vertical line has the same relationship to a horizontal line that a rectangle standing on its end has to a rectangle lying on its side.

2.

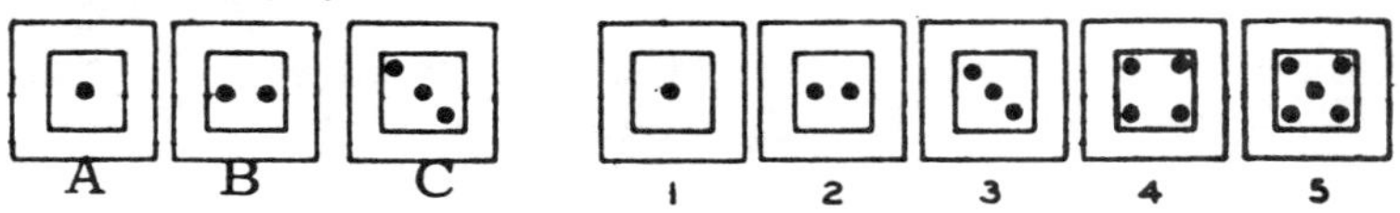

The second square has one more dot than the first square. Therefore the CORRECT answer is alternative 4, which has one more dot than the third square.

3.

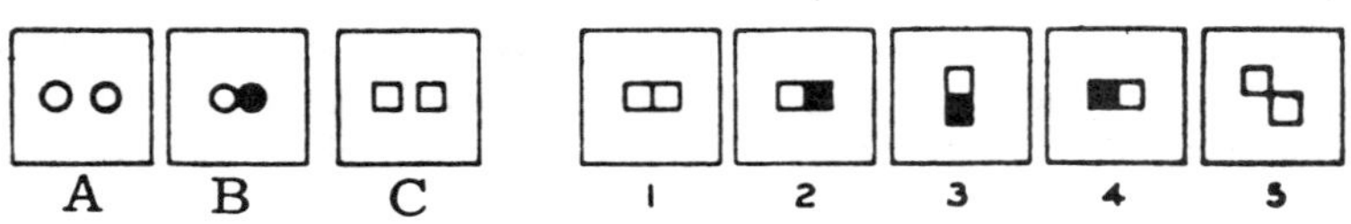

In the second drawing the circles are moved together and the circle on the right darkened. Therefore the CORRECT answer is 2, in which the squares are moved together and the right-hand square darkened.

4.

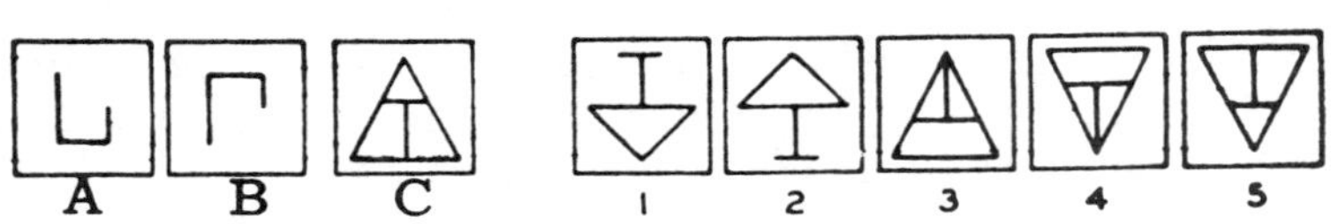

The CORRECT answer is 5. The second drawing is the inverted version of the first; alternative 5 is the inverted version of the third drawing.

5. 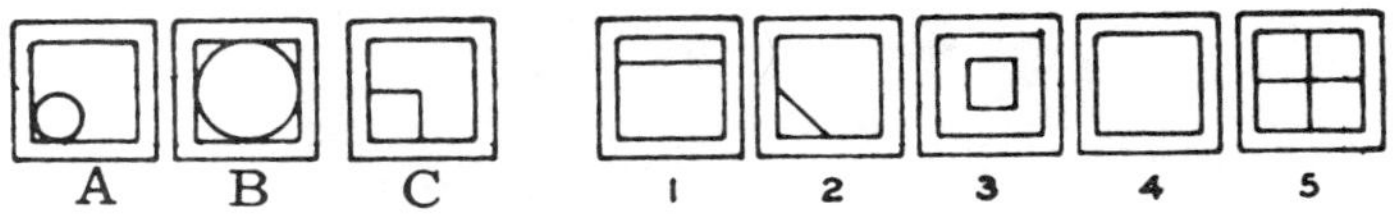

The CORRECT answer is 4. Drawing A has a small circle within a square; drawing B contains a circle completely filling the square. Drawing C has a small square within a square; in alternative 4, this small square has been magnified to its complete size within the square so that this magnified square coincides with the enclosing square, leaving the outline of only one square.

6. 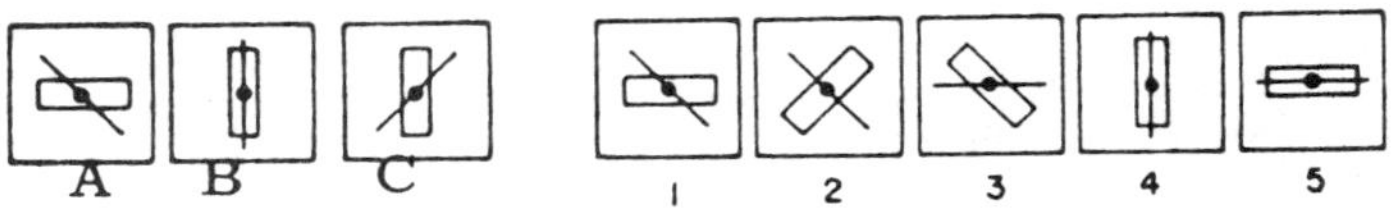

The CORRECT answer is 5. Drawing A appears in a horizontal position, with a diagonal line drawn through the center dot; drawing B appears in a vertical position, with a straight line drawn through the center dot. Drawing C is similar to drawing A, except that it appears in a vertical position; drawing 5 is similar to drawing B, except that it appears in a horizontal position. Our analogy may, therefore, be verbally expressed as

A:B:C:5.

SUGGESTIONS FOR ANSWERING THE FIGURE ANALOGY QUESTION

1. In doing the actual questions, there can be little practical gain in rationalizing each answer that you attempt. What is needed is a quick and ready perceptive sense in this matter.

2. The BEST way to prepare for this type of question is to do the "Tests" in figure analogies that follow. By this method, you will gain enough functional skill to enable you to cope successfully with this type of question on the Examination.

PLEASE NOTE -- In the tests which begin on page 5, after the sample questions, the three (3) drawings are unlabeled and the answers have four (4) choices instead of five (5) labeled A,B,C and D. They are to be answered in the same way.

SAMPLE TEST

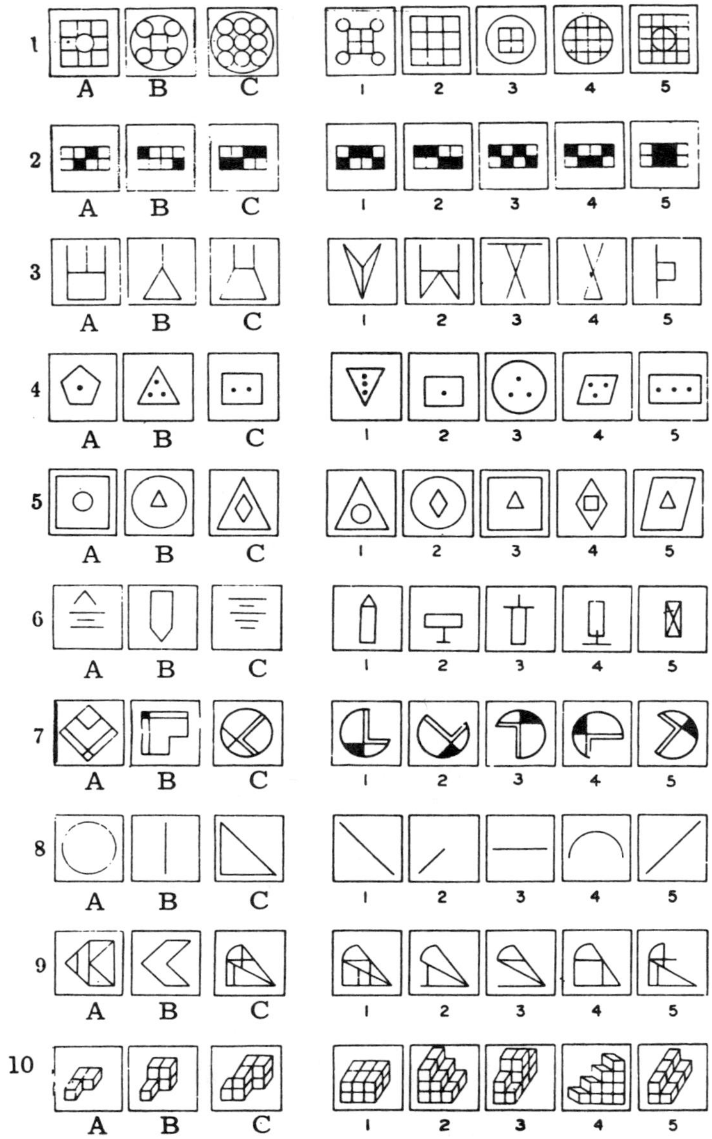

KEY(CORRECT ANSWERS)

1. 2
2. 2
3. 4
4. 1
5. 4
6. 3
7. 3
8. 2

EXPLANATION OF ANSWERS

1. In the second figure, the squares are changed to circles and the circles to squares.
2. In the second figure, the upper darkened area has moved two squares to left; the lower, two squares to right.
3. The second figure has a flat base, like the first.
4. The sum of sides and dots in the second figure equals that of the first.
5. The outside part of the second figure is the inside part of the first.
6. The second figure is constructed from the lines given in the first.
7. The second figure is obtained from the first by rotating it 135° clockwise, darkening the smaller area and deleting the larger.
8. The second figure is the bisector of the area of the first.
9. The second figure is obtained from the first by deleting all the vertical lines.
10. The second figure contains two blocks more than the first.

EXAMINATION SECTION

PROBLEM FIGURES

ANSWER FIGURES

1.

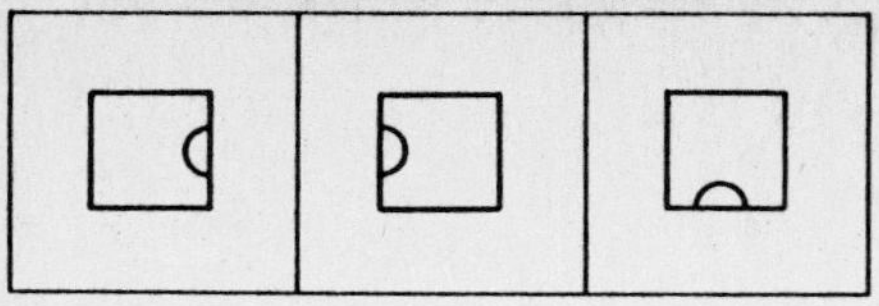

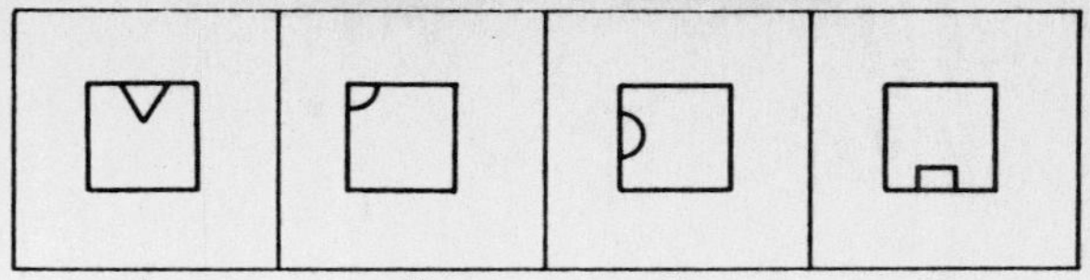

A B C D

2.

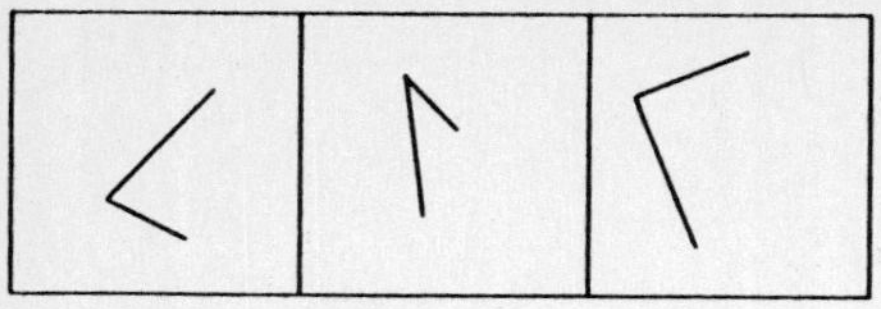

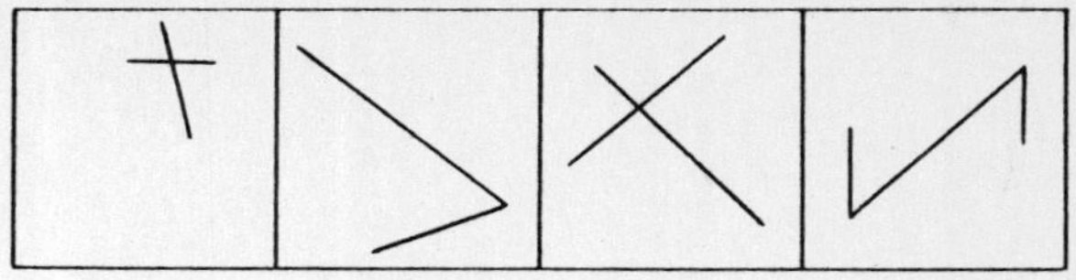

A B C D

3.

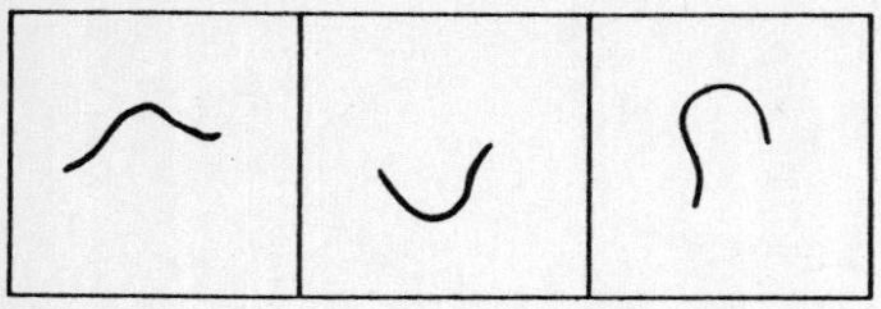

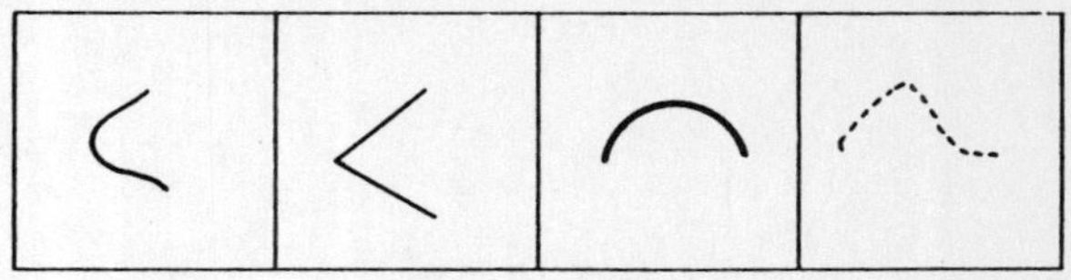

A B C D

4.

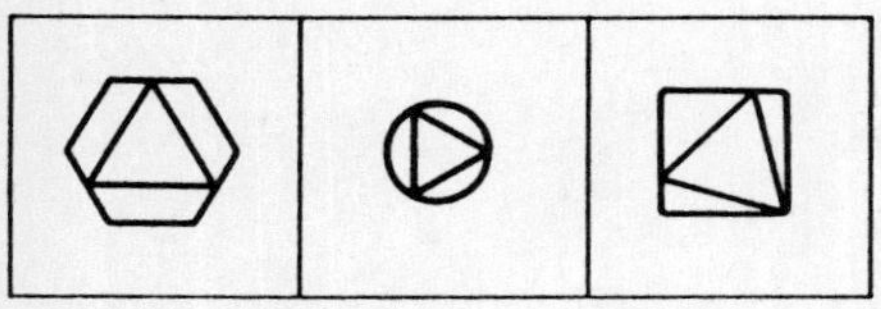

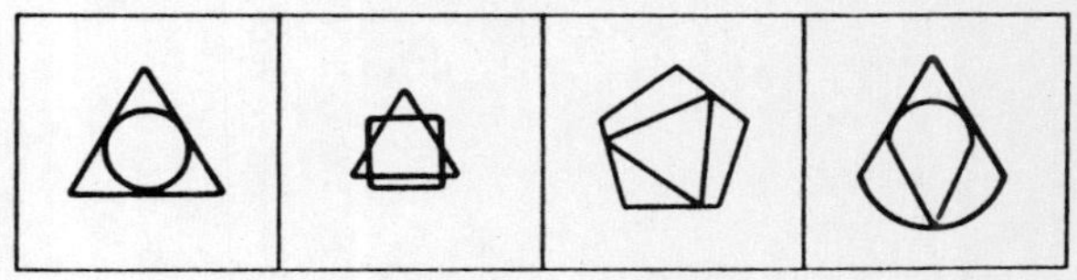

A B C D

5.

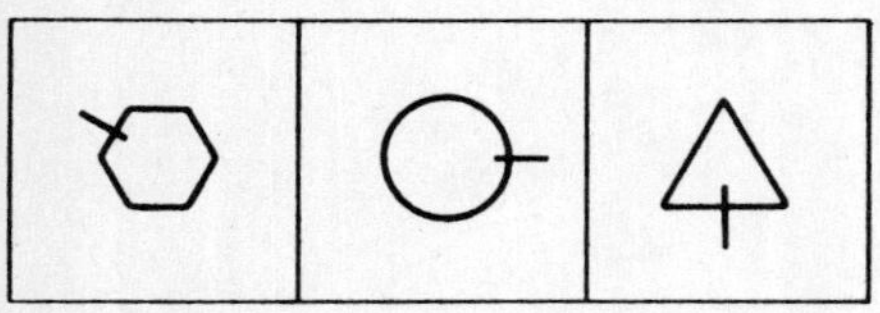

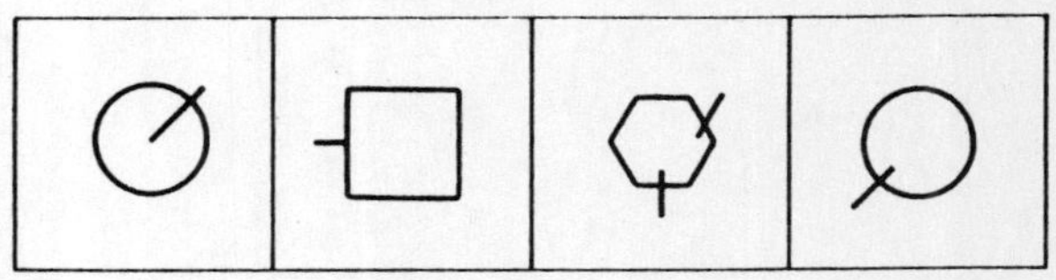

A B C D

6.

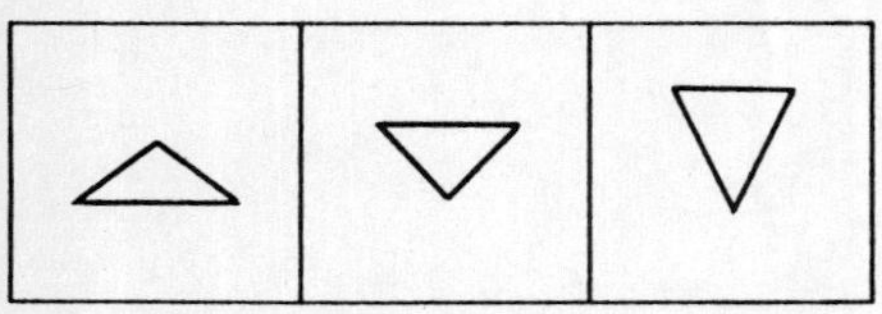

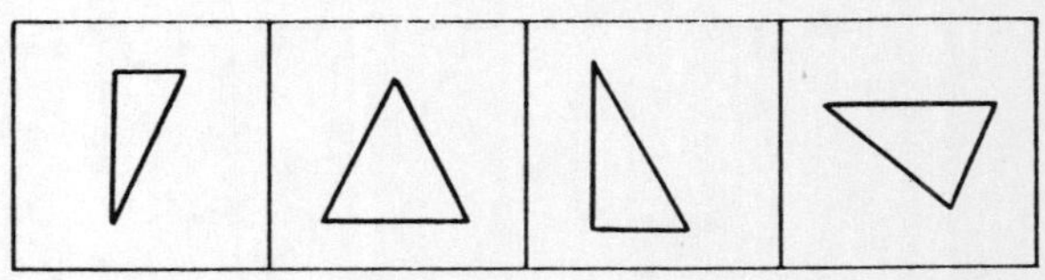

A B C D

7.

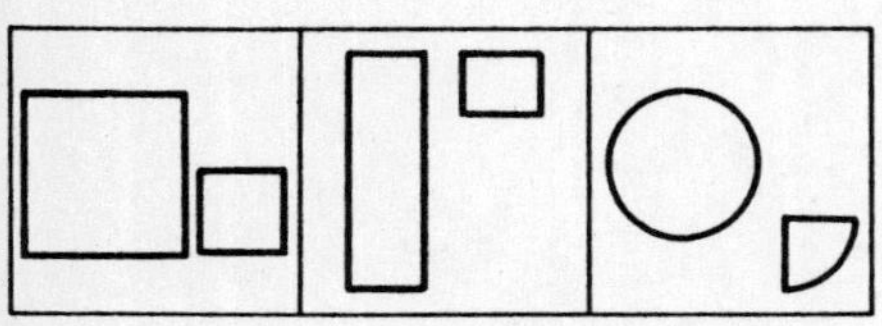

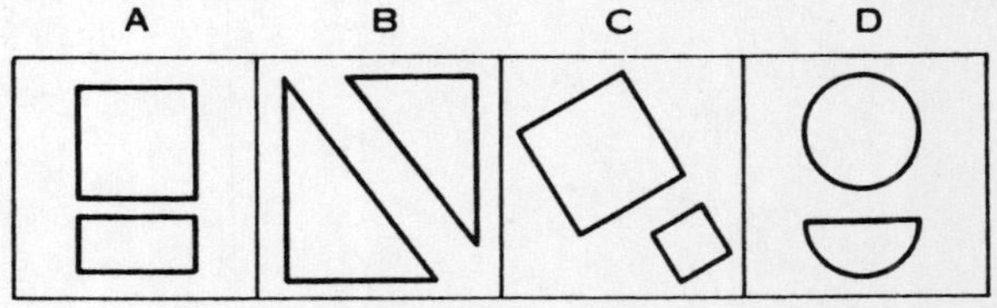

A B C D

8.

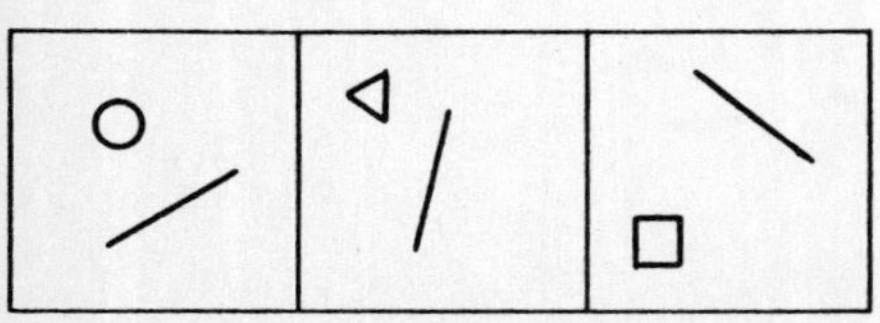

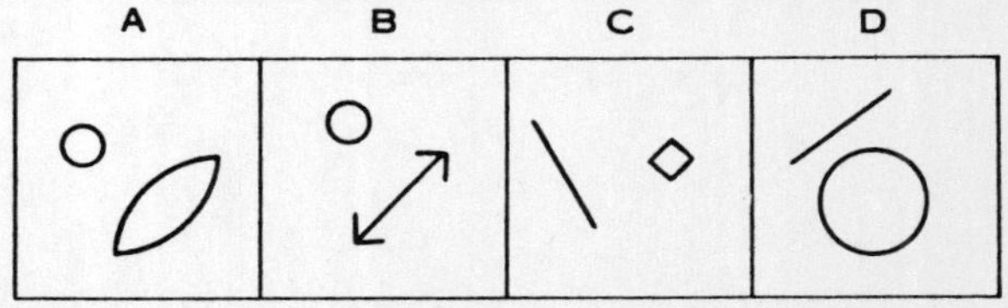

A B C D

9.

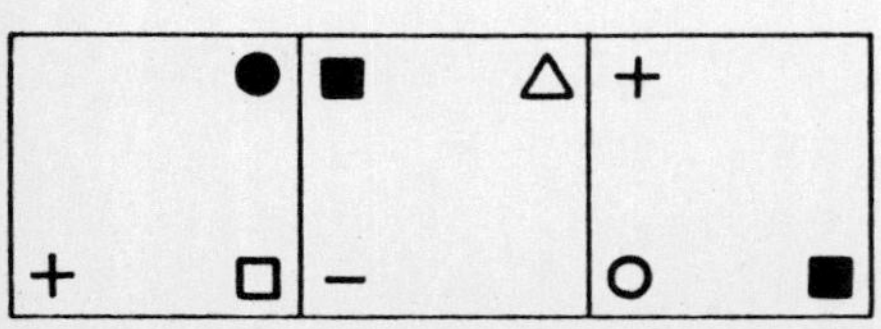

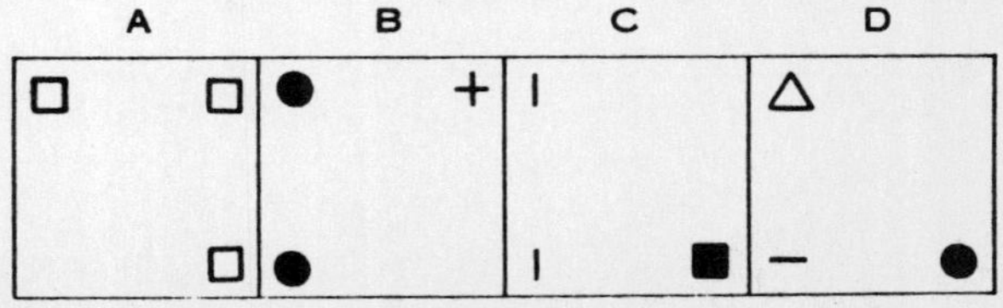

A B C D

10.

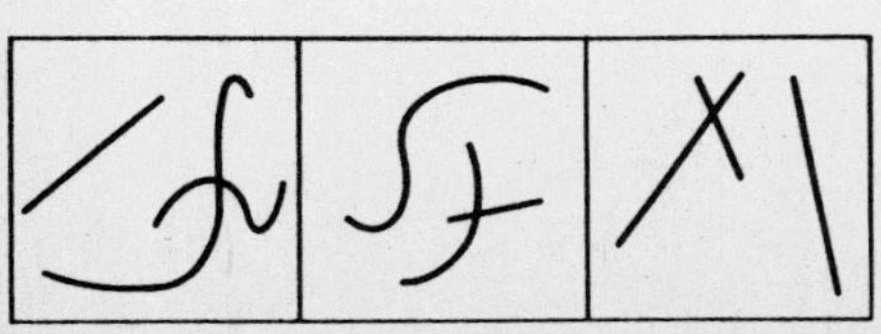

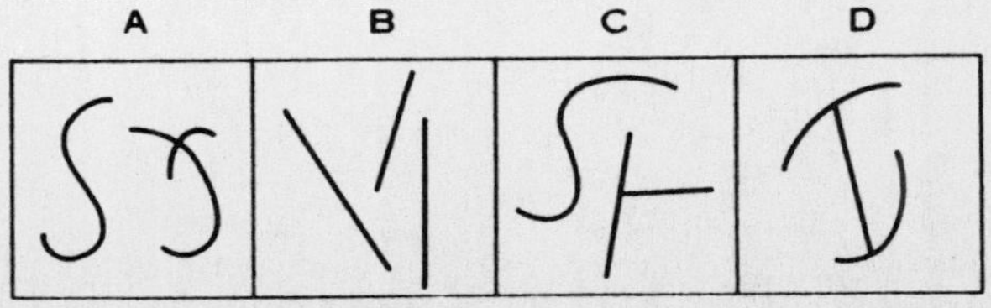

A B C D

PROBLEM FIGURES | ANSWER FIGURES

11.
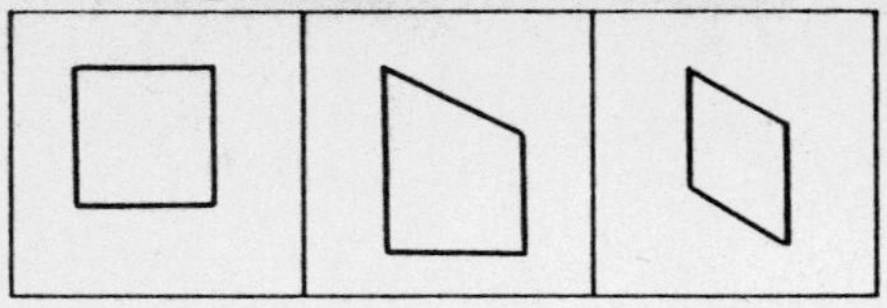
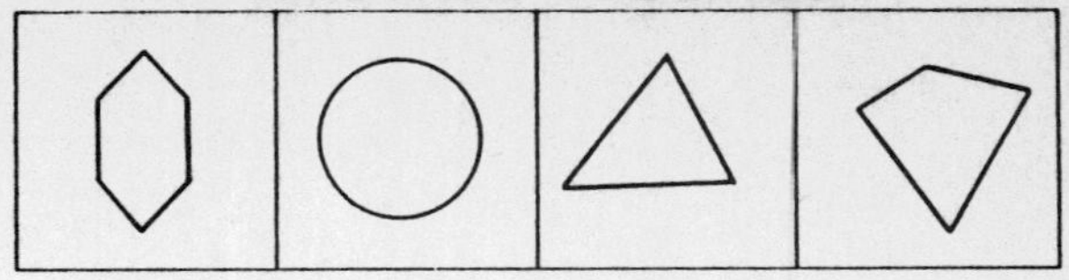
A B C D

12.
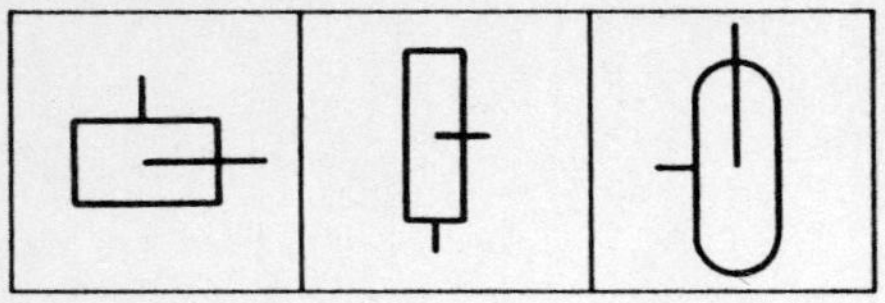
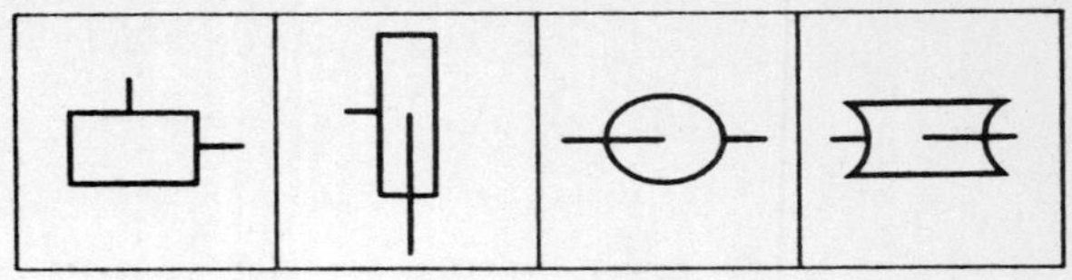
A B C D

13.
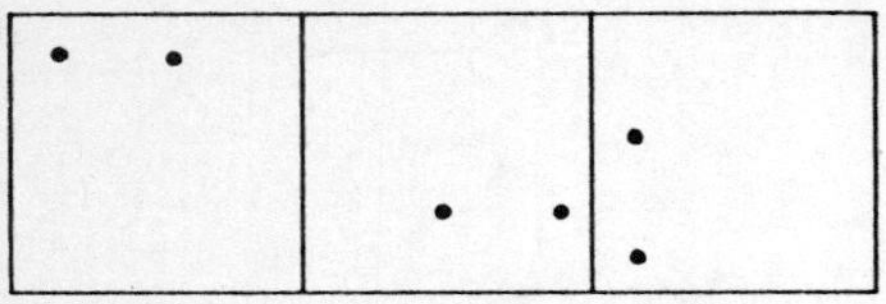
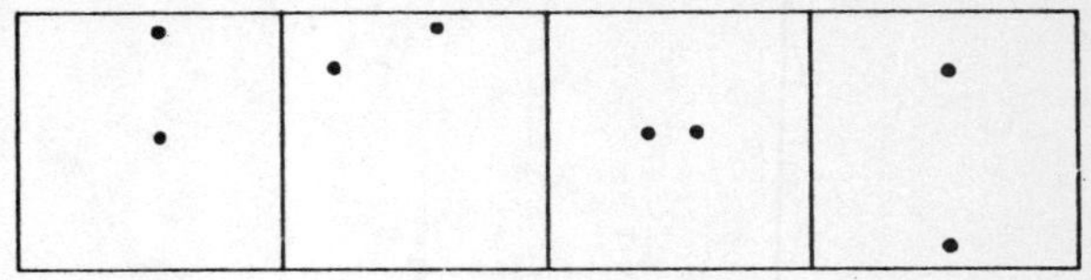
A B C D

14.
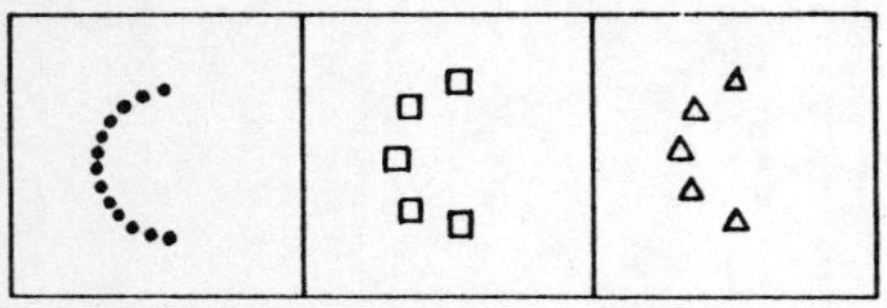
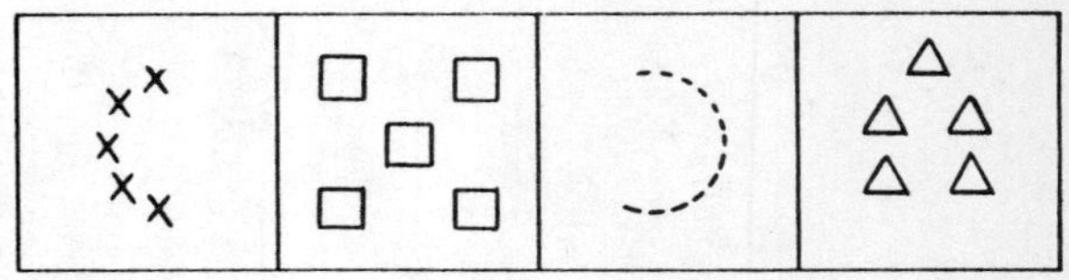
A B C D

15.
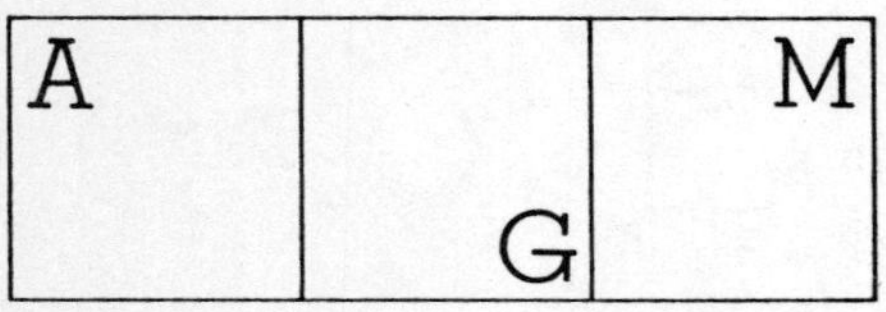

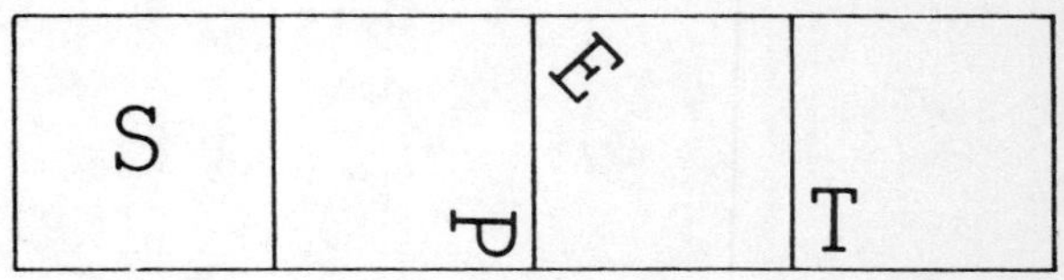

A B C D

16.
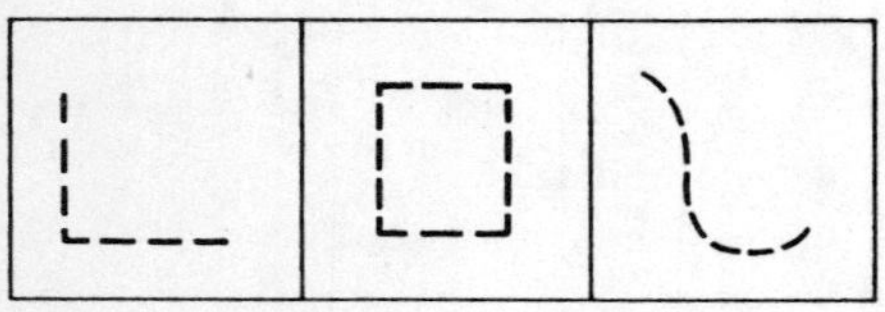
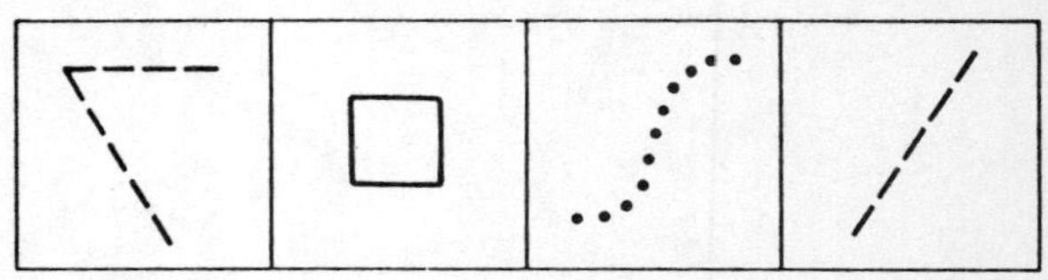
A B C D

17.
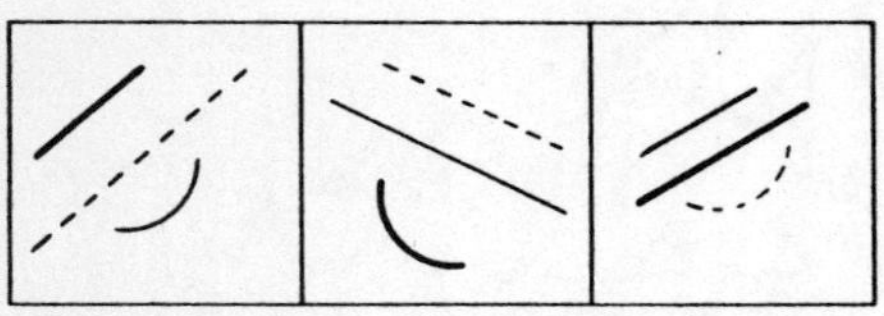
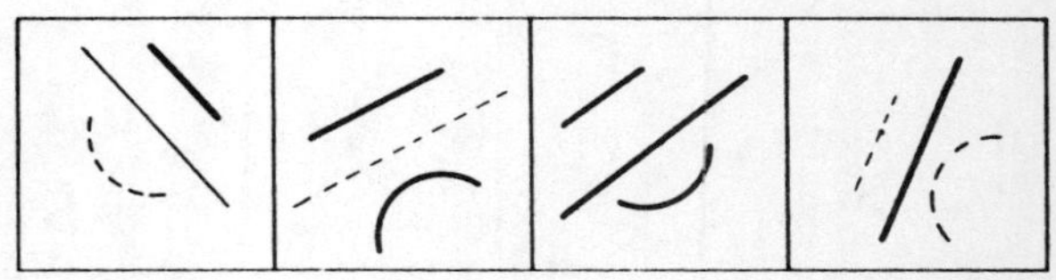
A B C D

18.
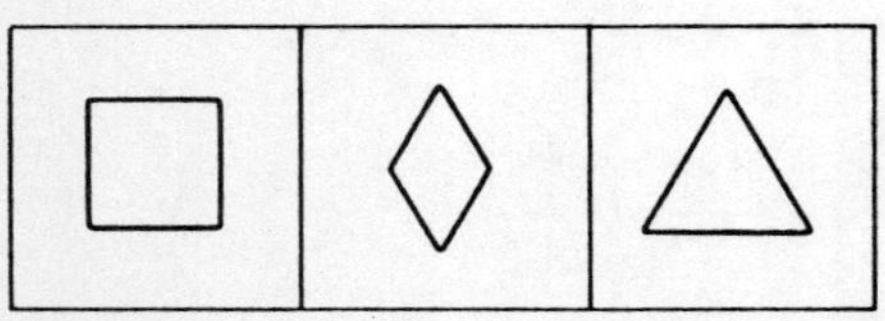
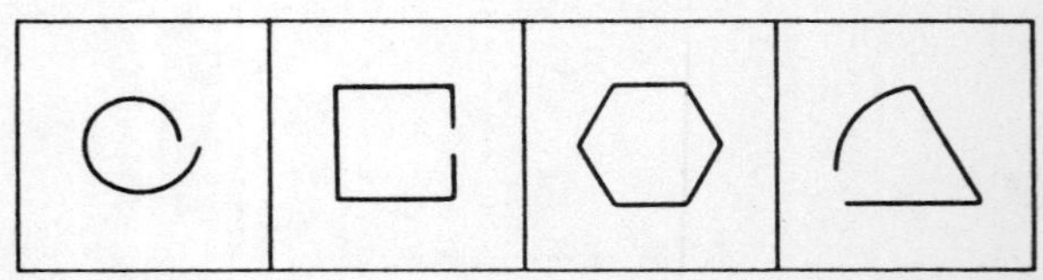
A B C D

19.
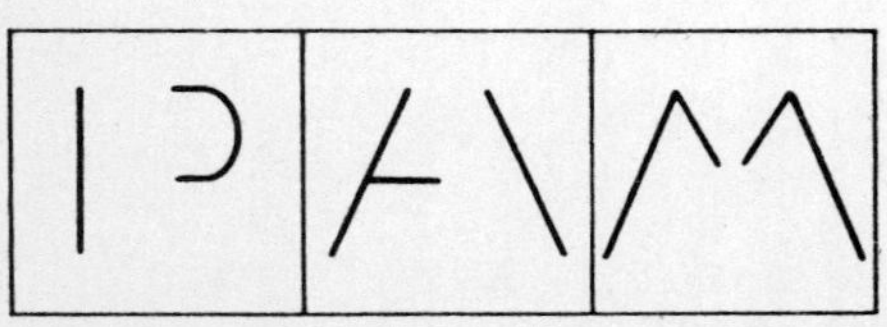
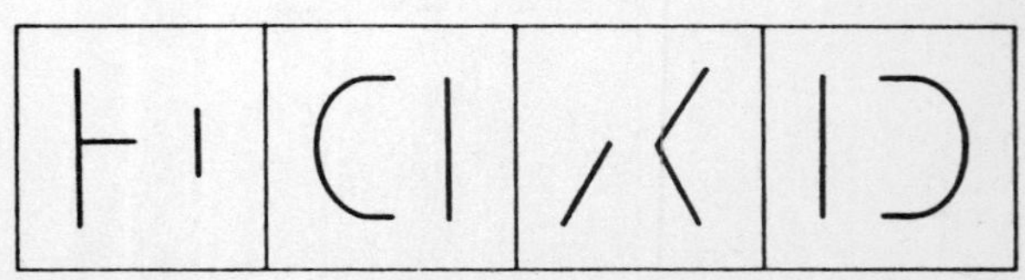
A B C D

20.
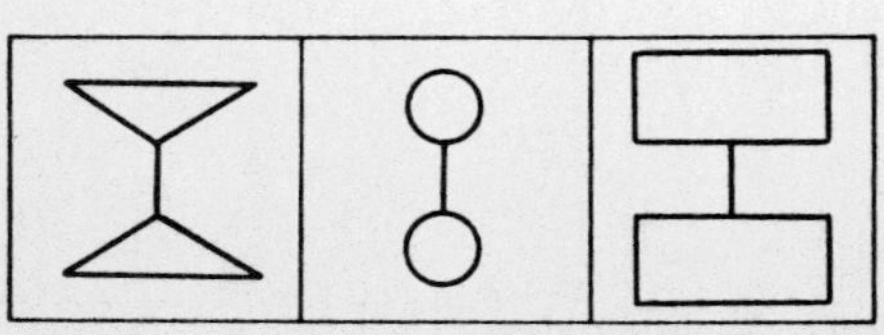
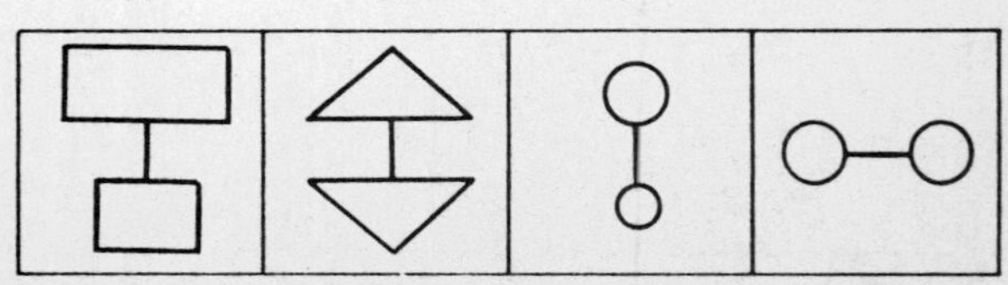
A B C D

PROBLEM FIGURES — ANSWER FIGURES

21.
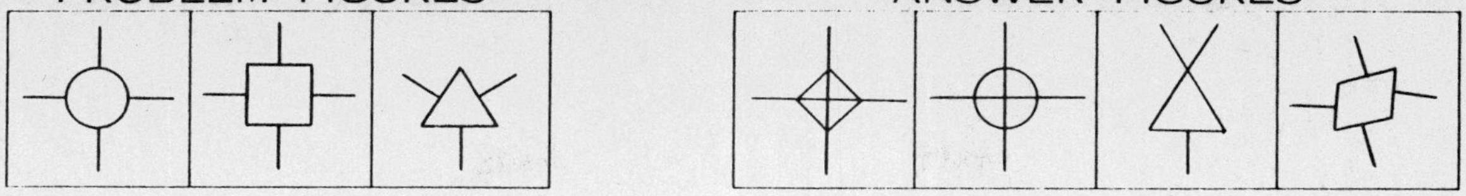
A B C D

22.
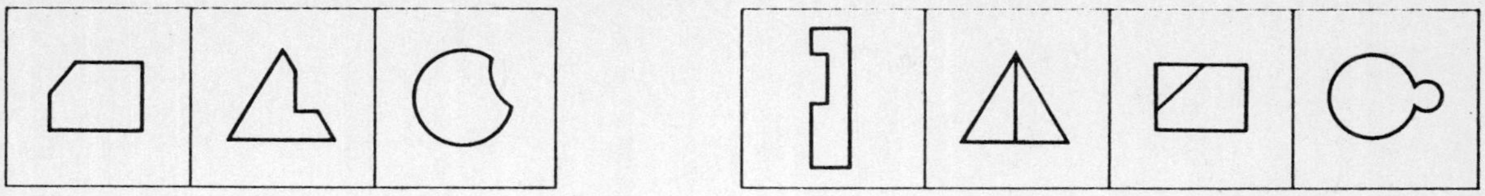
A B C D

23.
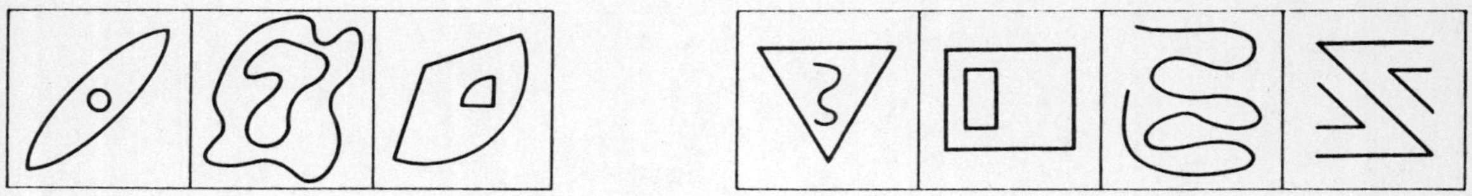
A B C D

24.
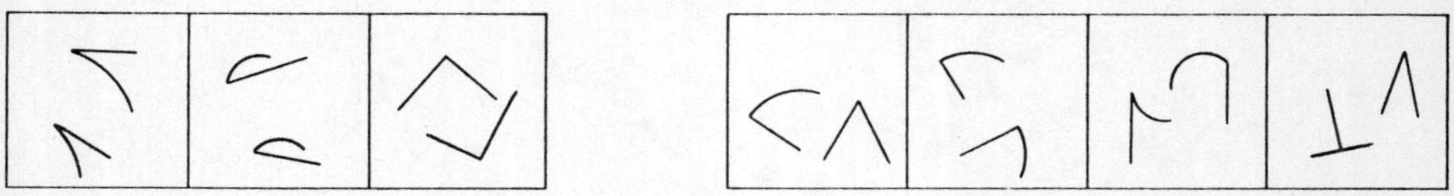
A B C D

25.
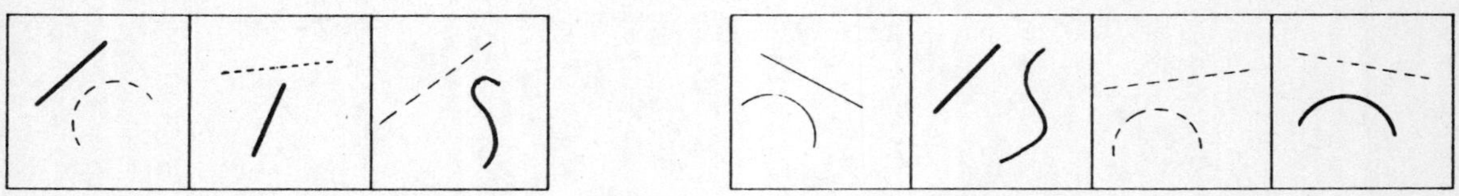
A B C D

26.
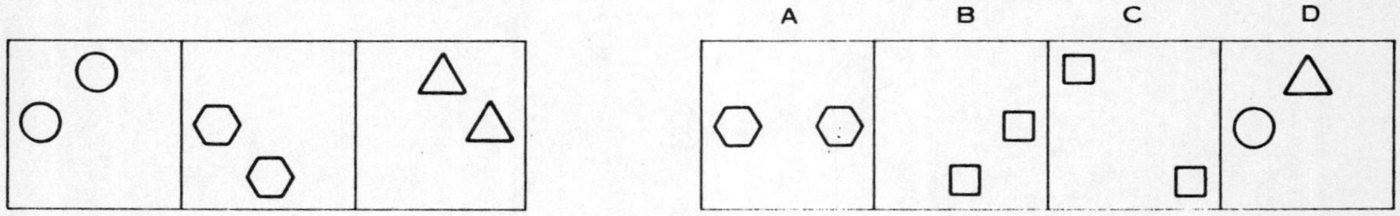
A B C D

27.
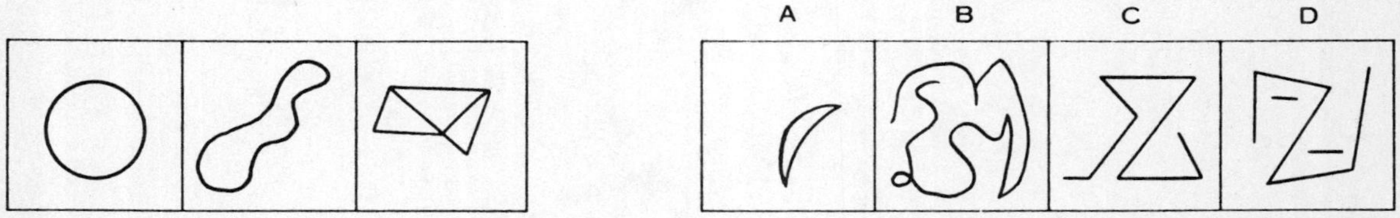
A B C D

28.
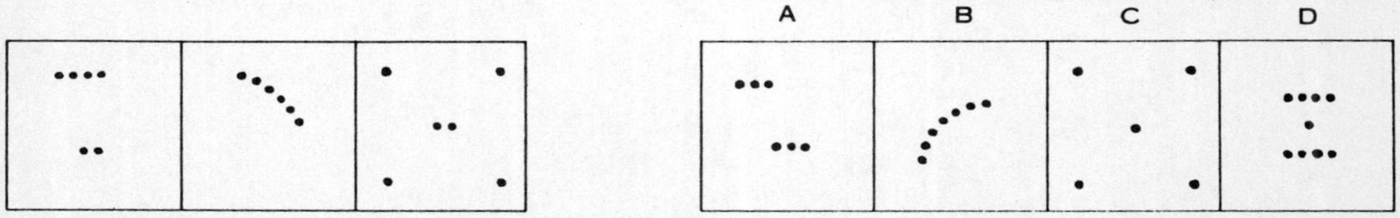
A B C D

29.
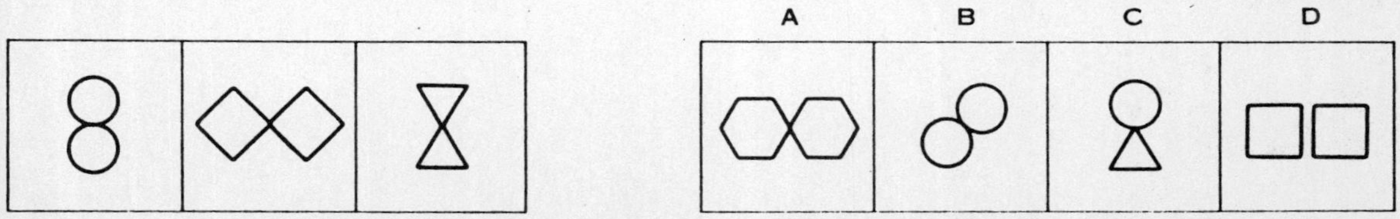
A B C D

30.
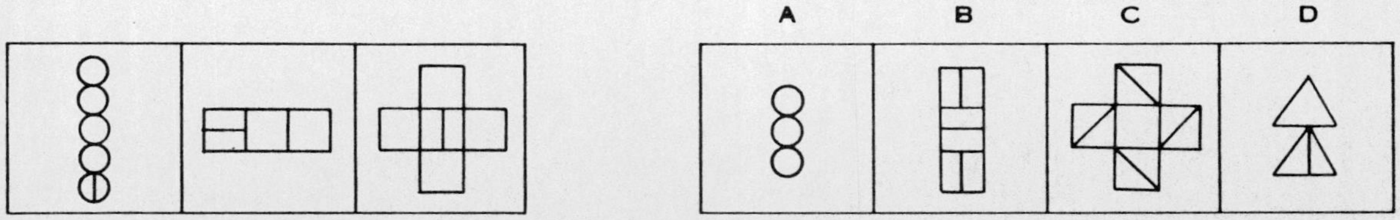
A B C D

PROBLEM FIGURES | ANSWER FIGURES

31.
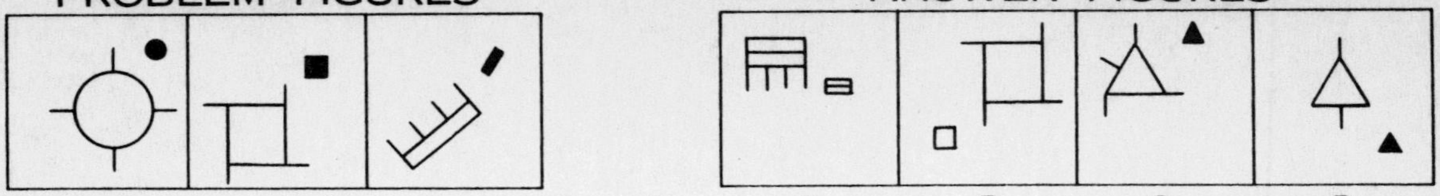
A B C D

32.
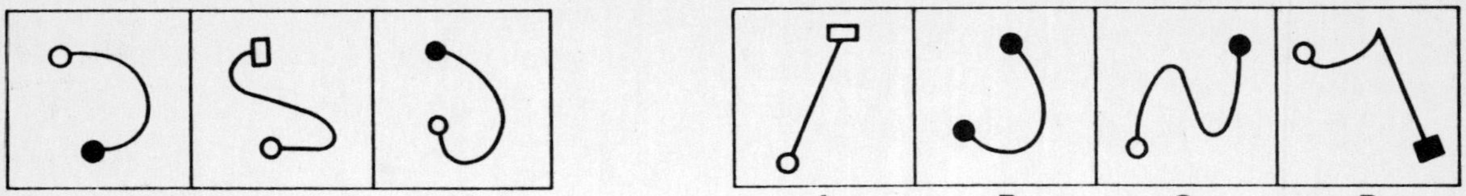
A B C D

33.
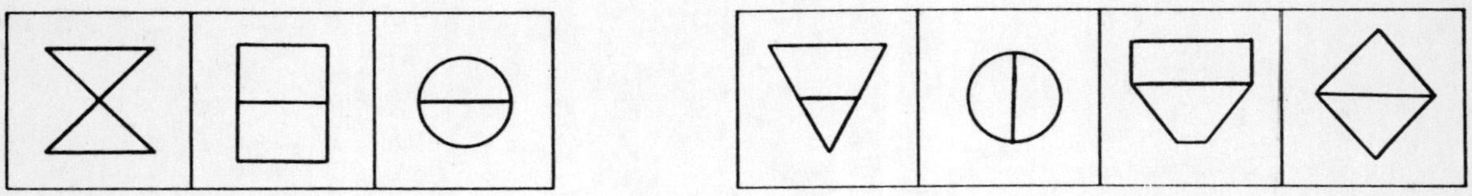
A B C D

34.
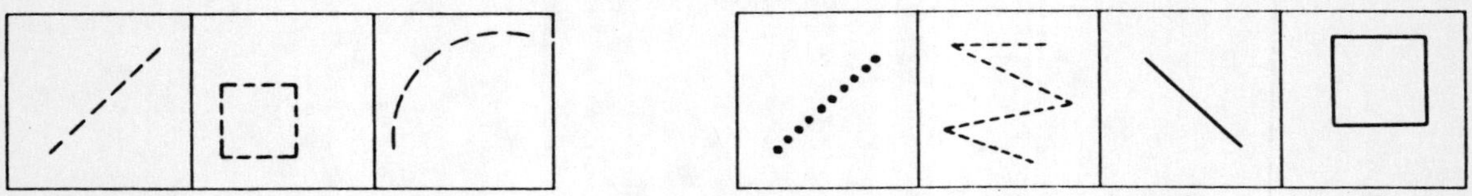
A B C D

35.
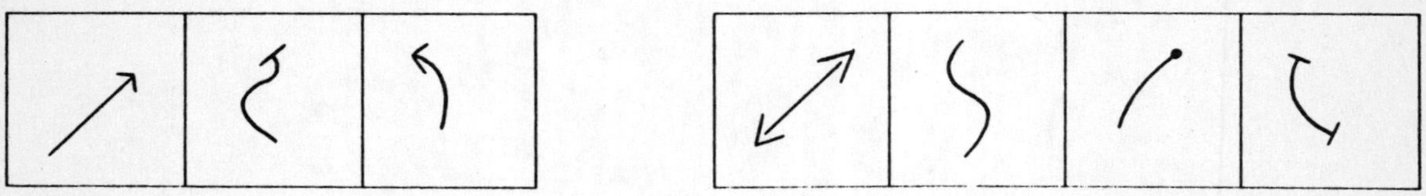
A B C D

36.
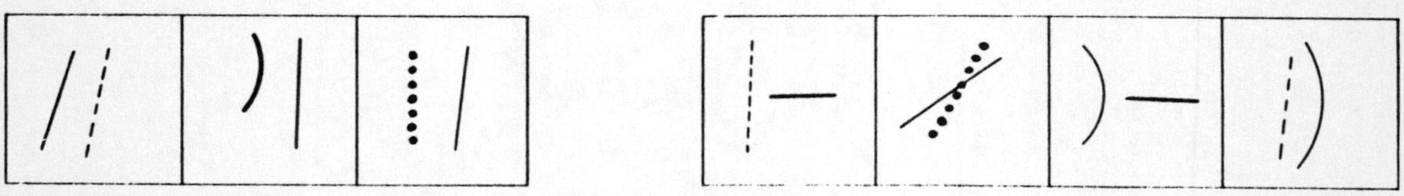
A B C D

37.
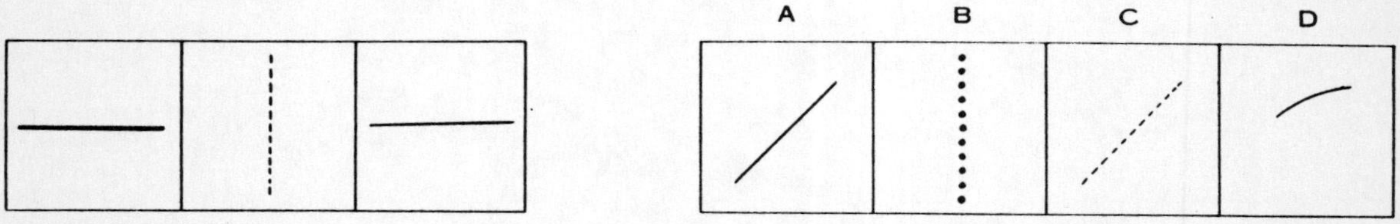
A B C D

38.
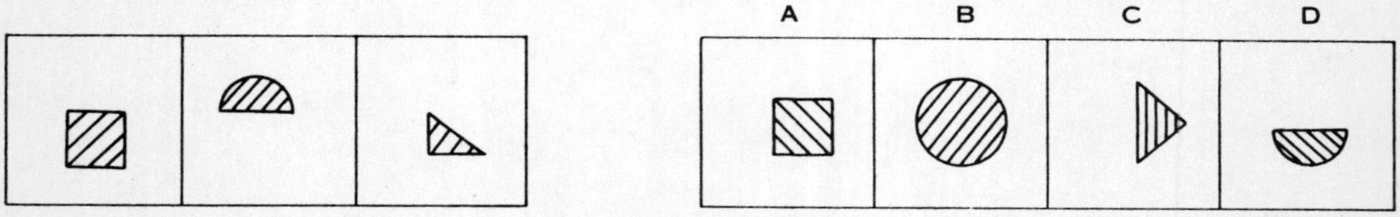
A B C D

39.
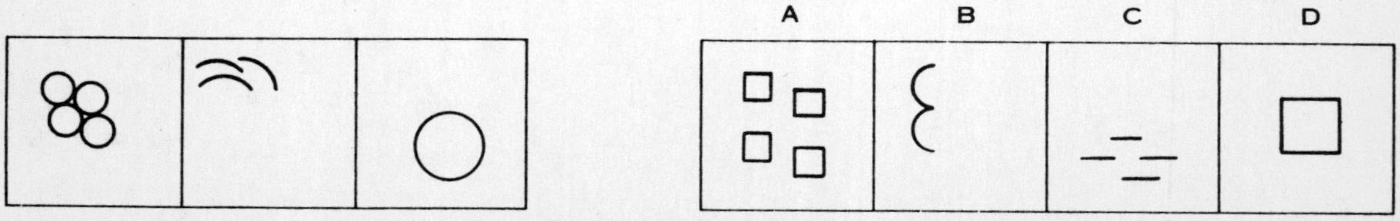
A B C D

40.
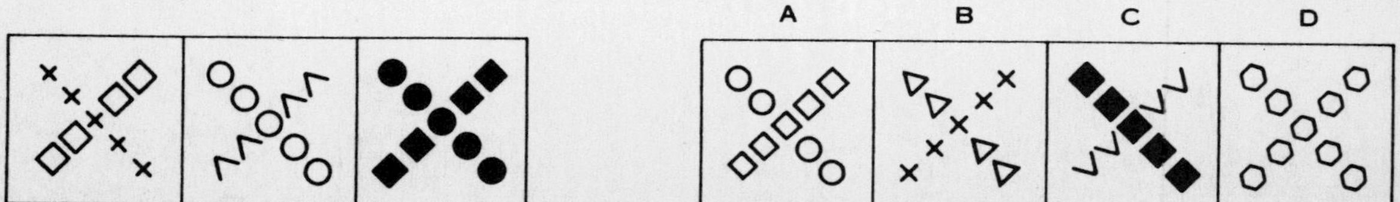
A B C D

PROBLEM FIGURES | ANSWER FIGURES

41. 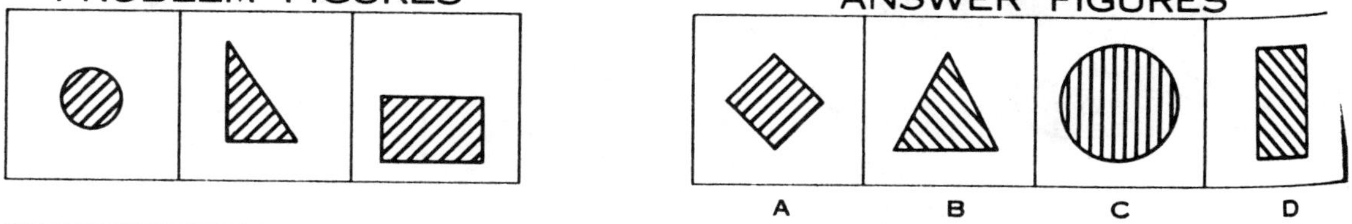

42. 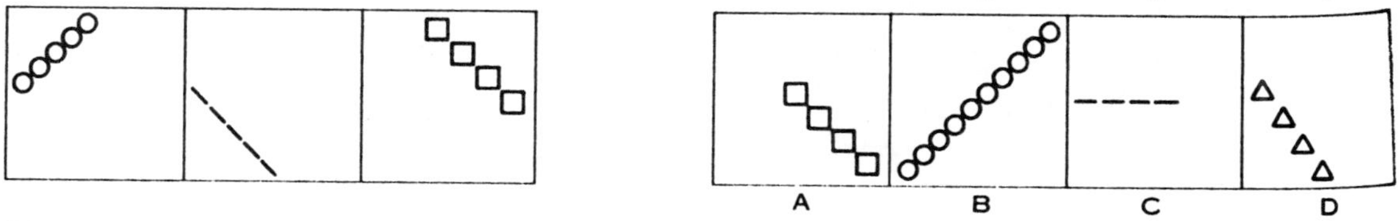

43. 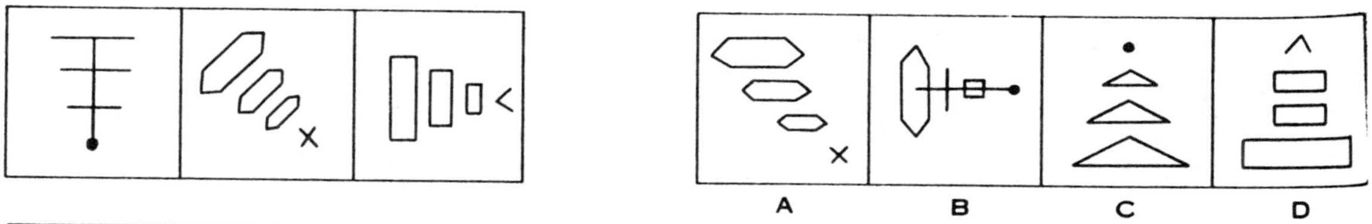

44. 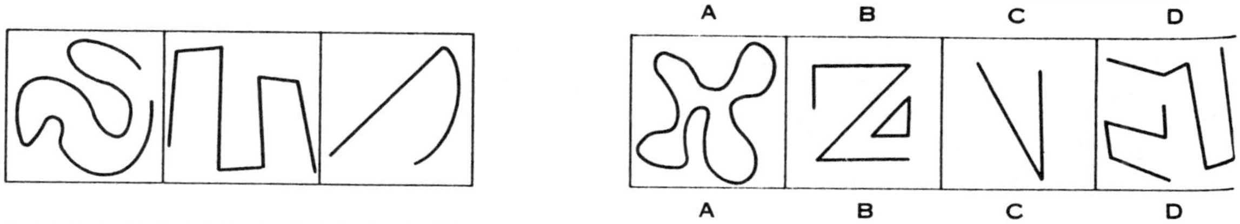

45. 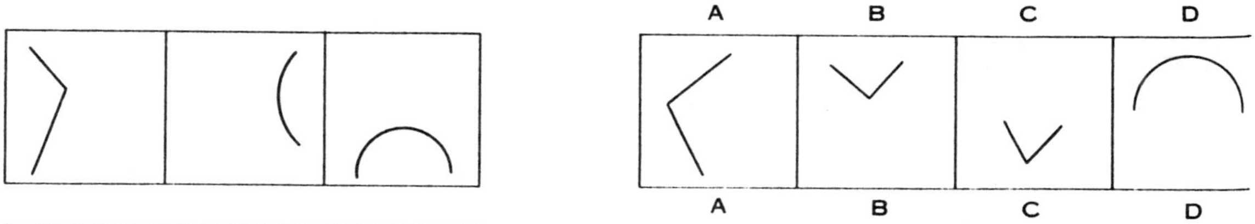

46. 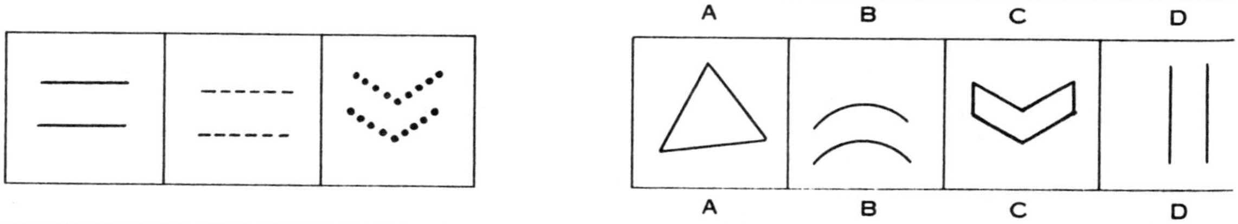

47. 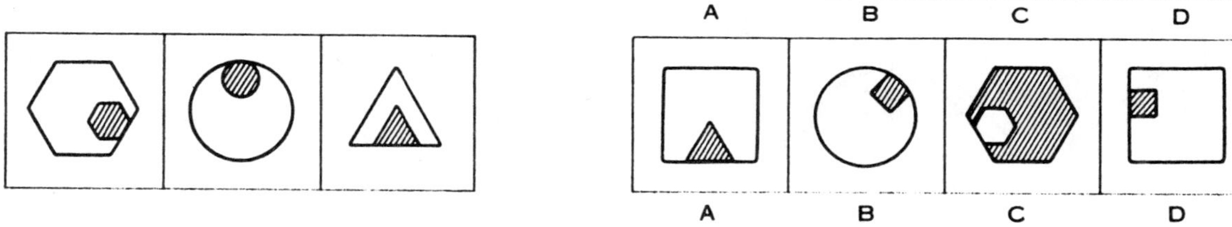

48. 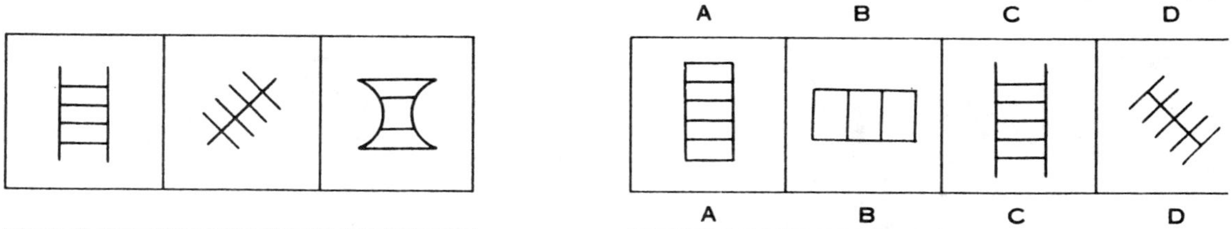

49. 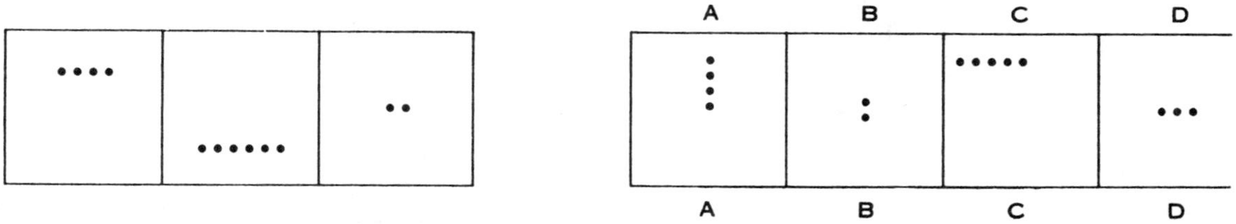

50. 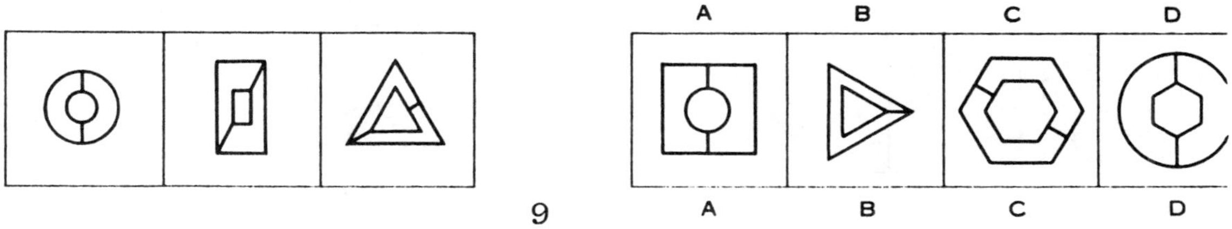

PROBLEM FIGURES | ANSWER FIGURES

51.
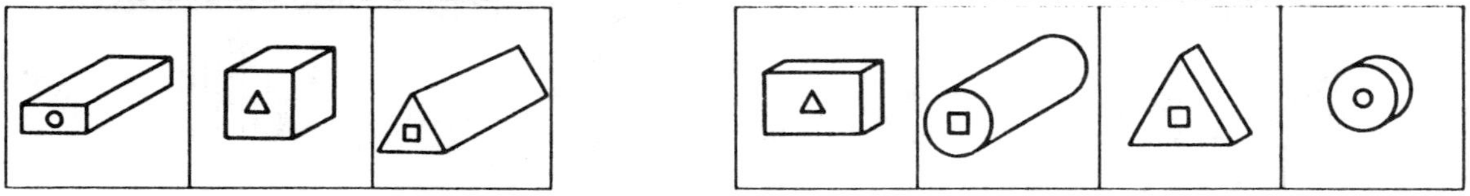
A B C D

52.
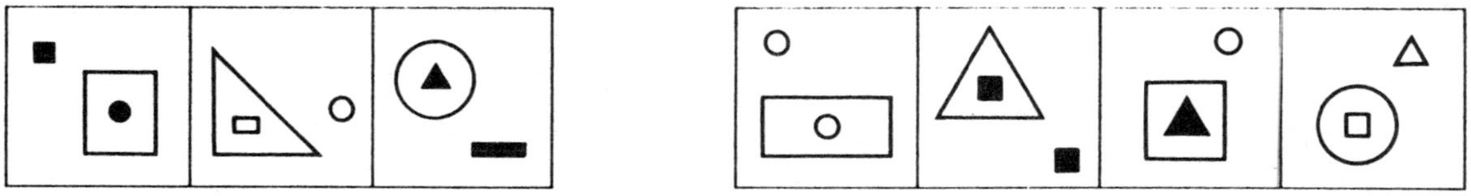
A B C D

53.
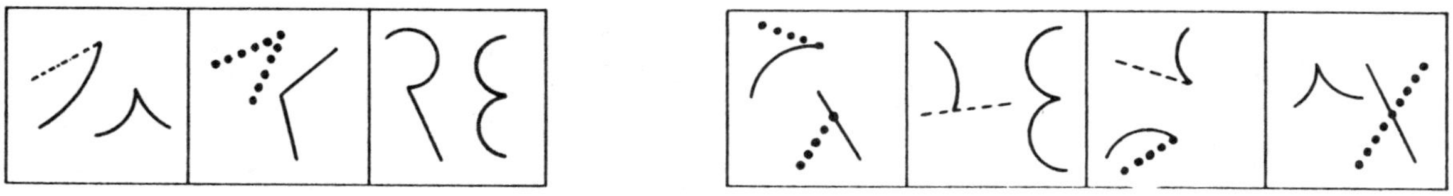
A B C D

54.
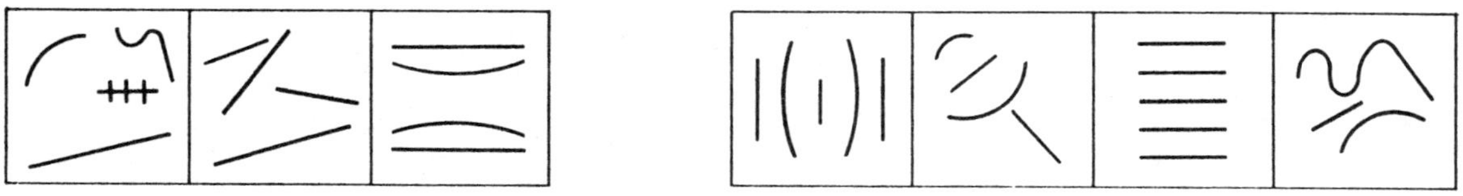
A B C D

55.
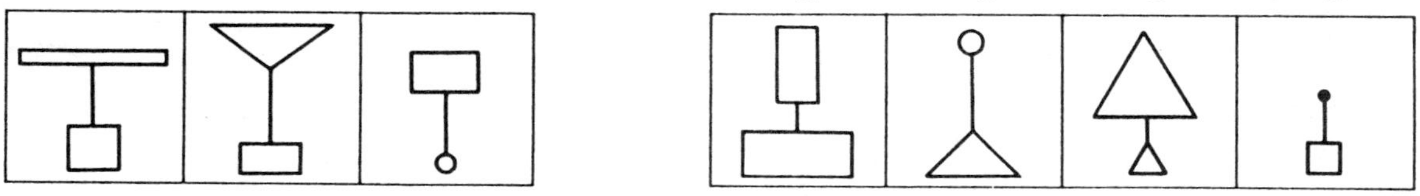
A B C D

56.
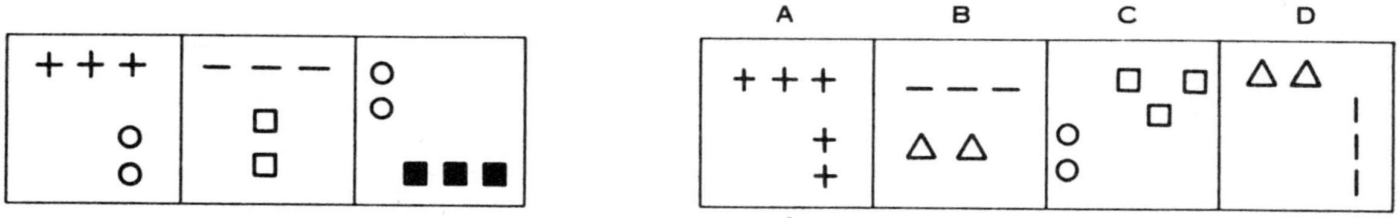
A B C D

57.
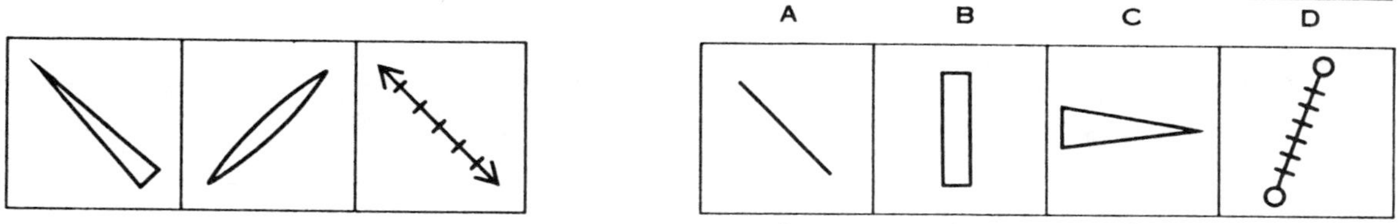
A B C D

58.
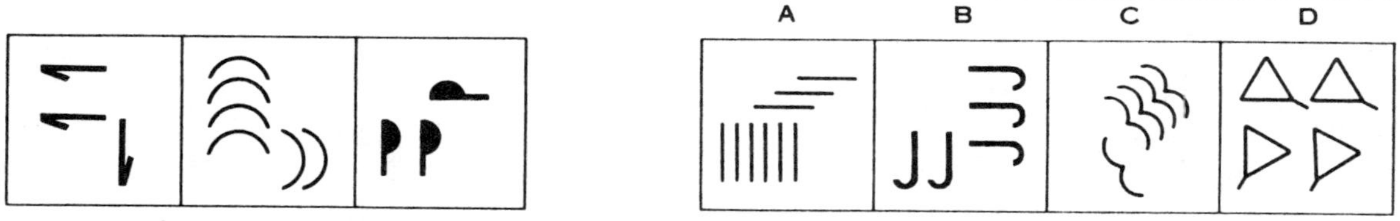
A B C D

59.
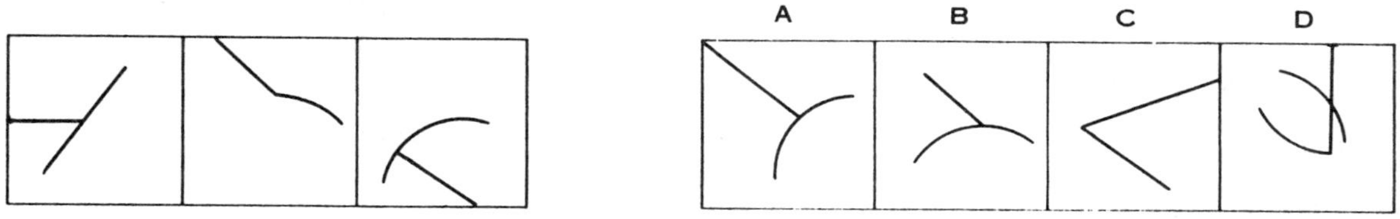
A B C D

60.
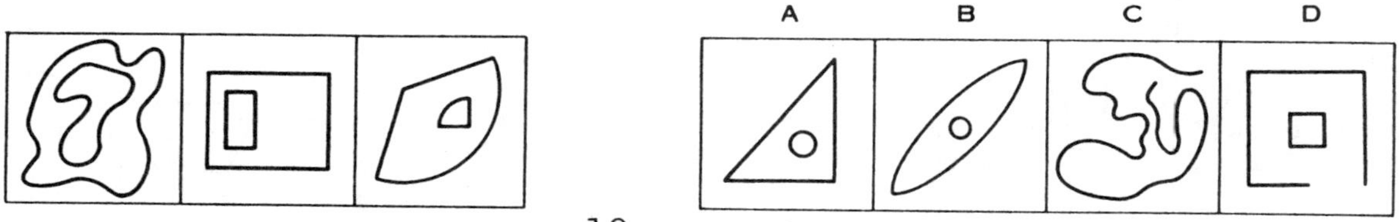
A B C D

KEY (CORRECT ANSWERS)

1.	C	21.	D	41.	A
2.	B	22.	A	42.	D
3.	A	23.	B	43.	C
4.	C	24.	B	44.	C
5.	D	25.	D	45.	B
6.	B	26.	B	46.	B
7.	C	27.	A	47.	D
8.	C	28.	A	48.	B
9.	D	29.	A	49.	D
10.	A	30.	D	50.	C
11.	D	31.	C	51.	B
12.	B	32.	C	52.	D
13.	A	33.	D	53.	C
14.	A	34.	B	54.	B
15.	D	35.	C	55.	C
16.	A	36.	D	56.	D
17.	A	37.	B	57.	A
18.	C	38.	B	58.	A
19.	D	39.	B	59.	C
20.	B	40.	C	60.	B

NUMBER SERIES PROBLEMS

COMMENTARY

Number series problems constitute an important means for measuring quantitative ability on the part of applicants for beginning and trainee positions as well as for regular, mid-level, and senior level positions.

In this method, numerical reasoning forms the primary technic for measuring mathematical ability.

This test measures your ability to think with numbers instead of words.

In each problem, you are given a series of numbers that are changing according to a rule - followed by five sets of 2 numbers each. Your problem is to figure out a rule that would make one of the five sets the next two numbers in the series.

The problems do not use hard arithmetic. The task is merely to see how the numbers are related to each other. The sample questions will explain several types in detail so that you may become familiar with what you have to do.

HINTS FOR ANSWERING NUMBER SERIES QUESTIONS

1. Do the ones that are easier for you *first*. Then go back and work on the others. Enough time is allowed for you to do all the questions, provided you don't stay too long on the ones you have trouble answering.
2. Sound out the series to yourself. You may hear the rule: 2 4 6 8 10 12 14 ... What are the next two numbers?
3. Look at the series carefully. You may see the rule: 9 2 9 4 9 6 9... What are the next two numbers?
4. If you can't hear it or see it, you may have to figure it out by writing down how the numbers are changing: 6 8 16 18 26 28 36 ... What are the next two numbers?

   $6^{+2}\ 8^{+8}\ 16^{+2}\ 18^{+8}\ 26^{+2}\ 28^{+8}$ 36... What are the next two numbers if this is +2 +8? 36 + 2 = 38 + 8 = 46 or 38 46. You would mark the letter of the answer that goes with 38 46.
5. If none of the answers given fits the rule you have figured out, try again. Try to figure out a rule that makes one of the five answers a correct one.
6. Don't spend too much time on any one question. Skip it and come back. A fresh look sometimes helps.

SAMPLE QUESTIONS

DIRECTIONS: In each of the questions in this test, there is at the top a series of numbers which follow some definite order and, below, five sets of two numbers each.

You are to look at the numbers in the series at the top and find out what order they follow. Then decide what the next two numbers in that series would be if the same order were continued. Next find these two numbers in one of the sets below. *PRINT THE LETTER OF THE CORRECT ANSWER IN THE SPACE AT THE RIGHT.*

1\. 1 2 3 4 5 6 7 ..... 1. ...

A. 1 2 B. 5 6 C. 8 9 D. 4 5 E. 7 8

How are these numbers changing? The numbers in this series are increasing by 1 or the rule is "add 1." If you apply this rule to the series, what would the next two numbers be? 7 + 1 = 8 + 1 = 9. Therefore, the CORRECT answer is 8 and 9, and you would select C. 8 9 as your answer.

2. 15 14 13 12 11 10 9 .... 2. ...
   A. 2 1 B. 17 16 C. 8 9 D. 8 7 E. 9 8

   The numbers in this series are decreasing by 1 or the rule is "subtract 1." If you apply that rule, what would the next two numbers be? 9 - 1 = 8 - 1 = 7. The CORRECT answer is 8 and 7, and you would select D. 8 7 as your answer.

3. 20 20 21 21 22 22 23 .... 3. ...
   A. 23 23 B. 23 24 C. 19 19 D. 22 23 E. 21 22

   In this series each number is repeated and then increased by 1. The rule is "repeat , add 1, repeat, add 1, etc." The series would be $20^{+0}20^{+1}21^{+0}21^{+1}22^{+0}22^{+1}23^{+0}23^{+1}24$. The CORRECT answer is 23 and 24, and you should have selected B. 23 24 as your answer.

4. 17 3 17 4 17 5 17 .... 4. ...
   A. 6 17 B. 6 7 C. 17 6 D. 5 6 E. 17 7

   If you can't find a single rule for all the numbers in a series, see if there are really two series in the problem. This series is the number 17 separated by numbers increasing by 1, starting with 3. If the series were continued for two more numbers, it would read 17 3 17 4 17 5 17 6 17. The CORRECT answer is 6 and 17, and you should have selected A. 6 17 for question 4.

5. 1 2 4 5 7 8 10 .... 5. ...
   A. 11 12 B. 12 14 C. 10 13 D. 12 13 E. 11 13

   The rule in this series is not easy to see until you actually set down how the numbers are changing: $1^{+1}2^{+2}4^{+1}5^{+2}7^{+1}8^{+2}10$. The numbers in this series are increasing first by 1 (that is, plus 1) and then by 2 (that is,plus 2). If the series were continued for two more numbers, it would read: 1 2 4 5 7 8 10 (plus 1) which is 11 (plus 2) which is 13. Therefore,the CORRECT answer is 11 and 13, and you should have selected E. 11 13 for question 5.

NOW READ AND WORK SAMPLE QUESTIONS 6 THROUGH 10 AND MARK YOUR ANSWERS IN THE SPACE PROVIDED AT THE RIGHT.

6. 21 21 20 20 19 19 18 .... 6. ...
   A. 18 18 B. 18 17 C. 17 18 D. 17 17 E. 18 19
7. 1 22 1 23 1 24 1 .... 7. ...
   A. 26 1 B. 25 26 C. 25 1 D. 1 26 E. 1 25
8. 1 20 3 19 5 18 7 .... 8. ...
   A. 8 9 B. 8 17 C. 17 10 D. 17 9 E. 9 18
9. 4 7 10 13 16 19 22 ... 9. ...
   A. 23 26 B. 25 27 C. 25 26 D. 25 28 E. 24 27
10. 30 2 28 4 26 6 24 .... 10. ...
   A. 23 9 B. 26 8 C. 8 9 D. 26 22 E. 8 22

EXPLANATIONS FOR QUESTIONS 6 THROUGH 10.

6. Each number in the series repeats itself and then decreases by 1 or minus 1; 21 (repeat) 21 (minus 1) which makes 20 (repeat) 20 (minus 1) which makes 19 (repeat) 19 (minus 1) which makes 18 (repeat) ? (minus 1) ? The CORRECT answer is B.
7. The number 1 is separated by numbers which begin with 22 and increase by 1; 1 22 1 (increase 22 by 1) which makes 23 1 (increase 23 by 1) which makes 24 1 (increase 24 by 1) which makes ? The CORRECT answer is C.

8. This is best explained by two alternating series - one series starts with 1 and increases by 2 or plus 2; the other series starts with 20 and decreases by 1 or minus 1. The CORRECT answer is D.

1↑ 3↑ 5↑ 7↑ ?
20 19 18 ?

9. This series of numbers increases by 3 (plus 3) beginning with the first number - 4 (plus 3) 7 (plus 3) 10 (plus 3) 13 (plus 3) 16 (plus 3) 19 (plus 3) 22 (plus 3) ? The CORRECT answer is D.

10. Look for two alternating series - one series starts with 30 and decreases by 2 (minus 2); the other series starts with 2 and increases by 2 (plus 2). The CORRECT answer is E.

30 ↑ 28 ↑ 26 ↑ 24 ↑ ?
2 4 6 ?

KEY (CORRECT ANSWERS)

1.	C	3.	B	5.	E	7.	C	9.	D
2.	D	4.	A	6.	B	8.	D	10.	E

NUMBER SERIES PROBLEMS

DIRECTIONS FOR THIS SECTION:

In each of the questions in this test, there is at the top a series of numbers which follow some definite order and, below, five sets of two numbers each.

You are to look at the numbers in the series at the top and find out what order they follow. Then decide what the next two numbers in that series would be if the same order were continued. Next find these two numbers in one of the sets below. *PRINT THE LETTER OF THE CORRECT ANSWER IN THE SPACE AT THE RIGHT.*

TEST 1

1. 5 6 20 7 8 19 9 .... 1. ...
   A. 10 18 B. 18 17 C. 10 17 D. 18 19 E. 10 11
2. 9 10 1 11 12 2 13 .... 2. ...
   A. 2 14 B. 3 14 C. 14 3 D. 14 15 E. 14 1
3. 4 6 9 11 14 16 19 .... 3. ...
   A. 21 24 B. 22 25 C. 20 22 D. 21 23 E. 22 24
4. 8 8 1 10 10 3 12 .... 4. ...
   A. 13 13 B. 12 5 C. 12 4 D. 13 5 E. 4 12
5. 14 1 2 15 3 4 16 .... 5. ...
   A. 5 16 B. 6 7 C. 5 17 D. 5 6 E. 17 5
6. 10 12 50 15 17 50 20 .... 6. ...
   A. 50 21 B. 21 50 C. 50 22 D. 22 50 E. 22 24
7. 1 2 3 50 4 5 6 51 7 8 .... 7. ...
   A. 9 10 B. 9 52 C. 51 10 D. 10 52 E. 10 50
8. 20 21 23 24 27 28 32 33 38 39 .... 8. ...
   A. 45 46 B. 45 52 C. 44 45 D. 44 49 E. 40 46
9. 17 15 21 18 10 16 19 .... 9. ...
   A. 20 5 B. 5 11 C. 11 11 D. 11 20 E. 15 14
10. 12 16 10 14 8 12 6 .... 10. ...
    A. 10 14 B. 10 8 C. 10 4 D. 4 10 E. 4 2

TEST 2

1. 10 11 12 10 11 12 10 .... — 1. ...
   A. 10 11 B. 12 10 C. 11 10 D. 11 12 E. 10 12
2. 4 6 7 4 6 7 4 — 2. ...
   A. 6 7 B. 4 7 C. 7 6 D. 7 4 E. 6 8
3. 7 7 3 7 7 4 7 .... — 3. ...
   A. 4 5 B. 4 7 C. 5 7 D. 7 5 E. 7 7
4. 3 4 10 5 6 10 7 .... — 4. ...
   A. 10 8 B. 9 8 C. 8 14 D. 8 9 E. 8 10
5. 6 6 7 7 8 8 9 .... — 5. ...
   A. 10 11 B. 10 10 C. 9 10 D. 9 9 E. 10 9
6. 3 8 9 4 9 10 5 .... — 6. ...
   A. 6 10 B. 10 11 C. 9 10 D. 11 6 E. 10 6
7. 2 4 3 6 4 8 5 .... — 7. ...
   A. 6 10 B. 10 7 C. 10 6 D. 9 6 E. 6 7
8. 11 5 9 7 7 9 5 .... — 8. ...
   A. 11 3 B. 7 9 C. 7 11 D. 9 7 E. 3 7
9. 12 10 8 8 6 4 4 .... — 9. ...
   A. 2 2 B. 6 4 C. 6 2 D. 4 6 E. 2 0
10. 20 22 22 19 21 21 18 .... — 10. ...
    A. 22 22 B. 19 19 C. 20 20 D. 20 17 E. 19 17

TEST 3

1. 5 7 6 10 7 13 8 .... — 1. ...
   A. 16 9 B. 16 10 C. 9 15 D. 10 15 E. 15 9
2. 13 10 11 15 12 13 17 .... — 2. ...
   A. 18 14 B. 18 15 C. 15 16 D. 14 15 E. 15 18
3. 30 27 24 21 18 15 12 .... — 3. ...
   A. 9 3 B. 9 6 C. 6 3 D. 12 9 E. 8 5
4. 3 7 10 5 8 10 7 .... — 4. ...
   A. 10 11 B. 10 5 C. 10 9 D. 10 10 E. 9 10
5. 12 4 13 6 14 8 15 .... — 5. ...
   A. 10 17 B. 17 10 C. 10 12 D. 16 10 E. 10 16
6. 21 8 18 20 7 17 19 .... — 6. ...
   A. 16 18 B. 18 6 C. 6 16 D. 5 15 E. 6 18
7. 14 16 16 18 20 20 22 .... — 7. ...
   A. 22 24 B. 26 28 C. 24 26 D. 24 24 E. 24 28
8. 5 6 8 9 12 13 17 .... — 8. ...
   A. 18 23 B. 13 18 C. 18 22 D. 23 24 E. 18 19
9. 1 3 5 5 2 4 6 6 3 .... — 9. ...
   A. 7 4 B. 5 5 C. 1 3 D. 5 7 E. 7 7
10. 12 24 15 25 18 26 21 .... — 10. ...
    A. 27 22 B. 24 22 C. 29 24 D. 27 27 E. 27 24

TEST 4

1. 8 9 9 8 10 10 8 .... — 1. ...
   A. 11 8 B. 8 13 C. 8 11 D. 11 11 E. 8 8
2. 10 10 11 11 12 12 13 .... — 2. ...
   A. 15 15 B. 13 13 C. 14 14 D. 13 14 E. 14 15
3. 6 6 10 6 6 12 6 .... — 3. ...
   A. 6 14 B. 13 6 C. 14 6 D. 6 13 E. 6 6

4. 17 11 5 16 10 4 15 .... — 4. ...
A. 13 9 B. 13 11 C. 8 5 D. 9 5 E. 9 3

5. 1 3 2 4 3 5 4 .... — 5. ...
A. 6 8 B. 5 6 C. 6 5 D. 3 4 E. 3 5

6. 11 11 10 12 12 11 13 .... — 6. ...
A. 12 14 B. 14 12 C. 14 14 D. 13 14 E. 13 12

7. 18 5 6 18 7 8 18 .... — 7. ...
A. 9 9 B. 9 10 C. 18 9 D. 8 9 E. 18 7

8. 7 8 9 13 10 11 12 14 13 14 .... — 8. ...
A. 15 16 B. 13 15 C. 14 15 D. 15 15 E. 13 14

9. 5 7 30 9 11 30 13 .... — 9. ...
A. 15 16 B. 15 17 C. 14 17 D. 15 30 E. 30 17

10. 5 7 11 13 17 19 23 .... — 10. ...
A. 27 29 B. 25 29 C. 25 27 D. 27 31 E. 29 31

TEST 5

1. 9 15 10 17 12 19 15 21 19 .... — 1. ...
A. 23 24 B. 25 23 C. 17 23 D. 23 31 E. 21 24

2. 34 37 30 33 26 29 22 .... — 2. ...
A. 17 8 B. 18 11 C. 25 28 D. 25 20 E. 25 18

3. 10 16 12 14 14 12 16 .... — 3. ...
A. 14 12 B. 10 18 C. 10 14 D. 14 18 E. 14 16

4. 11 12 18 11 13 19 11 14 .... — 4. ...
A. 18 11 B. 16 11 C. 20 11 D. 11 21 E. 17 11

5. 20 9 8 19 10 9 18 11 10 .... — 5. ...
A. 19 11 B. 17 10 C. 19 12 D. 17 12 E. 19 10

6. 28 27 26 31 30 29 34 .... — 6. ...
A. 36 32 B. 32 31 C. 33 32 D. 33 36 E. 35 36

7. 10 16 14 20 18 24 22 .... — 7. ...
A. 28 32 B. 27 26 C. 28 26 D. 26 28 E. 27 28

8. 9 9 7 8 7 7 9 10 5 .... — 8. ...
A. 5 11 B. 11 12 C. 5 9 D. 9 11 E. 5 5

9. 5 7 11 17 10 12 16 22 15 17 .... — 9. ...
A. 27 26 B. 19 23 C. 19 27 D. 21 23 E. 21 27

10. 12 19 13 20 14 21 15 .... — 10. ...
A. 16 17 B. 22 16 C. 16 22 D. 15 22 E. 15 16

TEST 6

1. 13 12 8 11 10 8 9 .... — 1. ...
A. 8 7 B. 6 8 C. 8 6 D. 8 8 E. 7 8

2. 13 18 13 17 13 16 13 .... — 2. ...
A. 15 13 B. 13 14 C. 13 15 D. 14 15 E. 15 14

3. 13 13 10 12 12 10 11 .... — 3. ...
A. 10 10 B. 10 9 C. 11 9 D. 9 11 E. 11 10

4. 6 5 4 6 5 4 6 .... — 4. ...
A. 4 6 B. 6 4 C. 5 4 D. 5 6 E. 4 5

5. 10 10 9 8 8 7 6 .... — 5. ...
A. 5 5 B. 5 4 C. 6 5 D. 6 4 E. 5 3

6. 20 16 18 14 16 12 14 .... — 6. ...
A. 16 12 B. 10 12 C. 16 18 D. 12 12 E. 12 10

7. 7 12 8 11 9 10 10 .... 7. ..
A. 11 9 B. 9 8 C. 9 11 D. 10 11 E. 9 10
8. 13 13 12 15 15 14 17 .... 8. ..
A. 17 16 B. 14 17 C. 16 19 D. 19 19 E. 16 16
9. 19 18 12 17 16 13 15 .... 9. ..
A. 16 12 B. 14 14 C. 12 14 D. 14 12 E. 12 16
10. 7 15 12 8 16 13 9 .... 10. ..
A. 17 14 B. 17 10 C. 14 10 D. 14 17 E. 10 14

TEST 7

1. 18 15 6 16 14 6 14 .... 1. ...
A. 12 6 B. 14 13 C. 6 12 D. 13 12 E. 13 6
2. 6 6 5 8 8 7 10 10 .... 2. ...
A. 8 12 B. 9 12 C. 12 12 D. 12 9 E. 9 9
3. 17 20 23 26 29 32 35 .... 3. ...
A. 37 40 B. 41 44 C. 38 41 D. 38 42 E. 36 39
4. 15 5 7 16 9 11 17 .... 4. ...
A. 18 13 B. 15 17 C. 12 19 D. 13 15 E. 12 13
5. 19 17 16 16 13 15 10 .... 5. ...
A. 14 7 B. 12 9 C. 14 9 D. 7 12 E. 10 14
6. 11 1 16 10 6 21 9 .... 6. ...
A. 12 26 B. 26 8 C. 11 26 D. 11 8 E. 8 11
7. 21 21 19 17 17 15 13 .... 7. ...
A. 11 11 B. 13 11 C. 11 9 D. 9 7 E. 13 13
8. 23 22 20 19 16 15 11 .... 8. ...
A. 6 5 B. 10 9 C. 6 1 D. 10 6 E. 10 5
9. 17 10 16 9 14 8 11 .... 9. ...
A. 7 11 B. 7 7 C. 10 4 D. 4 10 E. 7 4
10. 11 9 14 12 17 15 20 18 23 .... 10. ...
A. 21 24 B. 26 21 C. 21 26 D. 24 27 E. 26 29

TEST 8

1. 13 4 5 13 6 7 13 .... 1. ...
A. 13 8 B. 8 13 C. 8 9 D. 8 8 E. 7 8
2. 10 10 9 11 11 10 12 .... 2. ...
A. 13 14 B. 12 11 C. 13 13 D. 12 12 E. 12 13
3. 6 6 8 10 10 12 14 .... 3. ...
A. 14 14 B. 14 16 C. 16 16 D. 12 14 E. 10 10
4. 8 1 9 3 10 5 11 .... 4. ...
A. 7 12 B. 6 12 C. 12 6 D. 7 8 E. 6 7
5. 30 11 24 12 19 14 15 17 12 21 10 .... 5. ...
A. 23 8 B. 25 8 C. 26 9 D. 24 9 E. 25 9
6. 24 30 29 22 28 27 19 26 25 15 24 .... 6. ...
A. 14 23 B. 19 18 C. 23 22 D. 25 11 E. 23 10
7. 7 5 9 7 11 9 13 .... 7. ...
A. 11 14 B. 10 15 C. 11 15 D. 12 14 E. 10 14
8. 9 10 11 7 8 9 5 .... 8. ...
A. 6 7 B. 7 8 C. 5 6 D. 6 4 E. 7 5
9. 8 9 10 10 9 10 11 11 10 11 12 .... 9. ...
A. 11 12 B. 12 10 C. 11 11 D. 12 11 E. 11 13
10. 5 6 8 9 12 13 17 18 23 24 .... 10. ...
A. 30 31 B. 25 31 C, 29 30 D. 25 30 E. 30 37

TEST 9

1. 8 9 10 8 9 10 8 ....
   A. 8 9 B. 9 10 C. 9 8 D. 10 8 E. 8 10 — 1. ...
2. 3 4 4 3 5 5 3 ....
   A. 3 3 B. 6 3 C. 3 6 D. 6 6 E. 6 7 — 2. ...
3. 7 7 3 7 7 4 7 ....
   A. 7 7 B. 7 8 C. 5 7 D. 8 7 E. 7 5 — 3. ...
4. 18 18 19 20 20 21 22 ....
   A. 22 23 B. 23 24 C. 23 23 D. 22 22 E. 21 22 — 4. ...
5. 2 6 10 3 7 11 4 ....
   A. 12 16 B. 5 9 C. 8 5 D. 12 5 E. 8 12 — 5. ...
6. 11 8 15 12 19 16 23 ....
   A. 27 20 B. 24 20 C. 27 24 D. 20 24 E. 20 27 — 6. ...
7. 16 8 15 9 14 10 13 ....
   A. 12 11 B. 13 12 C. 11 13 D. 11 12 E. 11 14 — 7. ...
8. 4 5 13 6 7 12 8 ....
   A. 9 11 B. 13 9 C. 9 13 D. 11 9 E. 11 10 — 8. ...
9. 3 8 4 9 5 10 6 11 7 ....
   A. 7 11 B. 7 8 C. 11 8 D. 12 7 E. 12 8 — 9. ...
10. 18 14 19 17 20 20 21 ....
    A. 22 24 B. 14 19 C. 24 21 D. 21 23 E. 23 22 — 10. ...

TEST 10

1. 6 9 10 7 11 12 8 ....
   A. 9 10 B. 9 13 C. 16 14 D. 13 14 E. 14 15 — 1. ...
2. 7 5 3 9 7 5 11 ....
   A. 13 12 B. 7 5 C. 9 7 D. 13 7 E. 9 9 — 2. ...
3. 7 9 18 10 12 18 13 ....
   A. 18 14 B. 15 18 C. 14 15 D. 15 14 E. 14 18 — 3. ...
4. 2 6 4 8 6 10 8 ....
   A. 12 10 B. 6 10 C. 10 12 D. 12 16 E. 6 4 — 4. ...
5. 7 9 12 14 17 19 22 ....
   A. 25 27 B. 23 24 C. 23 25 D. 24 27 E. 26 27 — 5. ...
6. 3 23 5 25 7 27 9 ....
   A. 10 11 B. 27 29 C. 29 11 D. 11 28 E. 28 10 — 6. ...
7. 18 17 16 14 13 12 10 ....
   A. 9 8 B. 6 7 C. 8 6 D. 8 7 E. 10 9 — 7. ...
8. 5 7 8 10 11 13 14 16 ....
   A. 18 19 B. 17 18 C. 18 20 D. 17 19 E. 19 20 — 8. ...
9. 28 27 25 24 22 21 19 ....
   A. 18 16 B. 17 16 C. 18 17 D. 17 15 E. 20 18 — 9. ...
10. 2 2 4 6 6 8 10 ....
    A. 12 12 B. 12 14 C. 10 10 D. 10 8 E. 10 12 — 10. ...

KEY (CORRECT ANSWERS)

	TEST 1	TEST 2	TEST 3	TEST 4	TEST 5
1.	A	D	A	D	A
2.	C	A	D	D	E
3.	A	D	B	A	B
4.	B	E	E	E	C
5.	D	C	E	C	D
6.	D	B	C	E	C
7.	B	C	D	B	C
8.	A	A	A	D	A
9.	B	E	D	D	E
10.	C	C	E	B	B

	TEST 6	TEST 7	TEST 8	TEST 9	TEST 10
1.	D	E	C	B	D
2.	A	B	B	D	C
3.	E	C	B	E	B
4.	C	D	A	A	A
5.	C	A	C	E	D
6.	B	C	E	E	C
7.	C	B	C	D	A
8.	A	E	A	A	D
9.	B	B	D	E	A
10.	A	C	A	E	E

EXAMINATION SECTION

TEST 1

DIRECTIONS: Each question or incomplete statement is followed by several suggested answers or completions. Select the one that BEST answers the question or completes the statement. *PRINT THE LETTER OF THE CORRECT ANSWER IN THE SPACE AT THE RIGHT.*

1. What is the sum of 7 and -8? 1.____
   A. -56 B. -15 C. 1
   D. 15 E. Not given

2. Multiply -3 by -15. 2.____
   A. 45 B. 12 C. -12 D. -18 E. -45

3. Two integers differ by 3. Their sum is 51. One of the integers is 3.____
   A. 21 B. 23 C. 24 D. 25 E. 26

4. Solve for t: $12(\frac{7}{3}) = \frac{1}{3}(t)$. 4.____
   A. $\frac{7}{12}$ B. 19 C. 43 D. 84 E. 252

5. What quantity is one-half of x? 5.____
   A. 2x B. $\frac{1}{2} - x$ C. $\frac{1}{2} + x$
   D. $\frac{1}{2x}$ E. Not given

6. When does 3 - b equal b - 3? 6.____
   A. Only when b = -3 B. Only when b = 3
   C. Only when b = 0 D. For all values of b
   E. For no values of b

7. 3 - (-8) = 7.____
   A. 11 B. 5 C. -5 D. -11 E. -24

8. If x > 7, what is TRUE about the quantity (x+2)? It is 8.____
   A. equal to 5 B. greater than 9
   C. equal to 9 D. greater than 14
   E. equal to 14

9. What is the sum of $a^2 + 3b^2 + 3a^2 + b^2$? 9.____
   A. $15a^2b^2$ B. $8a^2b^2$ C. $8a^4b^4$
   D. $4(a^2+b^2)$ E. $4a^4 + 4b^4$

10. One number plus one-half of a SECOND number equals 36. What is the second number? 10.____
A. 27
B. 18
C. 12
D. 9
E. Cannot be determined without more information

11. Bananas are 10 cents a pound. For p pounds and q ounces of bananas, Mary MUST pay ____ cents. 11.____

A. $10(p + \frac{q}{16})$ B. $10(p + 16q)$ C. $10(16p + q)$

D. $10p + \frac{q}{16}$ E. $10(p+q)$

12. In the problem 11 + 8 + 23 = 42, 8 is called a(n) 12.____
A. addend B. subtrahend C. dividend
D. sum E. difference

13. $\frac{2}{3} \div \frac{2}{3} =$ 13.____

A. $\frac{4}{9}$ B. $\frac{9}{4}$ C. 1 D. $\frac{4}{6}$ E. $\frac{2}{3}$

14. Which number is the LARGEST? 14.____
A. 4.5 B. 4.4449 C. .459
D. .057399 E. 1.000

15. $2.4 \div 6 =$ 15.____
A. .4 B. 2.8 C. 8.4 D. 14.4 E. 40

16. In the fraction $\frac{11}{16}$, 16.____

A. 11 is the denominator
B. 16 is the numerator
C. 11 and 16 are both numerators
D. both are denominators
E. 16 is the denominator

17. $-8 - (-7) =$ 17.____
A. -15 B. -1 C. 1 D. 15

18. $5x^3 - 2x^3 + 3x^3 =$ 18.____
A. $-30x^3$ B. $3x^3$ C. $6x^3$ D. $3 + 3x^3$

19. If $16 * \frac{1}{2} = 8$, the operation * could be which operation? 19.____
A. Addition B. Subtraction
C. Multiplication D. Division

20. If $3y - 6 = 5y$, then $y =$ 20.___
A. -3 B. -2 C. 2 D. 3

21. If $p = 0$, the expression $r + p(r+s) + 1 =$ 21.___
A. r B. $r+1$ C. $r+s+1$ D. $2r+1$

22. $6x^2 - 8xy$ is the product of $2x$ and 22.___
A. $3x-4y$ B. $3x-4$ C. $4x-6y$ D. $3x-8xy$

23. $(x+2y)(2x-y) =$ 23.___
A. $2x^2 - 2y^2$ B. $2x^2 + 3xy - 2y^2$
C. $2x^2 + 3xy + 2y^2$ D. $2x^2 + 5xy + 2y^2$

24. For which of the following values of x is $\sqrt{x^2-1}$ NOT a real number? 24.___
A. -3 B. -2 C. -1 D. 0

25. 25.___

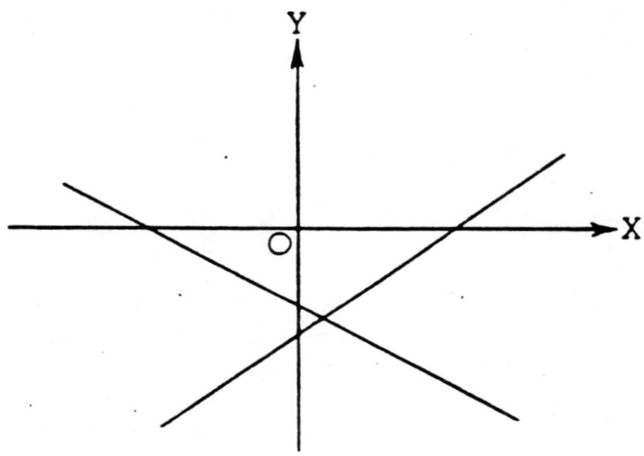

In the figure above, which of these (x,y) pairs could be the common solution of the two linear equations represented on the graph?
A. (1,-4) B. (1,4) C. (-1,-4) D. (4,1)

KEY (CORRECT ANSWERS)

1. E	6. B	11. A	16. E	21. B
2. A	7. A	12. A	17. B	22. A
3. C	8. B	13. C	18. C	23. B
4. D	9. D	14. A	19. C	24. D
5. E	10. E	15. A	20. A	25. A

SOLUTIONS TO PROBLEMS

1. $7 + (-8) = -1$

2. $(-3)(-15) = 45$

3. Let x = 1st integer, x + 3 = 2nd integer. Then, $x + x + 3 = 51$. Solving, $x = 24$ (The other integer is 27)

4. $12(\frac{7}{3}) = \frac{1}{3}t$. $28 = \frac{1}{3}t$. So, $t = (28)(3) = 84$

5. One-half of x is written as $\frac{1}{2}x$ or $\frac{x}{2}$

6. If $3 - b = b - 3$, then $-2b = -6$. Solving, $b = 3$

7. $3 - (-8) = 3 + 8 = 11$

8. Since $x > 7$, then $x + 2 > 9$

9. $a^2 + 3b^2 + 3a^2 + b^2 = 4a^2 + 4b^2 = 4(a^2+b^2)$

10. The given statement can be written as $x + \frac{1}{2}y = 36$. Neither number can be found solely from this equation.

11. The cost of p pounds = 10p. The cost of q ounces = $10 \cdot q/16$. Total cost is $10p + 10q/16 = 10(p + \frac{q}{16})$

12. In $11 + 8 + 23 = 42$, 8 is an addend.

13. $\frac{2}{3} \div \frac{2}{3} = \frac{2}{3} \cdot \frac{3}{2} = 1$

14. 4.5 is larger than the other selections.

15. $2.4 \div 6 = .4$

16. For the fraction $\frac{11}{16}$, 16 is the denominator.

17. $-8 - (-7) = -8 + 7 = -1$

18. $5x^3 - 2x^3 + 3x^3 = 6x^3$

19. Since $(16)(\frac{1}{2}) = 8$, the * could be a multiplication operation.

20. $3y - 6 = 5y$. Then, $-6 = 2y$, so $y = -3$

21. $r + p(r+s) + 1 = r + 0(r+s) + 1 = r + 1$

22. $6x^2 - 8xy$ can be written as $(2x)(3x-4y)$

23. $(x+2y)(2x-y) = 2x^2 + 4xy - xy - 2y^2 = 2x^2 + 3xy - 2y^2$

24. For $\sqrt{x^2-1}$ to NOT be a real number, $x^2 - 1 < 0$. Then, $x^2 < 1$, so $-1 < x < 1$. Choice D, with $x = 0$, satisifes this inequality.

25. Since the intersection occurs where x is positive and y is negative, only choice A (1,-4) would be correct.

—

TEST 2

DIRECTIONS: Each question or incomplete statement is followed by several suggested answers or completions. Select the one that BEST answers the question or completes the statement. *PRINT THE LETTER OF THE CORRECT ANSWER IN THE SPACE AT THE RIGHT.*

Questions 1-4.

DIRECTIONS: In answering Questions 1 to 4, use the following information.

An operation involves the addition of integers 1, 2, 3, ... up to some final integer A. This operation we might represent by the special symbol A*. From this definition A*, we can see that 4* = 1 + 2 + 3 + 4 = 10.

1. What is the value of 3*? 1. ____
   A. 3 B. 5 C. 7 D. Not given

2. What is the sum of 5* and 7*? 2. ____
   A. 24 B. 42 C. 43 D. Not given

3. If B* - 5* = 13, what does B* equal? 3. ____
   A. 28 B. 18 C. 8 D. Not given

4. What is another way of representing 8 + 7 + 6? 4. ____
   A. 8* B. 8* - 5* C. 8* - 6* D. Not given

Questions 5-8.

DIRECTIONS: Use the definition below in answering Questions 5 to 8.

The symbol $\begin{vmatrix} A & B \\ C & D \end{vmatrix}$ means A times D minus B times C. That is, the product of B and C is subtracted from the product of A and D.

5. What is the value of $\begin{vmatrix} 3 & 1 \\ 2 & 3 \end{vmatrix}$? 5. ____
   A. 2 B. 3 C. 7 D. Not given

6. If $\begin{vmatrix} 1 & 2 \\ 3 & 6 \end{vmatrix} = \begin{vmatrix} 2 & 2 \\ 3 & A \end{vmatrix}$, what does A equal? 6. ____
   A. 3 B. 5 C. 6 D. Not given

7. If $\begin{vmatrix} 4 & D \\ D & 5 \end{vmatrix} = 11$, what does D equal? 7. ____
   A. 3 B. 6 C. 9 D. Not given

8. What is the value of $\begin{vmatrix} 3 & H \\ 2 & H \end{vmatrix}$? 8.____

A. 1 B. 5 C. H D. Not given

9. Solve for y: $6 - y = 10$. 9.____
A. 16 B. 4 C. -4
D. -16 E. Not given

10. What is the sum of $8a^3$ and $6a^3$? 10.____
A. $14a^3$ B. $14a^6$ C. $48a^3$ D. $48a^6$ E. $48a^9$

11. One-fourth of the quantity $(2r+12)$ equals 25. Find the value of r. 11.____
A. $6\frac{1}{2}$ B. 26 C. 44
D. 56 E. Not given

12. Divide $15m^2n^4$ by $3mn^2$. 12.____
A. $5mn$ B. $5mn^2$ C. $5m^2n^2$
D. $5m^3n^6$ E. Not given

13. Subtract: 13.____

$$\begin{array}{r} 6a^2 + 5b^3 - 3c \\ \underline{5a^2 + 4b^3 - 2c} \end{array}$$

A. $a^2 + b^3 - 5c$ B. $a^2 + 9b^3 - c$ C. $a^2 + 9b^3 - 5c$
D. $11a^2 + 9b^3 - 5c$ E. Not given

14. What is the value of $5(7b-9) + 3$? 14.____
A. $12b - 11$ B. $12b + 17$ C. $35b + 48$
D. $35b - 42$ E. Not given

15. Mr. Smith leaves home on a business trip at 8 A.M. He averages 45 miles an hour. Mr. Smith's son, John, leaves home at 9 A.M. trying to catch him. 15.____
The MINIMUM speed John can average and still catch his father by noon is ____ miles per hour.
A. 70 B. 60 C. 55 D. 50 E. 40

16. What is the sum of $3x^2$ and $5y^2$? 16.____
A. $8xy^2$ B. $8x^2y^2$ C. $15x^2y^2$
D. $3x^2 + 5y^2$ E. Not given

17. Write in simplified form: $a(2x-7y+1) + a$. 17.____
A. $2ax - 7ay + 2a$ B. $2ax - 7ay$ C. $2ax - 7ay + 1 + a$
D. $-5axy + 2a$ E. $2a + 2x - 7y + 1$

18. -3 is a solution for which of these equations? 18.____
A. $x^2 = -9$ B. $x^3 = 27$ C. $-5x = -15$
D. $5x^2 + 3x = 36$ E. $2x^2 + 6x + 1 = 0$

19. $a^2 + b^2 - a(a-b) =$ 19.____
A. $a^2 + b^2 + ab$ B. $2a^2 + b^2 - ab$ C. $2a^2 + b^2 + ab$
D. $b^2 - ab$ E. $b^2 + ab$

20. 20.

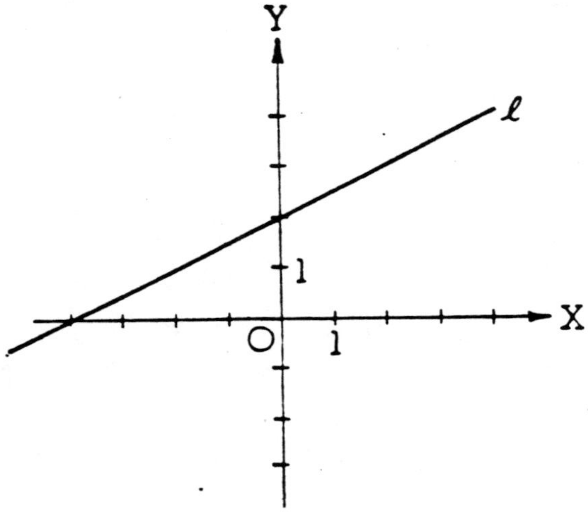

What is the slope of line l above?

A. 2 B. $\frac{1}{2}$ C. $-\frac{1}{2}$ D. -2

21. In which diagram could the shaded region represent $\{(x,y): x > 2 \text{ and } y < -1\}$? 21.

A.

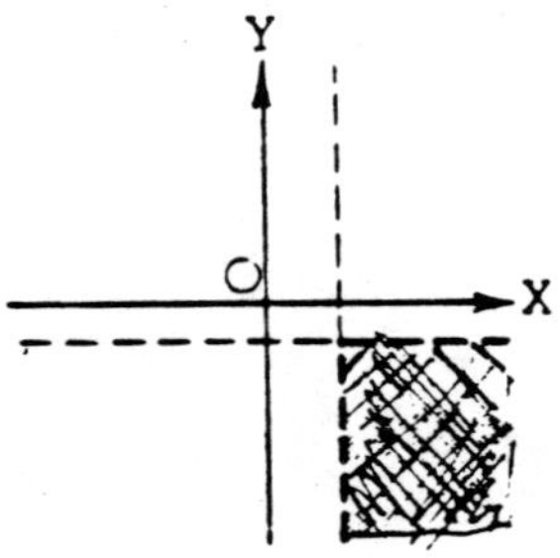

B.

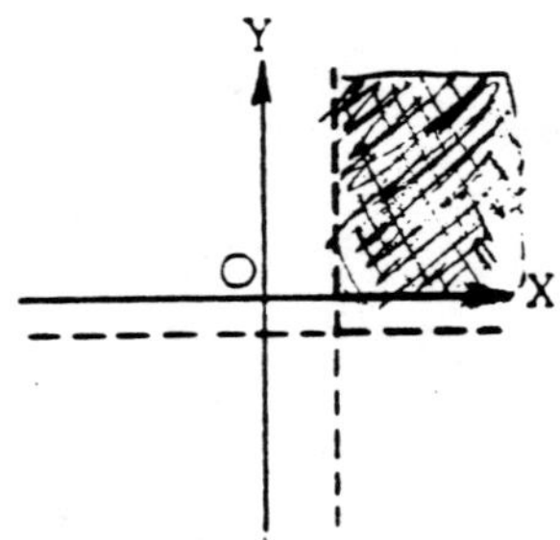

C.

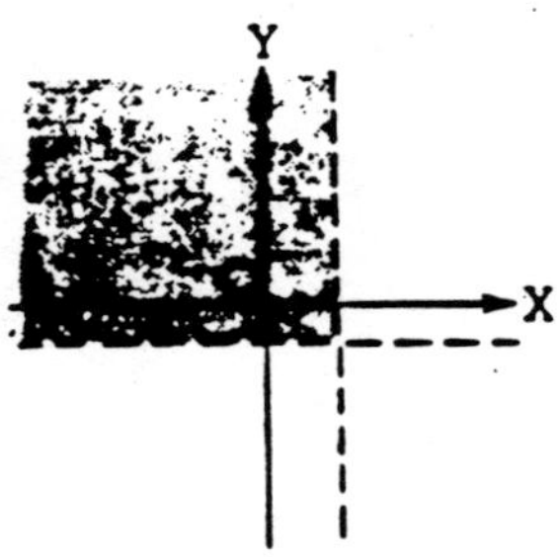

D.

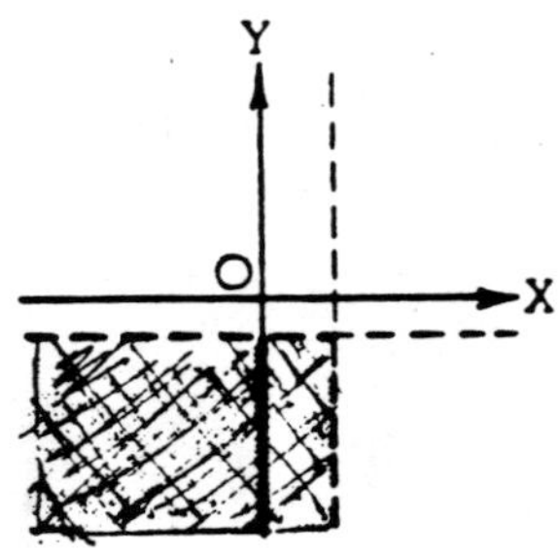

22. If $x > 1$ and $\frac{x^n}{x^2} = x^3$ for all x, then n = 22.

A. 1 B. 2 C. 5 D. 6

23. What is the solution set of the equation $x^2 - x = 0$? 23.

A. {0} B. {0,1} C. {0,1,2} D. {-1,0,1}

24. John states that $\frac{x^2-1}{x-1} = x + 1$ for all numbers x. 24.____

Which value of x shows that John is WRONG?

A. $x = 0$ B. $x = \frac{1}{2}$ C. $x = 1$ D. $x = 2$

25. Which of these is the graph of the inequality $x - 2 \geq 0$? 25.____

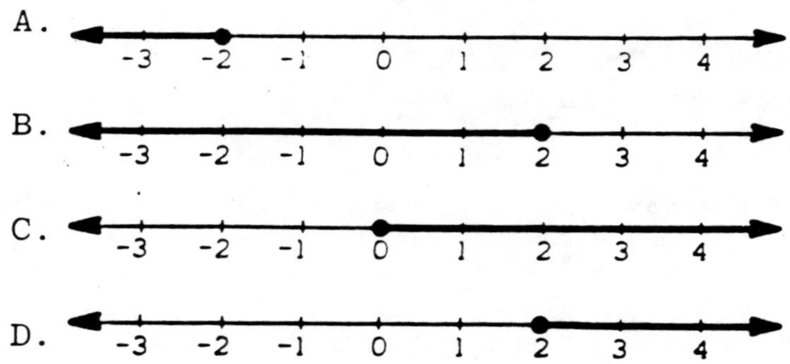

KEY (CORRECT ANSWERS)

1. D
2. C
3. A
4. B
5. C

6. A
7. A
8. C
9. C
10. A

11. C
12. B
13. E
14. D
15. B

16. D
17. A
18. D
19. E
20. B

21. A
22. C
23. B
24. C
25. D

SOLUTIONS TO PROBLEMS

1. $3* = 3 + 2 + 1 = 6$

2. $5* + 7* = (1+2+3+4+5) + (1+2+3+4+5+6+7) = 15 + 28 = 43$

3. $B* - 5* = 13$. Since $5* = 15$, $B* = 13 + 15 = 28$

4. $8 + 7 + 6 = (8+7+6+5+4+3+2+1) - (5+4+3+2+1) = 8* - 5*$

5. $\begin{vmatrix} 3 & 1 \\ 2 & 3 \end{vmatrix} = (3)(3) - (2)(1) = 9 - 2 = 7$

6. $\begin{vmatrix} 1 & 2 \\ 3 & 6 \end{vmatrix} = \begin{vmatrix} 2 & 2 \\ 3 & A \end{vmatrix}$ Then, $6 - 6 = 2A - 6$, $0 = 2A - 6$. Solving, $A = 3$

7. $\begin{vmatrix} 4 & D \\ D & 5 \end{vmatrix} = 11$ Then, $2D - D^2 = 11$. So, $D^2 = 9$ and D could equal 3 or -3

8. $\begin{vmatrix} 3 & H \\ 2 & H \end{vmatrix} = 3H - 2H = H$

9. $6 - y = 10$. Then, $-y = 4$, so $y = -4$

10. $8a^3 + 6a^3 = 14a^3$

11. $\frac{1}{4}(2r+12) = 25$. Then, $2r + 12 = 100$. Simplifying, $2r = 88$. Solving, $r = 44$.

12. $15m^2n^4 \div 3mn^2 = 5mn^2$

13. $(6a^2+5b^3-3c) - (5a^2+4b^3-2c) = a^2 + b^3 - c$

14. $5(7b-9) + 3 = 35b - 45 + 3 = 35b - 42$

15. Mr. Smith travels a total of $(45)(4) = 180$ miles. Since John must cover the same distance in 3 hours, his minimum speed must be $180 \div 3 = 60$ mph.

16. Since $3x^2$ and $5y^2$ are unlike terms, their sum can only be written as $3x^2 + 5y^2$

17. $a(2x-7y+1) + a = 2ax - 7ay + a + a = 2ax - 7ay + 2a$

18. -3 is a solution of $5x^2 + 3x = 36$, since $5(-3)^2 + 3(-3) = 45 - 9 = 36$

19. $a^2 + b^2 - a(a-b) = a^2 + b^2 - a^2 + ab = b^2 + ab$

20. From the points (0,2) and (-4,0), the slope is $\frac{0-2}{-4-0} = \frac{1}{2}$

21. The graph of $x > 2$ and $y < -1$ must lie to the right of $x = 2$ and below $y = -1$, as in choice A.

22. $x^n \div x^2 = x^3$. Then, $n - 2 = 3$, so $n = 5$

23. $x^2 - x = 0$. Then, $x(x-1) = 0$. Solving, $x = 0$ or $x = 1$

24. If $x = 1$, then $\frac{x^2-1}{x-1} = \frac{0}{0}$ = undefined

25. If $x - 2 \geq 0$, then $x \geq 2$. The single variable graph would be a dot on 2 and an arrow to the right of 2.

TEST 3

DIRECTIONS: Each question or incomplete statement is followed by several suggested answers or completions. Select the one that BEST answers the question or completes the statement. *PRINT THE LETTER OF THE CORRECT ANSWER IN THE SPACE AT THE RIGHT.*

Questions 1-3.

DIRECTIONS: In answering Questions 1 to 3, use the following definitions.

A vector may be represented by a row of numbers inside parentheses. An example of a vector is (1,3,7). The numbers 1, 3, and 7 are called the elements of the vector. A vector may have any number of elements.

The following is an example of vector addition: (4,5,6) + (1,2,3) = (5,7,9). The first elements of the added vectors are 4 and 1, and the first element of the sum vector is 4 + 1 = 5. The other elements of the sum vector are found in the same manner. Vector subtraction is performed by subtracting comparable elements.

1. What vector is obtained by subtracting (14,42,18) from (67,59,83)? 1.____
   A. (53,17,65)
   B. (53,17,75)
   C. (53,27,75)
   D. Not given

2. Which of these operations is NOT defined in the introductory material? 2.____
   A. (7,8,3) - (7,8,3)
   B. (4,10,3) - (0,0,0)
   C. (9,5,2,1) - (3,4,1,1)
   D. (4,6,2) - (5,3,1,7)

3. Which of these defines in symbolic form the addition of vectors with three elements? 3.____
   A. (a,b,c) + (d,e,f) = (a+b+c,d+e+f)
   B. (a,b,c) + (d,e,f) = (a,b,c,d,e,f)
   C. (a,b,c) + (d,e,f) = (a+b+c+d+e+f)
   D. (a,b,c) + (d,e,f) = (a+d,b+e,c+f)

Questions 4-8.

DIRECTIONS: Questions 4 to 8 are based on the following:

Vector multiplication is shown by an example.
(1,2,3) × (4,6,5) = 1 × 4 + 2 × 6 + 3 × 5 = 4 + 12 + 15 = 31.
Another example is (1,1) × (2,2) = 4

4. What is the product of (3,7,11) and (1,2,2)? 4.____
   A. 28
   B. 39
   C. 40
   D. Not given

5. What is the product of (3,3,3,3) and (4,5,4,3)? 5.____
   A. 38 B. 48 C. 53 D. Not given

6. What is the product of (17,4) and (0,0)? 6.____
   A. 21 B. 1 C. 0 D. Not given

7. When D = 4, what does $(D,7) \times (1,D)$ equal? 7.____
   A. 4 B. 28 C. 32 D. Not given

8. If $(2,4) \times (3,C) = 18$, what does C equal? 8.____
   A. 3 B. 6 C. 9 D. Not given

9. What value of m makes $6 - 3m = 15$ a TRUE statement? 9.____
   A. -9 B. -7 C. -3 D. 3 E. 7

10. Let $y = \frac{2}{1+x}$, where $x > 0$. Then, 10.____

    A. as x increases, y increases
    B. as x decreases, y decreases
    C. as x increases, y decreases
    D. when $0 < x < 1$, y is less than 1
    E. when $x > 1$, y is greater than 1

11. $(x^3)^2$ equals 11.____
    A. x^5 B. x^6 C. x^8 D. x^9 E. x^{32}

12. What is $7 + \frac{1}{4-y}$ when $y = -4$? 12.____

    A. 7 B. $7\frac{1}{8}$ C. $7\frac{1}{4}$

    D. 8 E. Not defined

13. What is the value of $3a^2$ when $a = -6$? 13.____
    A. -18 B. -36 C. 36 D. 108 E. -108

14. The perimeter of a square is 4e. 14.____
    What is the area of another square whose sides are twice as long as the sides of the first square?
    A. 8e B. $4e^2$ C. $16e^2$
    D. $64e^2$ E. Not given

15. If $x > 3$ and $y < 0$, then the value of $\frac{x}{y}$ is 15.____

    A. greater than 3 B. 3 C. between 0 and 3
    D. 0 E. less than 0

16. One-third of a certain number minus one-eighth of the same number equals 5. 16.____
    What is the number?
    A. 1 B. 8 C. 24
    D. 48 E. Not given

17. Solve for y: $5 - 4y = 2$. 17.___

A. $-\frac{7}{4}$ B. $-\frac{2}{5}$ C. $\frac{2}{5}$

D. $\frac{3}{4}$ E. Not given

18. What is the value of d^2d^x when x is an integer and d is any real number? 18.___

A. $d^{(x+2)}$ B. d^{x^2} C. $d2^x$

D. d^{2x} E. Not given

19. What is $\frac{5}{3-x}$ when $x = 3$? 19.___

A. 0 B. $\frac{5}{6}$ C. $\frac{5}{3}$

D. 5 E. Not defined

20. The sum of three numbers is 50, and x is the average of the first two numbers. 20.___
Identify the BEST expression for the third number.

A. $25 - x$ B. $50 - x$ C. $50 - 2x$ D. $\frac{50 + x}{2}$

21. $\frac{3}{x-1} - \frac{2}{x} =$ 21.___

A. $\frac{1}{x-1}$ B. $\frac{1}{x(x-1)}$ C. $\frac{x-2}{x(x-1)}$ D. $\frac{x+2}{x(x-1)}$

22. The meter in a certain taxi registers a minimum fare for distances up to 0.5 kilometer and $0.30 for each 0.5 kilometer thereafter. The *total* fare for a 4-kilometer ride is $2.85. 22.___
What is the fare for the FIRST 0.5 kilometer?
A. $0.45 B. $0.65 C. $0.75 D. $0.85

23. The annual income of a corporation increased 70 percent during the past year. 23.___
What is the ratio of its present income to its income a year ago?
A. $\frac{1}{70}$ B. $\frac{7}{10}$ C. $\frac{10}{7}$ D. $\frac{17}{10}$

24. $(x^2-5x+3) - (x^2-6x+4) =$ 24.___
A. $x - 1$ B. $x + 7$
C. $-11x - 7$ D. $x^2 - 11x + 7$

25. 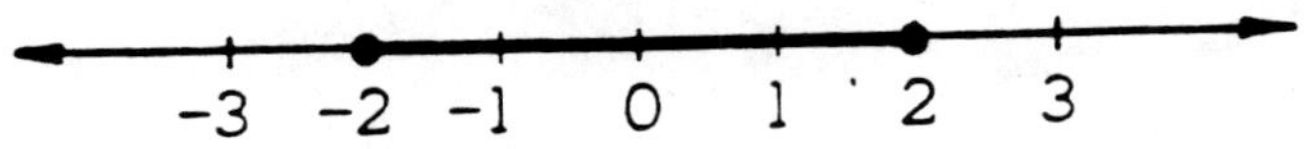 25.___

If the graph above represents $\{x : x^2 - k \leq 0\}$, then k =
A. 4 B. 2 C. -2 D. -4

KEY (CORRECT ANSWERS)

1. A
2. D
3. D
4. B
5. B

6. C
7. C
8. A
9. C
10. C

11. B
12. B
13. D
14. B
15. E

16. C
17. D
18. A
19. E
20. C

21. D
22. C
23. D
24. A
25. A

SOLUTIONS TO PROBLEMS

1. (67, 59, 83) - (14, 42, 18) = (53, 17, 65)

2. (4,6,2) - (5,3,1,7) is undefined since the two vectors do not have the same number of elements.

3. (a,b,c) + (d,e,f) = (a+d, b+e, c+f)

4. (3,7,11) × (1,2,2) = 3 + 14 + 22 = 39

5. (3,3,3,3) × (4,5,4,3) = 12 + 15 + 12 + 9 = 48

6. (17,4) × (0,0) = 0 + 0 = 0

7. (4,7) × (1,4) = 4 + 28 = 32

8. 6 + 4C = 18. Then, 4C = 12. Solving, C = 3

9. 6 - 3M = 15. Then, -3M = 9. Solving, M = -3

10. With $y = \frac{2}{1+x}$, x > 0, as x increases, y decreases. For example, when x = 1, y = 1. When x = 2, $y = \frac{2}{3}$

11. $(x^3)^2 = x^3 \cdot x^3 = x^6$

12. $7 + \frac{1}{4-(-4)} = 7 + \frac{1}{8} = 7\frac{1}{8}$

13. $3(-6)^2 = (3)(36) = 108$

14. If perimeter is 4e, each side of the original square is e. The new square will have each side of length 2e. Thus, the area of the new square is $(2e)^2 = 4e^2$

15. If x > 3 and y < 0, then $\frac{x}{y}$ must be negative (positive ÷ negative = negative). Thus, $\frac{x}{y} < 0$

16. Let x = number. Then, $\frac{1}{3}x - \frac{1}{8}x = 5$. Simplifying, $\frac{5}{24}x = 5$. So, $x = 5 \div \frac{5}{24} = 24$

17. $5 - 4y = 2$. Then, $-4y = -3$. Solving, $y = \frac{3}{4}$

18. $d^2 \cdot d^x = d^{2+x}$ or $d^{(x+2)}$

19. If x = 3, $\frac{5}{3-x} = \frac{5}{0}$ = undefined

20. If x = average of two numbers, their sum must be 2x. Since all three numbers add up to 50, the 3rd number is 50 - 2x.

21. $\frac{3}{x-1} - \frac{2}{x} = \frac{3x}{x(x-1)} - \frac{2(x-1)}{x(x-1)} = \frac{x+2}{x(x-1)}$

22. Let x = fare for the first .5 km. Then, x + .30(7) = 2.85. Solving, x = .75

23. Let x = income one year ago, so that x + .70x = 1.70x = current income. Then, $1.70x/x = 1.7/1 = \frac{17}{10}$

24. $(x^2-5x+3) - (x^2-6x+4) = x - 1$

25. For $x^2 - 4 \leq 0$, the solution is $-2 \leq x \leq 2$, which is the given graph. So, k = 4

TEST 4

DIRECTIONS: Each question or incomplete statement is followed by several suggested answers or completions. Select the one that BEST answers the question or completes the statement. *PRINT THE LETTER OF THE CORRECT ANSWER IN THE SPACE AT THE RIGHT.*

1. Factor $t^2 - 8t + 16$. 1.___
   A. (t-8)(t-2) B. (t-4)(t-4) C. (t-4)(t+4)
   D. (t+4)(t+4) E. Not given

2. Rich and Drew have 11 marbles to share. Rich takes more than 4. 2.___
   How many does Drew get?
   A. More than 7 B. 7 C. Less than 7
   D. 6 E. Less than 6

3. $(5x-3)(7x+4) =$ 3.___
   A. $12x + 1$ B. $35x^2 - 12$ C. $12x + 2x + 1$
   D. $35x^2 - x - 12$ E. $35x^2 - 41x - 12$

4. For any real number p, which of the following is TRUE? 4.___
   A. $p^2 \leq 0$ B. $p^2 \geq 0$ C. $p^3 \geq 0$
   D. $p^2 \leq p$ E. $p^2 \geq p$

5. A track star practices t hours each day. He alternates running and walking, spending one-half his time on each. He runs at 16 miles per hour and walks at 3 miles per hour. During practice, he covers _____ miles. 5.___
   A. 9.5t B. 11t C. 19t D. 22t E. 38t

6. $\frac{5u}{4} = 2 - \frac{u}{3}$. What is the value of u? 6.___
   A. $\frac{2}{19}$ B. $\frac{1}{3}$ C. $1\frac{5}{19}$
   D. $1\frac{11}{19}$ E. Not given

7. For non-zero x and y, when does $x \div y = y \div x$? 7.___
   A. Only when $y = 1$
   B. Only when $x = -y$
   C. When $x = y$ or $x = -y$
   D. For all non-zero values of x and y
   E. For no values of x and y

8. If $5 + x < 3$, then 8.___
   A. $x > 8$ B. $x < 8$ C. $x < 2$ D. $x > -2$ E. $x < -2$

9. The quantity $\frac{1}{-x}$, where $x \neq 0$, is the same as 9.____

A. $\frac{1}{x}$ B. $\frac{-1}{x}$ C. $-x$ D. x E. $-(\frac{1}{-x})$

10. Which is a solution to the equation $x^4 = 625$? 10.____

A. -5 B. 25 C. 125 D. $156\frac{1}{4}$ E. 2500

11. To cut a ribbon into 7 equal lengths would require _____ separate cuts. 11.____

A. $3\frac{1}{2}$ B. 6 C. 7 D. 8 E. 14

12. ____ are both factors of 12. 12.____

A. 10,2 B. 9,3 C. 4,3 D. 12,0 E. 8,4

13. In the problem $63 \div 7 = 9$, 7 is called the 13.____

A. quotient B. dividend C. divisor
D. product E. sum

14. $\frac{124}{24}$ reduces completely to 14.____

A. $\frac{12}{2}$ B. 6 C. $5\frac{1}{6}$ D. $5\frac{4}{24}$ E. $\frac{1}{6}$

15. If $\frac{x}{4} = 12$, $x =$ 15.____

A. 48 B. 4 C. 3 D. $\frac{1}{3}$ E. $\frac{1}{4}$

16. Solve the formula $T = b + \frac{km}{3}$ for **k**. 16.____

A. $k = 3T - 3b - m$ B. $k = \frac{T - b - m}{3}$

C. $k = \frac{T - b}{3} - m$ D. $k = \frac{3(T-b)}{m}$

E. $k = \frac{3T + 3b}{m}$

17. If $\frac{2x-1}{3} = 5$, then $2x + 1 =$ 17.____

A. 7 B. 13 C. 16 D. 17

18. A shelf contains a total of 180 science, math and English books. There are twice as many English books as math books and three times as many math books as science books. How many English books are on the shelf? 18.____

A. 60 B. 72 C. 108 D. 120

19. If $|x-3| = 4$, then the solution set of x is 19.____
A. {-1} B. {7} C. {-1,7} D. {1,-1}

20. If 2 is a root of the equation $3x^2 + ax - 12 = 0$, then a = 20.____
A. -12 B. 0 C. 6 D. 12

21. $\begin{cases} x-8y = 2 \\ x+4y = 5 \end{cases}$ 21.____
What is the value of x that satisfies the system of equations above?
A. 0 B. 2 C. 4 D. 6

22. $(y-3)(y+2) - (y-3) =$ 22.____
A. $(y+3)(y-1)$ B. $(y-3)(y+1)$ C. $(y-3)(y+3)$ D. $(y+3)(y+1)$

23. $\sqrt{16^3} =$ 23.____
A. $4\sqrt{3}$ B. 24 C. 64 D. 512

24. If $x \neq 0$, then $\frac{15x^3+3x}{3x} =$ 24.____
A. $15x^3$ B. $15x^3 + 1$ C. $5x^2 + 3x$ D. $5x^2 + 1$

25. Line l shown at the right is the graph of the equation y = 25.____
A. $-\frac{3}{2}x - 3$ B. $-\frac{2}{3}x + 2$
C. $\frac{3}{2}x - 3$ D. $\frac{2}{3}x + 2$

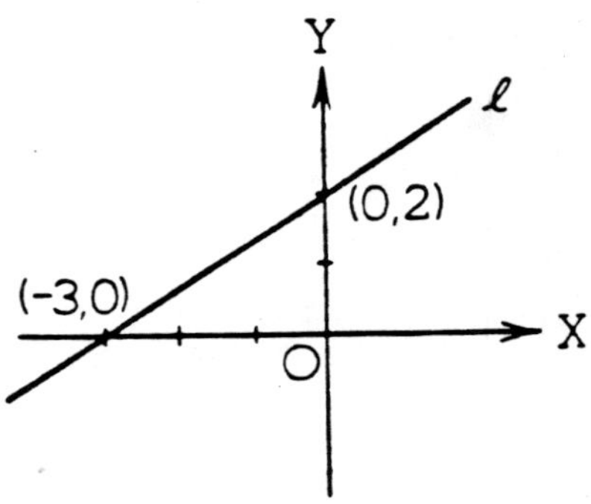

KEY (CORRECT ANSWERS)

1. B
2. C
3. D
4. B
5. A

6. C
7. C
8. E
9. B
10. A

11. B
12. C
13. C
14. C
15. A

16. D
17. D
18. C
19. C
20. B

21. C
22. B
23. C
24. D
25. D

SOLUTIONS TO PROBLEMS

1. The factoring of $t^2 - 8t + 16$ is $(t-4)(t-4)$

2. Since Rich takes more than 4 marbles, Drew will have less than 11 - 4 or less than 7 marbles.

3. $(5x-3)(7x+4) = 35x^2 + 20x - 21x - 12 = 35x^2 - x - 12$

4. For any real p, $p^2 \geq 0$ always

5. t/2 hours are spent running and t/2 hours are spent walking. Total distance (in miles) is $16(t/2) + 3(t/2) = 9.5t$

6. $5u/4 = 2 - u/3$. Multiply equation by 12 to get: $15u = 24 - 4u$. Then, $19u = 24$, so $u = 24/19 = 1\ 5/19$.

7. If $x \div y = y \div x$, then $x^2 = y^2$. This is true if $x = y$ or if $x = -y$

8. $5 + x < 3$. Then, $x < -2$

9. $\frac{1}{-x} = \frac{-1}{x}$, provided $x \neq 0$.

10. $x^4 = 625$. Then, $x = \pm \sqrt[4]{625} = 5$ or -5

11. Since the first cut would provide 2 equal lengths, 6 cuts would be needed for 7 equal lengths.

12. 4 and 3 are both factors of 12, since both divide evenly into 12.

13. $63 \div 7 = 9$. The 7 is called the divisor.

14. $\frac{124}{24}$ can be reduced to $5\frac{1}{6}$

15. $\frac{x}{4} = 12$. Multiply both sides by 4 to get $x = 48$

16. $T = b + \frac{km}{3}$. Then, $3T = 3b + Km$. Subtracting 3b, $3T - 3b = Km$ Finally, $K = (3T-3b)/m$ or $3(T-b)/m$

17. $\frac{2x-1}{3} = 5$. Then, $2x - 1 = 15$, so $x = 8$. Thus, $2x + 1 = 2(8) + 1 = 17$

18. Let x = number of science books, 3x = number of math books, and 6x = number of English books. Then, $x + 3x + 6x = 180$. Solving, $x = 18$. The number of English books is $6(18) = 108$

19. If $|x-3| = 4$, then $x - 3 = 4$ or $x - 3 = -4$. The solution set is $\{7,-1\}$

20. $3(2^2) + 2a - 12 = 0$. Then, $12 + 2a - 12 = 0$. Thus, $a = 0$

21. Double the 2nd equation to read $2x + 8y = 10$ and now add the 1st equation. The result is $3x = 12$, so $x = 4$

22. $(y-3)(y+2) - (y-3) = y^2 - y - 6 - y + 3 = y^2 - 2y - 3 = (y-3)(y+1)$

23. $\sqrt{16^3} = (\sqrt{16})^3 = 4^3 = 64$

24. $(15x^3 + 3x)/3x = 5x^2 + 1$, provided $x \neq 0$

25. The slope is $(2-0)/(0-(-3)) = \frac{2}{3}$ and the y-intercept is (0,2). Thus, $y = \frac{2}{3}x + 2$

EXAMINATION SECTION

TEST 1

DIRECTIONS: Each question or incomplete statement is followed by several suggested answers or completions. Select the one that BEST answers the question or completes the statement. *PRINT THE LETTER OF THE CORRECT ANSWER IN THE SPACE AT THE RIGHT.*

1. Monday I read *a* pages of a book, Tuesday I read *b* pages, Wednesday I read *c* pages. How many pages did I read altogether? 1.____
   A. abc B. a+b+c C. 3abc D. Not given

2. If the number of days in March is represented by *d*, indicate the number of days in January. 2.____
   A. d-1 B. d-2 C. d-3 D. Not given

3. A man 45 years old has a son who is *y* years younger. Indicate the age of the son. 3.____
   A. y-45 B. 45-y C. 45y D. Not given

4. Ray wants to buy a gun which costs *x* dollars. He has *y* dollars, but that is NOT enough. How many dollars more does he need? 4.____
   A. y-x B. xy C. x-y D. Not given

5. Represent the integer next greater than the one represented by *m*. 5.____
   A. m B. m+1 C. 1-m D. Not given

6. What is the volume of a room which is *r* feet wide, *s* feet long, and *t* feet high? 6.____
   A. rst B. r+s+t C. r+st D. Not given

7. One day a boy caught *f* fish, then gave away *a* of them. The next day, he caught *b* more, but sold half of them. How many fish had he left? 7.____
   A. fa-b B. $fa-\frac{1}{2}b$ C. $f-a+\frac{1}{2}b$ D. Not given

8. Indicate the number of days in *r* weeks. 8.____
   A. 7r B. $\frac{r}{7}$ C. r+7 D. Not given

9. John and James have *x* marbles between them, and each has as many as the other. How many has each? 9.____
   A. 2x B. $\frac{2}{x}$ C. $\frac{x}{2}$ D. Not given

10. If a certain number is represented by *x* and we give *x* a value of 5, what would be the value of $x + 2$? 10.____
    A. 10 B. 5x+2 C. 7 D. Not given

Questions 11-15.

DIRECTIONS: Use the following code to answer Questions 11 to 15.

┘ = 1, ⊔ = 2, └ = 3, ⊐ = 4, □ = 5, ⊏ = 6,
┐ = 7, ⊓ = 8, ┌ = 9. (Therefore, ┐ └. ⊔ is 673.2.)

11. ┘┌⊓⊏ = 11.___

A. 1927 B. 1986 C. 3784 D. 3926 E. 9683

12. ┘□ × └ = 12.___

A. └□ B. ⊐□ C. ┌└

D. ┘┘□ E. ┘⊔└

13. □⊐ + ⊔□ = 13.___

A. 63 B. 65 C. 74 D. 79 E. 141

14. ⊔⊓ ÷ ┐ = 14.___

A. └ B. ⊓ C. ┌ D. ⊐ E. ⊔

15. 45 ÷ 18 = 15.___

A. ┘.□ B. □.⊔ C. └.└

D. ⊔.⊔ E. ⊔.□

16. $\frac{5}{7} \div \frac{2}{3} =$ 16.___

A. $\frac{7}{10}$ B. $\frac{10}{21}$ C. $1\frac{8}{21}$ D. $1\frac{1}{14}$ E. $3\frac{1}{3}$

17. The lowest common denominator for $\frac{2}{3}, \frac{1}{4}, \frac{7}{9}$ is 17.___

A. 9 B. 12 C. 16 D. 36 E. 108

18. The basic formula for the volume of a box is V = 18.___

A. lwh B. $\frac{1}{3}$lwh

C. 6lwh D. $\pi r^2 h$

E. 2(lw+lh+wh)

19. 24 yards = 19.____
   A. 72 ft.   B. 72 in.   C. 8 yds.   D. 8 ft.   E. 1 rod

20. $\sqrt{36}$ = 20.____
   A. 1   B. 6   C. 18   D. 36   E. 136

21. Subtract $9x^2y^3$ from $4x^2y^3$. 21.____
   A. -5   B. -5xy   C. $-5x^2y^3$
   D. $-5x^4y^6$ E. Not given

22. The equation 5x + 7 = 2 + 3x is equivalent to which of the following? 22.____
   A. 8x = 9   B. 8x = -9   C. 5x = -5   D. 2x = 5   E. 2x = -5

23. Multiply: (x+7)(x-2). 23.____
   A. $x^2 - 14$ B. $x^2 + 5x - 14$ C. $x^2 + 5x + 14$
   D. $x^2 + 9x - 14$ E. $x^2 - 9x + 14$

24. Solve for x: 5x + 7 = 9. 24.____
   A. $\frac{2}{5}$ B. $\frac{5}{2}$ C. $\frac{16}{5}$
   D. -3   E. Not given

25. A quantity, P, is determined by the formula $\frac{1}{2}h(a^2+b)$. If h = 5, a = 3, and b = 7, what does P equal? 25.____
   A. 40   B. 52   C. 80
   D. 160   E. Not given

KEY (CORRECT ANSWERS)

1. B
2. D
3. B
4. C
5. B

6. A
7. C
8. A
9. C
10. C

11. B
12. B
13. D
14. D
15. E

16. D
17. D
18. A
19. A
20. B

21. C
22. E
23. B
24. A
25. A

SOLUTIONS TO PROBLEMS

1. The sum of a, b, and c is represented as $a + b + c$

2. d = number of days in March = number of days in January

3. The son's age is $45 - y$

4. If x is larger than y, their difference is shown as $x-y$

5. If m is an integer, the next integer must be $m+1$

6. Volume = (width)×(length)×height = rst

7. After one day, the boy had f-a fish. On the second day, he caught b fish but, after giving away $\frac{1}{2}$b fish, had $\frac{1}{2}$b fish left for that day. His 2-day total was $f - a + \frac{1}{2}b$

8. r weeks means $(r)(7) = 7r$ days

9. Each of them has half of $x = \frac{x}{2}$ marbles

10. $x + 2 = 5 + 2 = 7$

11. 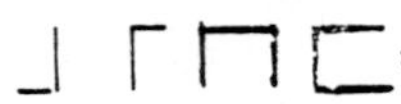 = 1986

12. 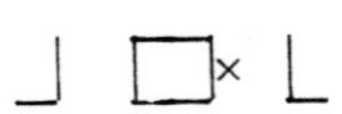 = 15 × 3 = 45 = 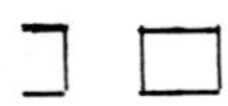

13. 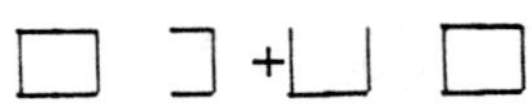 = 54 + 25 = 79

14. 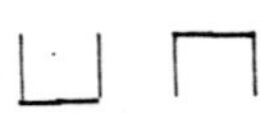 ÷ 7 = 28 ÷ 7 = 4 = 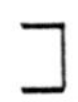

15. 45 ÷ 18 = 2.5 = 

16. $\frac{5}{7} \div \frac{2}{3} = (\frac{5}{7})(\frac{3}{2}) = \frac{15}{14} = 1\frac{1}{14}$

17. The lowest common denominator for 3, 4, and 9 is 36

18. The volume of a box $V = Lwh$, where L = length, w = width, and h = height

19. 24 yards = (24)(3) = 72 feet

20. $\sqrt{36} = 6$, since $6^2 = 36$

21. $4x^2y^3 - 9x^2y^3 = -5x^2y^3$

22. $5x + 7 = 2 + 3x$ can be written as $2x = -5$ by subtracting $3x + 7$ from both sides of the equation

23. $(x+7)(x-2) = x^2 + 7x - 2x - 14 = x^2 + 5x - 14$

24. $5x + 7 = 9$. Then, $5x = 2$, so $x = \frac{2}{5}$

25. $P = \frac{1}{2}h(a^2+b) = (\frac{1}{2})(5)(9+7) = \frac{5}{2}(16) = 40$

TEST 2

DIRECTIONS: Each question or incomplete statement is followed by several suggested answers or completions. Select the one that BEST answers the question or completes the statement. *PRINT THE LETTER OF THE CORRECT ANSWER IN THE SPACE AT THE RIGHT.*

1. $2.4 \times 6 =$ 1.___
   A. 1.8 B. 8.4 C. 14.4 D. 40 E. 144

2. In the problem 2 + 9 + 12 + 24 = 47, 47 is called the 2.___
   A. addend B. subtrahend C. dividend
   D. sum E. difference

3. In the fraction $\frac{21}{26}$, 3.___
   A. 21 is the denominator
   B. 26 is the numerator
   C. both are numerators
   D. neither is the denominator
   E. 26 is the denominator

4. To cut a board into 5 equal lengths would require ____ separate cuts. 4.___
   A. 3 B. $3\frac{1}{2}$ C. 4 D. 5 E. 6

5. In the problem 21 - 3 = 18, 18 is called the 5.___
   A. subtrahend B. minuend C. difference
   D. quotient E. product

6. $\frac{5}{7} - \frac{2}{3} =$ 6.___
   A. $\frac{3}{4}$ B. $\frac{3}{10}$ C. $\frac{7}{10}$ D. $\frac{1}{21}$ E. $\frac{3}{21}$

7. The LOWEST common denominator of $\frac{3}{5}$, $\frac{4}{5}$, and $\frac{2}{5}$ is 7.___
   A. 120 B. 24 C. 15 D. 10 E. 5

8. In the problem $7 \times 8 = 56$, 56 is called the 8.___
   A. product B. quotient C. multiplier
   D. multiplicand E. sum

9. ____ are both factors of 10. 9.___
   A. 10,0 B. 8,2 C. 2,5 D. 6,4 E. 7,3

10. $\sqrt{64} =$ 10.___
   A. 0 B. 1 C. 8 D. 32 E. 128

11. Which number is SMALLEST? 11.___
   A. 4.5 B. 4.449 C. .459
   D. .057399 E. 1.000

12. Of these two formulas: $A = \frac{1}{2}bh$ and $A = bh$, the 12.___
   A. first gives the area of a rectangle
   B. first gives the area of a triangle
   C. first gives the area of a trapezoid
   D. second gives the perimeter of a rectangle
   E. second gives the perimeter of a triangle

13. If you earn $40.00 and save $8.00 of it, what percent do you save? 13.___
   A. $\frac{1}{5}$ B. 5 C. 8 D. 20 E. 32

14. Reduce $\frac{\frac{36}{2}}{\frac{12}{4}}$ to simplest terms. 14.___
   A. 5 B. $\frac{15}{3}$ C. $\frac{1}{5}$ D. $\frac{3}{15}$ E. 6

15. I = PRT is a formula for 15.___
   A. increment B. investment C. interest
   D. insurance E. none of the above

16. Take any number (your age will do); add ten to it; double the answer; subtract the number you started with; add twenty to that answer; again subtract your starting number; square that answer. 16.___
The final answer is
   A. your age B. 80 C. 160
   D. 1600 E. 1960

Questions 17-18.

DIRECTIONS: Use the following code to answer Questions 17 and 18.

Let $\square$ stand for the number of boys in the class. Let $\circ$ stand for the number of girls in the class.

17. $\square - \circ$ = the 17.___
   A. sum of boys and girls
   B. total of boys and girls
   C. total ages of the class
   D. excess of boys over girls
   E. excess of girls over boys

18. The ratio of boys to the TOTAL enrollment in the class would be 18.___
   A. $\frac{\circ}{\square}$ B. $\frac{\square}{\circ}$ C. $\circ + \square$
   D. $\frac{\square}{\circ + \square}$ E. $\frac{\circ}{\square + \circ}$

19. Perimeters are ALWAYS measured in 19.___
A. volume B. area C. linear measure
D. square measure E. cubic measure

20. 5 × 30% of 30 = 20.___
A. 30 B. 40 C. 45 D. 50 E. 150

Questions 21-30.

DIRECTIONS: Each of Questions 21 to 30 presents a TRUE statement about counting numbers which are represented by the letters x, y, k, m, or s. You are to tell what MUST happen to x if certain changes are made in y, k, m, or s and the statement is to remain TRUE. If there is not enough information given to decide what happens to x, choose answer D, "cannot tell".

21. $x = y + 8$ 21.___
If y were made greater, what MUST happen to x?
A. Remain the same B. Become greater
C. Become less D. Cannot tell

22. $x = y + m$ 22.___
If m were to be made 1 greater and y were to be made 1 less, what MUST happen to x?
A. Remain the same B. Become greater
C. Become less D. Cannot tell

23. $y = x + m$ 23.___
If m were made greater, what MUST happen to x so that y would remain the same?
A. Remain the same B. Become greater
C. Become less D. Cannot tell

24. $x = ym$ 24.___
If y were made greater and m were made less, what MUST happen to x?
A. Remain the same B. Become greater
C. Become less D. Cannot tell

25. $x = y + \frac{m}{s}$ 25.___

If m were made less and y and s did not change, what MUST happen to x?
A. Remain the same B. Become greater
C. Become less D. Cannot tell

26. $k = xm$ 26.___
If m were made less and k remained the same, what MUST happen to x?
A. Remain the same B. Become greater
C. Become less D. Cannot tell

27. $x = y - m$ 27.___
If m were made greater and y remained the same, what MUST happen to x?
A. Remain the same B. Become greater
C. Become less D. Cannot tell

28. $x = y + m - k$ 28.____
If y, m, and k were made equal to each other, what MUST happen to x?
A. Remain the same B. Become greater
C. Become less D. Cannot tell

29. $x = y + \frac{m}{s}$ 29.____
If s were made less and y and m did not change, what MUST happen to x?
A. Remain the same B. Become greater
C. Become less D. Cannot tell

30. $x = \frac{y}{m}$ 30.____
Given that y and m are always equal, what MUST happen to x if y and m are made greater in the same proportion?
A. Remain the same B. Become greater
C. Become less D. Cannot tell

KEY (CORRECT ANSWERS)

1. C	11. D	21. B
2. D	12. B	22. A
3. E	13. D	23. C
4. C	14. E	24. D
5. C	15. C	25. C
6. D	16. D	26. B
7. E	17. D	27. C
8. A	18. D	28. D
9. C	19. C	29. B
10. C	20. C	30. A

SOLUTIONS TO PROBLEMS

1. $2.4 \times 6 = 14.4$

2. In $2 + 9 + 12 + 24 = 47$, 47 is called the sum

3. In $\frac{21}{26}$, 26 is the denominator

4. Since 1 cut makes 2 equal lengths, 4 cuts would make 5 equal lengths

5. In $21 - 3 = 18$, 18 is called the difference

6. $\frac{5}{7} - \frac{2}{3} = \frac{15}{21} - \frac{14}{21} = \frac{1}{21}$

7. Since all fractions have a denominator of 5, then 5 is the lowest common denominator

8. In $7 \times 8 = 56$, 56 is called the product

9. 2 and 5 are both factors of 10 since 10 divides evenly by each of them

10. $\sqrt{64} = 8$, since $8^2 = 64$

11. .057399 is the smallest in this group of numbers

12. The formula $A = \frac{1}{2}bh$ represents the area of a triangle

13. $\$8/\$40 = \frac{1}{5} = 20\%$

14. $\frac{36}{2} \div \frac{12}{4} = 18 \div 3 = 6$

15. I = PRT is a formula for interest. (Incidentally, P = principal, R = rate, and T = time)

16. Let x = initial number. Following directions, we get: $x + 10$, $2x + 20$, $x + 20$, $x + 40$, 40, 1600

17. $\square - 0$ = the difference between number of boys and the number of girls = excess of boys over girls

18. Total enrollment is $\square + 0$. The ratio of boys to this total $= \frac{\square}{0 + \square}$

19. Perimeters are always a linear measure

20. $5 \times 30\%$ of $30 = (5)(9) = 45$

21. $x = y + 8$. As y increases, so will x increase

22. $x = y + m$. By changing m to m+1 and y to y-1, $x = y-1 + m+1 = y + m$. Thus, x remains the same

23. $y = x + m$. If m is increased and x were decreased, by the same amount, then y remains the same

24. $x = ym$. If y increases and m decreases, the change in x is unknown

25. $x = y + \frac{m}{s}$. By decreasing m and leaving y and s alone, x becomes less

26. $k = xm$. If m decreases and k remains unchanged, then x becomes greater

27. $x = y - m$. If m increases and y remains unchanged, then x becomes less

28. $x = y + m - k$. If $y = m = k$, $x = y = m = k$, but the change in x is unknown

29. $x = y + \frac{m}{s}$. If s decreases and y, m remain unchanged, x becomes greater.

30. $x = \frac{y}{m}$. If $m = y$, and both m and y change equally, then x remains the same. (In fact, $x = 1$)

TEST 3

DIRECTIONS: Each question or incomplete statement is followed by several suggested answers or completions. Select the one that BEST answers the question or completes the statement. *PRINT THE LETTER OF THE CORRECT ANSWER IN THE SPACE AT THE RIGHT.*

1. 24 ft. = 1.___
   A. 72 ft. B. 72 in. C. 8 yds. D. 8 ft. E. 1 rod

2. The formula for the area of a circle is A = 2.___
   A. πr^2 B. $\frac{1}{2}\pi r^2$ C. $2\pi r$
   D. $2\pi r^2$ E. none of the above

3. $\frac{24}{124}$ reduces to 3.___
   A. $\frac{1}{6}$ B. $\frac{2}{12}$ C. $\frac{6}{31}$ D. $\frac{6}{1}$ E. $\frac{1}{5}$

4. Of these two formulas: P = a+b+c and P = 2a+2b, the 4.___
   A. first gives the area of a rectangle
   B. first gives the area of a triangle
   C. first gives the perimeter of a triangle
   D. second gives the perimeter of a trapezoid
   E. second gives the area of a trapezoid

5. 4 × 20% of 25 = 5.___
   A. 10 B. 20 C. 4.8 D. 80 E. 200

6. Distances are measured in units of 6.___
   A. volume B. area C. linear measure
   D. square measure E. cubic measure

7. In the problem 56 ÷ 7 = 8, 8 is called the 7.___
   A. quotient B. dividend C. divisor
   D. product E. sum

8. If $\frac{x}{2}$ = 12, x = 8.___
   A. $\frac{1}{6}$ B. $\frac{1}{2}$ C. 2 D. 6 E. 24

9. Melons are selling at 3 for 25¢. Each weighs 2 lbs. How much would 54 lbs. cost? 9.___
   A. 75¢ B. $1.62 C. $2.25 D. $4.50 E. $9.00

10. Take any number; double it; add ten; subtract twice the number you started with; double the answer; square this answer; subtract one hundred. 10.___
    The answer is
    A. 90 B. 100 C. 300
    D. 500 E. impossible

Questions 11-14.

DIRECTIONS: Use the following code and rules to answer Questions 11 to 14.

Code	Rules for addition
0 = 0	0 + 0 = 0
I = 1	0 + I = I
I0 = 2	I + I = I0 (Put down 0, carry I to the next column left.)
II = 3	
I00 = 4	
I0I = 5	Example:
II0 = 6	I0 (2)
III = 7	+ II (3)
I000 = 8	I0I (5)

11. 3 + 4 can then be written 11.____
A. I + II B. II + I00 C. 0 + I00
D. I0I + III E. I000 + I0

12. I00 + I = 12.____
A. 3 B. 4 C. 5 D. 6 E. 7

13. 9 would be 13.____
A. II00 B. I00I C. II0I D. IIII E. I0000

14. III + I0I = 14.____
A. I000 B. I00I C. I0II D. II00 E. II0I

15. Reduce $\dfrac{\frac{24}{4}}{\frac{18}{9}}$ to simplest terms. 15.____

A. $\frac{1}{3}$ B. 3 C. $\frac{6}{2}$ D. 4 E. $1\frac{1}{6}$

16. If you spend $21.00 from your savings account of $28.00, what percent have you spent? 16.____
A. $\frac{3}{4}$ B. 21 C. 25 D. 70 E. 75

17. A cube has 6 sides that are squares. 17.____
Besides, it has ____ edges and ____ corners.
A. 6; 6 B. 8; 8 C. 6; 8
D. 8; 6 E. none of the above

18. $\frac{2}{3} \div \frac{3}{2}$ = 18.____
A. $\frac{4}{9}$ B. $\frac{9}{4}$ C. 1 D. $\frac{4}{6}$ E. $\frac{2}{3}$

19. The formula for the area of a sphere (ball) is A = 19.___
A. lwh B. πr^2 C. $\frac{1}{2}$bh D. prt E. $4\pi r^2$

20. If *y* represents an even number, represent the next greater even number. 20.___
A. y+2 B. y+1 C. 2y+1 D. Not given

21. If one load of coal costs *c* dollars, what will be the cost of *b* loads of such coal? 21.___
A. b-c B. b+c C. $\frac{b}{c}$ D. Not given

22. How much money is in Joe's bank account when *y* dollars are deposited and *x* dollars withdrawn if the previous balance was *k* dollars? 22.___
A. y-xk B. k+y-x C. y-k+x D. Not given

23. Three boys decide to run a refreshment stand. The equipment costs *r* dollars. The father of one of the boys gave them $20.00. 23.___
Indicate how many dollars each boy will have to pay if the remaining expense is to be divided evenly among them.
A. $\frac{r-20}{3}$ B. $\frac{r+20}{3}$ C. $\frac{20r}{3}$ D. Not given

24. How many hours will it take a person to go *m* miles if he goes *r* miles in one hour? 24.___
A. mr B. $\frac{r}{m}$ C. $\frac{m}{r}$ D. Not given

25. If the product of two numbers is 24 and one of the numbers is *m*, what is the other number? 25.___
A. 24m B. 24+m C. 24-m D. Not given

26. If the quotient of two numbers is *y* and the divisor is *m*, represent the dividend. 26.___
A. $\frac{y}{m}$ B. my C. $\frac{m}{y}$ D. Not given

27. Indicate the number of cents in *m* dimes and 2 pennies. 27.___
A. 12 B. m+2 C. 10m D. Not given

28. A book, a pencil, and a tablet together cost *y* cents. The pencil cost *m* cents, and the tablet cost twice as much as the pencil. 28.___
What did the book cost?
A. y-3m B. 2m-y C. 3m D. Not given

29. One roll of telephone wire will reach *f* feet. 29.___
How many rolls of such wire are needed to reach *t* feet?
A. t-f B. $\frac{t}{f}$ C. tf D. Not given

30. One number is 7 less than another number. If 5 times the greater number is subtracted from 8 times the other, the difference is 25.
What is the GREATER number? 30. ____

A. 27
B. 20
C. 9
D. 2
E. Not given

KEY (CORRECT ANSWERS)

1. C	11. B	21. D
2. A	12. C	22. B
3. C	13. B	23. A
4. C	14. D	24. C
5. B	15. B	25. D
6. C	16. E	26. B
7. A	17. E	27. D
8. E	18. A	28. A
9. C	19. E	29. B
10. C	20. A	30. A

SOLUTIONS TO PROBLEMS

1. 24 ft = 24 ÷ 3 = 8 yds

2. The area of a circle is given by $A = \pi r^2$, where $\pi \approx \frac{22}{7}$ and r = radius

3. $\frac{24}{124}$ reduces to $\frac{6}{31}$ by dividing numerator and denominator by 4

4. P = a + b + c represents the perimeter of a triangle, where a, b, and c represent the sides

5. 4 × 20% of 25 = (4)(.20)(25) = 20

6. Distances are measured in units of linear measure

7. In 56 ÷ 7 = 8, 8 is called the quotient

8. $\frac{x}{2} = 12$. Multiply both sides by 2 to get x = 24

9. 54 ÷ 2 = 27. If 3 melons cost 25¢, then 27 melons cost (9)(.25) = $2.25

10. Let x = original number. Following instructions, we get: 2x, 2x+10, 10, 20, 400, 300

11. 3 + 4 = II + IOO

12. IOO + I = 4 + 1 = 5

13. 9 would be written as IOOI

14. III + IOI = 7 + 5 = 12 = IIOO

15. $\frac{24}{4} \div \frac{18}{9} = 6 \div 2 = 3$

16. $21 ÷ $28 = .75 = 75%

17. A cube has 12 edges and 8 corners

18. $\frac{2}{3} \div \frac{3}{2} = \frac{2}{3} \cdot \frac{2}{3} = \frac{4}{9}$

19. The formula for the area of a sphere is $A = 4\pi r^2$, where r = radius. Incidentally, this area is called surface area.

20. If y is an even number, the next largest even number is $y + 2$

21. One load costs c dollars. Thus, b loads cost bc dollars

22. Starting with a balance of k dollars, depositing y dollars, and withdrawing x dollars, yields a result of $k + y - x$ dollars

23. The remaining expense is r-20. If this is divided evenly 3 ways, each boy will have to pay $(r-20)/3$

24. A rate of r miles per hour means a distance of m miles requires $\frac{m}{r}$ hours

25. If m is one number and two numbers multiply to give 24, then the other number is $\frac{24}{m}$

26. If y = quotient, m = divisor, then my = dividend

27. m dines and 2 pennies is equivalent to 10m+2 cents

28. Since the pencil costs m cents, the tablet costs 2m cents. Now, the book must have cost $y - m - 2m = y - 3m$ cents

29. If one roll of wire reaches f feet, then $\frac{t}{f}$ rolls are needed to reach t feet

30. Let x = larger number, x-7 = smaller number. Then, we get $8(x-7) - 5x = 25$. Simplifying, $8x - 56 - 5x = 25$. This reduces to $3x = 81$, so $x = 27$

MATHEMATICS

EXAMINATION SECTION

TEST 1

DIRECTIONS:
Each question or incomplete statement is followed by several suggested answers or completions. Select the one that *BEST* answers the question or completes the statement. *PRINT THE LETTER OF THE CORRECT ANSWER IN THE SPACE AT THE RIGHT.*

1. x is what percent of 10? 1. ...
   A. 10x B. $\frac{x}{10}$ C. 100x D. 50x
   E. $\frac{10}{x}$
2. Write $\frac{1}{4}$ percent as a fraction. 2. ...
   A. 25/100 B. 1/400 C. 25/1000 D. 1/4
   E. 1/40
3. The number of students in a school increased from 100 to 300. What is the percent increase? 3. ...
   A. 150 B. 200 C. 250 D. 300
   E. 450
4. $\sqrt{.005}$ is what percent of $\sqrt{2}$? 4. ...
   A. 5 B. 10 C. 15 D. 20
   E. 25
5. What is 2/5 percent as a decimal? 5. ...
   A. .4 B. .04 C. .004 D. .0004
   E. .00004
6. One worker picks 25 percent as many bushels as all the other workers combined. This worker picks 20 bushels. How many bushels were picked by all the workers? 6. ...
   A. 100 B. 90 C. 80 D. 75 E. 70
7. A man bought a suit for $45 during a 10-percent-discount sale. How much money did he save? 7. ...
   A. $14 B. $3.50 C. $5 D. $4.50 E. $7
8. A factory turns out 400 cars each month. This is an increase of 25 percent over the previous months. How many cars were turned out the previous months? 8. ...
   A. 300 B. 320 C. 330 D. 350
   E. 400
9. 2/5 of 14 is what percent of 7? 9. ...
   A. 5 3/5 B. 125 C. 80 D. $87\frac{1}{2}$
   E. 90
10. What is $\frac{1}{2}$ percent written as a decimal? 10. ...
    A. .5 B. .05 C. .005 D. .0005 E. .50
11. In triangle ABC, angle A is 150 percent as large as angle B, and angle B is 50 percent of angle C. How many degrees are there in angle C? 11. ...
    A. 30 B. 40 C. 60 D. 80 E. 160
12. If each side of a square is increased by 50 percent, by what percent is the area increased? 12. ...
    A. 50 B. 100 C. 125 D. 150 E. 200
13. 1/3 is what percent of 3? 13. ...
    A. 33 1/3 B. 66 2/3 C. 11 1/9 D. 12 1/2
    E. 16 2/3

14. In one class 30 percent are boys and in another class, ½ as large, 40 percent are boys. Find the percentage of boys in both classes combined. 14. ...
A. 12½ B. 15 C. 25 D. 33 1/3 E. 50

15. $\frac{x}{250}$ = 2.4 percent. Find x. 15. ...
A. 3 B. 5 C. 6 D. 104 1/6 E. 600

KEY (CORRECT ANSWERS)

1. A
2. B
3. B
4. A
5. C

6. A
7. C
8. B
9. C
10. C

11. D
12. C
13. C
14. D
15. C

SOLUTIONS TO PROBLEMS

1. Let P = required percent. Then, $\frac{x}{10} = \frac{P}{100}$. Solving, P = 10x.

2. $\frac{1}{4}\% = \frac{1}{4} \div 100 = \frac{1}{400}$

3. Actual increase is 200. The percent increase = $(\frac{200}{100})(100) = 200$

4. Let x = required percent. $\sqrt{.005}/\sqrt{2} = x/100$. Then, $x = 100\sqrt{.0025} = 5$

5. $\frac{2}{5}\% = \frac{2}{5} \div 100 = .004$

6. Let x = number of bushels picked by all the other workers. Then, 20 = .25x, so x = 80. Now the number of bushels picked by all workers is 80 + 20 = 100.

7. Let x = original price. Then, \$45 = .90x, so x = \$50. The amount saved is \$50 − \$45 = \$5.

8. Let x = number of cars produced in previous months. Then, 400 = 1.25x, so x = 320.

9. $(\frac{2}{5})(14) = 5.6$. Let x = required percent. Then, 5.6/7 = x/100. Solving, x = 80.

10. $\frac{1}{2}\% = \frac{1}{2} \div 100 = \frac{1}{200} = .005$

11. Let x = ∠B, 2x = ∠C, 1.5x = ∠A. Then, x + 2x + 1.5x = 180°. Solving, x = 40°. So, ∠C = 2x = 80°.

12. Let x = original side of the square, so that 1.5x = enlarged side of the square. Then, x^2 = original area and $2.25x^2$ = enlarged area. The increase is $1.25x^2$, which is 125%.

13. Let x = required percent. $\frac{1}{3}/3 = x/100$, so $x = \frac{100}{9} = 11\frac{1}{9}$

14. Let 2x = size of 1st class, x = size of 2nd class. The number of boys in the 1st class is (.30)(2x) = .60x, whereas the number of boys in the 2nd class is .40x. The ratio of boys to the total enrollment in both classes combined is x/3x, which is $33\frac{1}{3}\%$.

15. x/250 = 2.4% = .024. Then, x = (250)(.024) = 6

TEST 2

DIRECTIONS:

Each question or incomplete statement is followed by several suggested answers or completions. Select the one that *BEST* answers the question or completes the statement. *PRINT THE LETTER OF THE CORRECT ANSWER IN THE SPACE AT THE RIGHT.*

1. If 3 men can do a job in 6 days, how long will it take 9 men to do the same job? 1. ...
   A. 2 days B. 54 days C. 8 days D. 27 days E. 6 days
2. It takes one minute to fill a tank 3/5 full. How much longer will it take to fill up the tank? 2. ...
   A. 5 seconds B. 10 seconds C. 20 seconds
   D. 30 seconds E. 40 seconds
3. The ratio of the legs of a right triangle is 1 : 3. If the area is 6, what is the length of the hypotenuse? 3. ...
   A. 8 B. $\sqrt{40}$ C. $\sqrt{12}$ D. 30
   E. None of these
4. If 3 pencils cost x cents, how many pencils can be bought for 30 cents 4. ...
   A. $\frac{90}{x}$ B. $\frac{x}{90}$ C. $\frac{30}{x}$ D. $\frac{x}{30}$ E. 90x
5. If one kilometer equals 5/8 of a mile, how many kilometers are there in 40 miles? 5. ...
   A. 25 B. 30 C. 35 D. 40 E. 64
6. If it takes 3 minutes to fill a pool 4/5 full, how much longer (in seconds) will it take to fill up the tank? 6. ...
   A. 12 B. 15 C. 30 D. 45 E. 50
7. If one inch equals 2.54 centimeters, then 8 centimeters equals approximately how many inches? 7. ...
   A. 2.7 B. 2.9 C. 3.1 D. 3.3 E. 3.5
8. A 100-yard dash is run in 10 seconds. What is the approximate speed in miles per hour? 8. ...
   A. 7 B. 9 C. 20 D. 25 E. 30
9. 8 men can complete a job in 24 days. How long will it take 12 men working at the same rate to do the job? 9. ...
   A. 10 days B. 12 days C. 14 days
   D. 16 days E. 20 days
10. If a map is drawn to the scale of 1 inch to 75 miles, what is the distance between 2 cities that are 4 3/4 inches apart on the map? 10. ...
    A. 340 1/3 B. 357 2/3 C. 370
    D. 344 E. 356 1/4
11. If *a* apples cost *b* cents, find the cost of *c* apples. 11. ...
    A. $\frac{bc}{a}$ B. $\frac{ac}{b}$ C. $\frac{ab}{c}$ D. $\frac{b}{ac}$ E. $\frac{c}{ab}$
12. Find the ratio of a yard to a foot. 12. ...
    A. 1:3 B. 3:1 C. 1:1 D. 12:1
    E. 2:1
13. Two girls buy a radio for $15, contributing amounts in the ratio of 5:4. How much was the smaller amount? 13. ...
    A. 1 2/3 B. 4 C. 5 D. 6 2/3 E 12

14. A gear with 48 teeth, rotating at 360 revolutions per minute, meshes with a gear of 72 teeth. How many revolutions per minute does the second gear make? 14. ...
   A. 180 B. 240 C. 277 D. 530 E. 432

15. A troop of 75 men have enough rations to last 4 days. if the troop is increased by 25 men, then how long will the same rations last? 15. ...
   A. $\frac{4}{3}$ days B. $\frac{3}{4}$ days C. 12 days
   D. 3 days E. 2 days

KEY (CORRECT ANSWERS)

1. A
2. E
3. B
4. A
5. E

6. D
7. C
8. C
9. D
10. E

11. A
12. B
13. D
14. B
15. D

SOLUTIONS TO PROBLEMS

1. The number of men is inversely proportional to the number of days. Let x = required number of days. Then, 3/9 = x/6. Solving, x = 2

2. 1 min./$\frac{3}{5}$ = x min./$\frac{2}{5}$. Solving, x = $\frac{2}{3}$ min. = 40 seconds.

3. Let x, 3x = lengths of the two. $(\frac{1}{2})(x)(3x) = 6$, so $3x^2 = 12$ and x = 2. The two legs are 2 and 6. Thus, the hypotenuse = $\sqrt{2^2 + 6^2} = \sqrt{40}$

4. Let p = number of pencils. 3/x = p/30, px = 90, so p = $\frac{90}{x}$

5. 40 miles = 40 ÷ $\frac{5}{8}$ = 64 kilometers

6. 3 min./$\frac{4}{5}$ = x min./$\frac{1}{5}$. Solving, x = $\frac{3}{4}$ min. = 45 seconds

7. 8 centimeters = 8 ÷ 2.54 ≈ 3.1 inches

8. 100 yards in 10 seconds means 36,000 yards per hour. Then, 36,000 yards = 36,000/1760 ≈ 20 miles. Thus, the speed is 20 mi/hr.

9. The number of men is inversely proportional to the number of days. Let x = required number of days. Then, 8/12 = x/24. Solving, x = 16.

10. $4\frac{3}{4}$ inches corresponds to $(75)(4\frac{3}{4}) = 356\frac{1}{4}$ miles

11. Let p = cost of c apples. a/b = c/p. Solving, p = $\frac{bc}{a}$

12. 1 yard : 1 foot = 3 feet : 1 foot = 3:1

13. Let 5x, 4x represent their respective contributions. Then, 5x + 4x = \$15. Solving, x = $\$1\frac{2}{3}$. The smaller amount is $(\$1\frac{2}{3})(4) = \$6\frac{2}{3}$

14. The number of teeth is inversely proportional to the number of revolutions per minute. Let x = required revolutions per minute. 48/72 = x/360. Solving, x = 240

15. The number of men is inversely proportional to the number of days. Let x = required number of days. 75/100 = x/4, so x = 3

TEST 3

DIRECTIONS:

Each question or incomplete statement is followed by several suggested answers or completions. Select the one that *BEST* answers the question or completes the statement. *PRINT THE LETTER OF THE CORRECT ANSWER IN THE SPACE AT THE RIGHT.*

1. A club goes on a boat ride for which the fare is 80 cents per adult and 60 cents per child. If there are 70 people on the ride, and the total cost is $47, *what* fractional part of the group is adults? 1. ...
   A. 2/35 B. 5/14 E. 4/7 D. 9/14 E. 3/4
2. A camping tent can be put up by 3 scout masters in 2 hours or by 5 boy scouts in 4 hours. *How many* hours will it take them to put up the tent if they all work together? 2. ...
   A. 1 B. 1 1/3 C. 2 1/3 D. 3 E. $3\frac{1}{2}$
3. A grocer has 60 baskets of peaches of which y baskets are spoiled. If he sells 3/4 of the remainder, *how many* baskets does he have left of the good peaches? 3. ...
   A. $\frac{15-y}{4}$ B. 15-y C. $15-\frac{y}{4}$ D. $\frac{y-15}{4}$ E. $\frac{y}{4} - 15$
4. A motorist drives 60 miles to his destination at 40 m.p.h. and returns at 30 m.p.h. Find his average speed in m.p.h. for the entire trip. 4. ...
   A. 28 B. 32 C. 34 2/7 D. $36\frac{1}{2}$ E. $43\frac{1}{4}$
5. The afternoon classes in a school begin at 1 p.m. and end at 3:52 p.m. There are 4 class-periods with 4 minutes between classes. *How many* minutes are there in each period? 5. ...
   A. 39 B. 40 C. 49 D. 59 E. 60
6. If a man paid $60 for a suit after receiving a discount of 10%, *how much* did he save? 6. ...
   A. $6 B. $6.50 C. $6.67 D. $6.75 E. $10
7. A high school football squad consists of 40 players. They arrange to play a 60-minute practice game with another team. If only 11 out of the 40 players participate at one time, and each is to play the same length of time, *how many* minutes would each play? 7. ...
   A. 12 B. $16\frac{1}{2}$ C. 18 D. 20 3/4 E. 22
8. If the base of a rectangle is increased by 30%, and the altitude decreased by 20%, by *what* percent is the area increased? 8. ...
   A. 4 B. 5 C. 10 D. 25 E. 50
9. If a flexible wire 220-feet long goes around a circle 5 times, approximately how many times will the same wire go around the square in which the circle is inscribed? (Use $\pi = 22/7$) 9. ...
   A. 2 3/4 B. $3\frac{1}{2}$ C. 4 D. $5\frac{1}{2}$ E. $6\frac{1}{4}$

10. A passenger ship traveling b miles an hour passes a freighter traveling c miles per hour. Fifteen minutes later the passenger ship reaches port.
How many hours after this will the freighter reach port? 10. ...
A. $\frac{4(b-c)}{c}$ B. $\frac{4(b-c)}{b}$ C. $\frac{b-c}{4c}$ D. $\frac{b-c}{4b}$ E. $\frac{c}{4(b-c)}$

11. If a-b = 5 and a+c = 6, *what* is the value of b in terms of c? 11. ...
A. c-1 B. c+1 C. 1-c D. c-11 E. 11 c

12. Twenty-five boys in a class have an average grade of 80. Fifteen girls in the same class have an average grade of 72. 12. ...
What is the average grade for the entire class?
A. 75 B. 76 C. 76.5 D. 77 E. 77.5

13. A line divides a square board into 2 equal triangles, each 200 square feet in area. 13. ...
How many feet are there in the length of the line?
A. $10\sqrt{2}$ B. $10\sqrt{3}$ C. $20\sqrt{2}$ D. $20\sqrt{3}$ E. 100

14. A 20-ounce solution of salt and water contains 3 ounces of salt. 14. ...
If 5 ounces of water are evaporated, *what* is the percent of salt in the new solution?
A. 12 B. 15 C. 20 D. 25 E. 33 1/3

15. If meat loses 20% of its weight when cooked, *how many* pounds of raw meat should be cooked to produce 2 lbs. of cooked meat? 15. ...
A. 2.25 B. 2.3 C. 2.5 D. 2.75 E. 3

16. *What* percent of 2 gallons is 6 pints? 16. ...
A. 30 B. 33 1/3 C. 37½ D. 137½ E. 300

17. *How many* inches are there in y yards? 17. ...
A. $\frac{y}{36}$ B. $\frac{y}{12}$ C. 3y D. 12y E. 36y

18. The missing number in the series: 2, 6, 12, 20, ?, 42, 56, 72, is: 18. ...
A. 30 B. 32 C. 36 D. 38 E. 40

19. If a car travels at 50 miles per hour, *how long* does it take at this rate to travel 1 mile? 19. ...
A. 50 seconds B. 70 seconds C. 72 seconds
D. 1 min. 15 sec. E. 1 min. 20 sec.

20. If m-x = m, *what* does x equal? 20. ...
A. o B. m C. $\frac{m}{2}$ D. 2m E. $\frac{2}{o}$

KEY (CORRECT ANSWERS)

1. B	6. C	11. C	16. C
2. B	7. B	12. D	17. E
3. C	8. A	13. C	18. A
4. C	9. C	14. C	19. C
5. B	10. C	15. C	20. A

SOLUTIONS TO PROBLEMS

1. Let x = number of adults, 30 - x = number of children. .80x = .60(30 - x) = $47. Solving, x = 25 adults, so there are 45 children. Now, 25/70 = $\frac{5}{14}$.

2. The rate for the scout masters is $\frac{1}{2}$ of the work in 1 hour. For the scouts, their rate is $\frac{1}{4}$ of the work in 1 hour. Let x = number of hours required working together. $\frac{1}{2}x + \frac{1}{4}x = 1$. Solving, x = 1 1/3

3. The grocer will sell $(\frac{3}{4})(60 - y) = 45 - \frac{3}{4}y$, where y = number of baskets with spoiled peaches. The number of baskets of good peaches left is $60 - y - (45 - \frac{3}{4}y) = 15 - \frac{y}{4}$.

4. Average speed = total distance ÷ total time = $(60 + 60)/(\frac{60}{40} + \frac{60}{30}) = 120/3\frac{1}{2} = 34\frac{2}{7}$

5. With 4 class-periods, there are three 4-minute breaks between classes, which is 12 minutes. From 1 PM to 3:52 PM represents 172 minutes. The actual number of minutes for each class period is (172 - 12)/4 = 40.

6. Let x = original price. Then, x - .10x = $60, so x = $66.67. The savings is $66.67 - $60 = $6.67.

7. Total player-minutes = (11)(60) = 660. Then, the number of minutes per player = 660 ÷ 40 = $16\frac{1}{2}$.

8. Let x, y represent the original base and height, so that 1.30x and .80y represent the new base and height. The original area = xy and the new area = (1.30)(.80)xy = 1.04xy. This is a 4% increase.

9. 220 ÷ 5 = 44 feet = circumference of circle. Then, the radius = 44 ÷ 2π = 7 feet. This implies that the side of the circumscribed square is 14 feet and its perimeter is 56 feet. Finally, 220 ÷ 56 $\approx$ 4.

10. In 15 minutes (= $\frac{1}{4}$ hour), the passenger ship travels $\frac{b}{4}$ miles to reach port. The freighter would need $\frac{b}{4} \div c = \frac{b}{4c}$ hours to travel $\frac{6}{4}$ miles. Thus, the extra time the freighter needs to reach port is $\frac{b}{4c} - \frac{1}{4} = \frac{b-c}{4c}$.

11. Subtracting $a - b = 5$ from $a + c = 6$ yields $c + b = 1$. Thus, $b = 1 - c$.

12. Average grade of entire class = $[(25)(80) + (15)(72)]/(25 + 15) = 3080/40 = 77$.

13. The area of the entire square is 400, and the line in question is a diagonal. Let x = length of this diagonal. Then, $\frac{1}{2}x^2 = 400$, so $x = \sqrt{800} = 20\sqrt{2}$.

14. The original solution had 17 ounces of water. The new solution will have 12 ounces of water and (still) 3 ounces of salt. The percent of salt is $(3/(3+12)(100) = 20$.

15. Let x = number of pounds of raw meat. Then, $x - .20x = 2$. Solving, $x = 2.5$.

16. 2 gallons = (2)(8) = 16 pints. Then, $\frac{6}{16} = 37\frac{1}{2}\%$.

17. Since 1 yard = 36 inches, y yards = $36y$ inches.

18. The differences between consecutive terms are 4, 6, 8, –, –, 14, 16. Then the difference between the 4th and 5th terms must be 10. Since the 4th term is 20, the 5th term must be 30. (Note: As a check, the difference between 30 and the 6th term should be 12. The 6th term is 42.)

19. At 50 mi/hour, the car requires $\frac{1}{50}$ hour to travel 1 mile. Now, $\frac{1}{50}$ hour = $1\frac{1}{5}$ minute = 72 seconds.

20. $m - x = m$. Then, $x = m - m = 0$

TEST 4

DIRECTIONS:
Each question or incomplete statement is followed by several suggested answers or completions. Select the one that *BEST* answers the question or completes the statement. *PRINT THE LETTER OF THE CORRECT ANSWER IN THE SPACE AT THE RIGHT.*

1. A part-time worker earns 3 times as much in September as in each of the other months. *What* part of his entire year's earnings does he earn in September? 1. ...
   A. 1/5 B. 3/14 C. 1/4 D. 3/11 E. 1/3
2. All the faces of a 4-inch cube have been painted. This is now cut into 1-inch cubes. The *number* of cubes that will show *no* paint at all is 2. ...
   A. 20 B. 8 C. 1 D. 4 E. 12
3. A 12-quart solution of alcohol and water is 10% alcohol. If 4 quarts of water are added, the solution becomes 3. ...
   A. 50% B. 40% C. 33-1/3% D. 7.5% E. 75%
4. It cost $3.60 for 2 adults and their child to attend the circus. If a child's ticket is half the price of an adult's ticket, *what* is the price of an adult's ticket? 4. ...
   A. $0.72 B. $0.90 C. $1.20 D. $1.44 E. $1.80
5. If the sides of a square are increased 100%, the increase in area is 5. ...
   A. 400% B. 200% C. 300% D. 100% E. 500%
6. A 100-yard dash run in 10 seconds is the *same* average speed in miles per hour approximately as 6. ...
   A. 5 B. 10 C. 20 D. 30 E. 40
7. A man bought 3 books for $1.50 and 2 books for $1.00 each. *What* was the average price per book? 7. ...
   A. $1.00 B. $1.10 C. $1.20 D. $1.25 E. $1.30
8. The missing number in the series: 2, 5, 10,17, ?, 37, 50, 65 is: 8. ...
   A. 22 B. 24 C. 26 D. 27 E. 29
9. If $y\sqrt{.04} = 1$, what is the value of y? 9. ...
   A. .05 B. .5 C. 5 D. 6.25 E. 50
10. The minimum temperatures for each day of one week were as follows: 7, 13, 5, -4, -8, 0, 3. *What* was the *average minimum* temperature for the week? 10. ...
    A. -2 2/3 B. -2 2/7 C. -2 D. 2 2/7 E. 2 2/3
11. A man sold a piece of land for $1500. If his profit was 200% of his cost, *how much* had the land cost him? 11. ...
    A. $500 B. $750 C. $1000 D. $1200 E. $1250
12. *What* is the area in square feet of a rectangular garden which is twice as long as it is wide if the fence around it is 240 feet long? 12. ...
    A. 2400 B. 3200 C. 4800 D. 7200 E. 12,800
13. *Which* of these quantities is the smallest? 13. ...
    A. 7/9 B. 9/11 C. 4/5 D. 5/7 E. .74
14. A baseball team has won 50 games out of 75 played. How many more games must the team win in succession to raise its record to 80%? 14. ...
    A. 10 B. 20 C. 22 D. 25 E. 50

15. A tank contains 500 gallons of gasoline. If the gasoline is withdrawn at the rate of x quarts a minute for 12 minutes, *how many* gallons of gasoline will remain? 15. ...
    A. 500-12x B. 500-6x C. 500-3x
    D. 12x E. 125x

KEY (CORRECT ANSWERS)

1. B
2. B
3. D
4. D
5. C

6. C
7. E
8. C
9. C
10. D

11. A
12. B
13. D
14. E
15. C

SOLUTIONS TO PROBLEMS

1. Let 3x = earnings in September, x = earnings in each of the other 11 months. Then, 11x + 3x = 14x = earnings for 1 year. Ratio of September's earnings to entire year's earnings = $3x/14x = \frac{3}{14}$.

2. There will be a total of 64 1-inch cubes of which the innermost 8 cubes will have no paint.

3. The amount of alcohol is still (.10)(12) = 1.2 quarts. Then, 1.2/16 = 7.5%.

4. Let x = price for each adult ticket, $\frac{1}{2}x$ = price for each child's ticket. $x + x + \frac{1}{2}x = \$3.60$. $2.5x = \$3.60$. Solving, x = \$1.44.

5. Let x = original side and 2x = new side. Original area = x^2 and new area = $4x^2$. The increase is $3x^2$, which means 300%.

6. 100 yards in 10 seconds means 36,000 yards per hour. Then, 36,000 yards = 36,000/1760 ≈ 20 miles. Thus, the speed is 20 mi/hour.

7. The average price per book = [(3)(\$1.50) + (2)(\$1.00)]/(3 + 2) = \$1.30.

8. The differences between consecutive terms are 3, 5, 7, _, _, 13, 15. The two blanks must be 9 and 11. Since the difference between the 4th and 5th terms is 9 and the 4th term is 17, the 5th term is 17 + 9 = 26.

9. $y\sqrt{.04} = 1$. Then, .2y = 1, so y = 5.

10. $(7 + 13 + 5 - 4 - 8 + 0 + 3)/7 = 16/7 = 2\frac{2}{7}$

11. Let x = cost. Profit = \$1500 - x = 2x. Solving, x = \$500

12. Let x = width, 2x = length. x + x + 2x + 2x = 240. Solving, x = 40 and 2x = 80. Area = (40)(80) = 3200 square feet.

13. Converting to decimals, answers A thru E appear as $.\overline{7}$, $.\overline{81}$, .8, .714, .74. Since .714 is the smallest, this corresponds to 5/7.

14. Let x = required number of wins. Then, (50 + x)/(75 + x) = .80. This leads to 50 + x = 60 + .80x. Solving, x = 50.

15. x quarts per minute means x gallons in 4 minutes. After 12 minutes, 3x gallons have been withdrawn from the tank. The number of gallons remaining is 500 - 3x.

TEST 5

DIRECTIONS:

Each question or incomplete statement is followed by several suggested answers or completions. Select the one that *BEST* answers the question or completes the statement. *PRINT THE LETTER OF THE CORRECT ANSWER IN THE SPACE AT THE RIGHT.*

1. A pool which holds 300 gallons of water can be filled by one pipe in 6 hours and emptied by another in 8 hours. *How many* hours will it take to fill it if *both* pipes are opened together? 1. ...
   A. 4 B. 7 C. 12 D. 14 E. 24
2. The floor of a kitchen 9 feet wide by 12 feet long is to be covered with linoleum which comes in a roll 27 inches wide. The *number* of yards of linoleum needed is: 2. ...
   A. 16 B. 24 C. 36 D. 48 E. 54
3. Four posts are set 15 feet apart along the edge of a field. How many feet is the first post from the last? 3. ...
   A. 30 B. 35 C. 45 D. 55 E. 60
4. During the second year of work a girl earned 5/4 as much as she did her first year. If she earned $3600 in the two years, *how much* did she earn the first year? 4. ...
   A. $1440 B. $1600 C. $1800 D. $2000 E. $2880
5. What fraction of 5 gallons is 3 quarts? 5. ...
   A. 3/20 B. 1/4 C. 4/15 D. 5/12 E. 3/5
6. A man gets 20 miles per gallon with grade X gasoline, which costs $1.00 per gallon; he gets 25 miles per gallon with grade Y, which costs $1.20 per gallon. *How much* does he save on a 1000-mile trip by using grade Y instead of grade X? 6. ...
   A. $1.25 B. $1.50 C. $1.75 D. $2.00 E. $2.25
7. How many twelfths are there in 83 1/3% of a pound? 7. ...
   A. 5 B. 10 C. 12 D. 14 E. 16
8. If there is 2.2 pounds in one kilogram and one kilogram equals 1000 grams, *how many* more grams are there in 8½ pounds than in 3 kilograms? 8. ...
   A. 824 B. 864 C. 1648 D. 1728 E. 4502
9. If, after receiving a discount of 12%, you pay $175 for a television set, the *original* price was: 9. ...
   A. $187.50 B. $192.50 C. $198.86 D. $200 E. $225
10. The 90 members of a certain organization contributed an average of 60 cents each toward a fund. If 2 of the members contributed $5.00 each, *how many* cents was the average contribution of the other 88 members? 10. ...
    A. 50 B. 56 C. 60 D. 61 E. 70
11. A person spent exactly one dollar in the purchase of 3-cent and 5-cent stamps. The number of 5-cent stamps he could *NOT* have bought is 11. ...
    A. 7 B. 14 C. 11 D. 8 E. 5
12. In the series 3, 7, 12, 18, 25, ..., the 10th term is 12. ...
    A. 88 B. 75 C. 63 D. 50 E. 86
13. 3/5 5/8 2/3 7/12. The fraction which is out of order is: 13. ...
    A. 3/5 B/ 5/8 C. 2/3 D. 7/12 E. None of these

14. At 3:20 p.m., *how many* degrees has the hour hand moved since noon? 14. ...

A. 200 B. 20 C. 10 D. 100 E. 120

15. (3/8) (1/8) = (?) (1/16) 15. ...

A. 1/8 B. 3/16 C. 3/8 D. 4/3 E. 3/4

KEY (CORRECT ANSWERS)

1. E
2. A
3. C
4. B
5. A

6. D
7. B
8. B
9. C
10. A

11. A
12. B
13. D
14. D
15. E

SOLUTIONS TO PROBLEMS

1. Let x = number of hours needed to fill the pool. $x/6 - x/8 = 1$. Then, $4x - 3x = 24$, so $x = 24$.

2. 9 feet ÷ 27 inches = 108 inches ÷ 27 inches = 4. Thus, 4 rolls of linoleum will be needed, each of which must extend to 12 feet = 4 yards. Total number of yards needed = (4)(4) = 16.

3. The distance from first post to last post is (15)(3) = 45 feet.

4. Let x and $\frac{5}{4}x$ represent her earnings in each of the first 2 years. Then, $x + \frac{5}{4}x = \$3600$. Solving, x = $1600

5. 3 quarts/5 gallons = 3 quarts/20 quarts = $\frac{3}{20}$

6. Using grade X, a trip of 1000 miles costs $(\frac{1000}{20})(\$1.00) = \$50$.
   Using grade Y, this same trip costs $(\frac{1000}{25})(\$1.20) = \$48$.
   The savings is $2.00.

7. $83\frac{1}{3}\%$ of a pound $= (\frac{5}{6})(16) = 13\frac{1}{3}$ ounces. $\frac{1}{12}$ of a pound $= 1\frac{1}{3}$ ounce
   Now, $13\frac{1}{3} \div 1\frac{1}{3} = 10$.

8. 8.5 lbs. = 8.5 ÷ 2.2 = $3.8\overline{63}$ kgms = $3863.\overline{63}$ gms, whereas 3 kgms = 3000 gms. The difference is about 864 gms.

9. Let x = original price. Then, $x - .12x = \$175$. Solving, x = $198.86

10. (90)(.60) = $54.00. $54.00 − (2)($5) = $44. Finally, $44 ÷ 88 = $0.50

11. He could NOT have bought 7 5-cent stamps since $1.00 − (7)(.05) = .65 and .65 is not divisible by 3 cents.

12. The difference between successive terms increases by 1, with the difference between the first two terms being 4. Since the fifth term is 25, the 10th term will be 25 + 8 + 9 + 10 + 11 + 12 = 75.

13. Since the first 3 fractions are in increasing order, $\frac{7}{12}$ is out of order because $\frac{7}{12} < \frac{2}{3}$.

14. The hour hand has moved $3\frac{1}{3}$ numbers = $(3\frac{1}{3}/12)(360°) = 100°$

15. $(\frac{3}{8})(\frac{1}{8}) = \frac{3}{64}$. Then, $\frac{3}{64} \div \frac{1}{16} = \frac{3}{4}$

TEST 6

DIRECTIONS:

Each question or incomplete statement is followed by several suggested answers or completions. Select the one that *BEST* answers the question or completes the statement. *PRINT THE LETTER OF THE CORRECT ANSWER IN THE SPACE AT THE RIGHT.*

1. One end of a ladder 26 feet long is placed 10 feet from the outer wall of a building. *How many* feet up the building will the ladder reach? 1. ...
   A. 14 B. 20 C. 22 D. 23 E. 24
2. A quart of ice cream will serve 6 adults or 8 children. If 39 adults have been served from a 10-quart container, *how many* children may then be served? 2. ...
   A. 28 B. 50 C. 29 D. 41 E. 43
3. Fifty students had an average of 80%. Thirty other students had an average of 86%. Find the average of *all* the students. 3. ...
   A. 81 B. $81\frac{1}{2}$ C. 82 D. $82\frac{1}{4}$ E. 83
4. A dealer paid 72¢ for a fountain pen listed at 90¢. *What* rate of discount did he receive? 4. ...
   A. 2% B. 5% C. 18% D. 20% E. 25%
5. A man makes a trip of 600 miles. He averages 40 m.p.h. for the first 200 miles. At *what* rate, in m.p.h., must he complete the trip to average 45 m.p.h. for the entire trip? 5. ...
   A. $47\frac{1}{2}$ B. 50 C. 47 D. $48\frac{1}{2}$ E. 48
6. The water which is 7" high in a fish tank $1\frac{1}{4}$ ft. by 8", is poured into a tank 13" x 20". *What* height will it reach in the larger tank? 6. ...
   A. .27" B. .31" C. 1.7" D. 3.2" E. 4.6"
7. .3% = ? 7. ...
   A. 3/1000 B. 3/100 C. 1/300 D. 3/10 E. 1/3
8. In one section of a test the first question is numbered 112 and the last 200. How many questions are there in this section of the test? 8. ...
   A. 88 B. 89 C. 87 D. 86 E. None of these
9. A block of wood 8" x 4" x 12" is to be cut into cubes. If the cubes are the largest that can be cut from this block, *how many* of them will there be? 9. ...
   A. 2 B. 4 C. 6 D. 8 E. 12
10. A 5-quart solution of sulphuric acid and water is 60% acid. If a gallon of water is added, *what* percent of the resulting solution is acid? 10. ...
    A. 20 B. 33 1/3 C. 40 D. 48 E. 50
11. A baseball team has won 50 games out of 75 played. It has 45 games still to play. *how many* of these must the team win to make its record for the season 60%. 11. ...
    A. 20 B. 22 C. 25 D. 30 E. None of these
12. If in any two-digit numbers, the tens-digit is represented by x and the units-digit by y, the number is represented by 12. ...
    A. x+y B. xy C. 10x + y D. 10y + x E. yx

13. *How many* pieces of cardboard 3" x 5" can be cut from a sheet 17" x 22" with the *minimum* amount of waste? 13. ...
A. 20 B. 21 C. 24 D. 25 E. None of these

14. If p pencils cost c cents, n pencils at the same rate will cost 14. ...
A. $\frac{pc}{n}$ cents B. $\frac{cn}{p}$ cents C. npc cents
D. $\frac{np}{c}$ cents E. $\frac{p}{nc}$ cents

15. If the population of a village was 300 before the war and is now 1200, *what* is the percentage of increase in population? 15. ...
A. 25% B. 75% C. 300% D. 400% E. 3%

KEY (CORRECT ANSWERS)

1. E
2. A
3. D
4. D
5. E

6. D
7. A
8. B
9. C
10. B

11. B
12. C
13. B
14. B
15. C

SOLUTIONS TO PROBLEMS

1. Let x = number of feet up the wall. Then, $x^2 + 10^2 = 26^2$. Solving, x = 24.

2. 10 quarts will serve 60 adults. Since 39 adults have been served, 21 more adults could be still served. Realizing that for every 6 adults, 8 children could be served, the equivalent of 21 adults is $21 \div \frac{6}{8} = 28$ children.

3. Average of all students = $[(50)(80) + (30)(86)]/(50 + 30) = 82\frac{1}{4}$

4. Discount = .90 − .72 = .18. Rate of discount = $\frac{.18}{.90} = 20\%$

5. Let x = rate for the remaining 400 miles. The time for this portion of the trip is 400/x hours. Then, 45 = average rate $= 600/[\frac{200}{40} + \frac{400}{x}]$. Simplifying, $5 + \frac{400}{x} = 13\frac{1}{3}$. Solving, x = 48

6. Volume in 1st tank = (7")(15")(8") = 840 cu.in. Let x = height in 2nd tank. Then, 840 = (13)(20)(x). Solving, x = 3.2

7. .3% = .3/100 = 3/1000

8. Number of questions = 200 − 111 = 89

9. (8)(4)(12) = 384 cubic inches. The largest possible side for each cube is 4 in. Each of these cubes has a volume of $(4)^3$ = 64 cu.in. Now, 384 ÷ 64 = 6

10. Amount of acid is (5)(.60) = 3 quarts. By adding a gallon of water, the new solution will contain 9 quarts. Finally, 3/9 = 33 1/3%.

11. Let x = number of additional games won. Then, (50 + x)/120 = .60 Solving, x = 22.

12. The number is represented as 10x + y. For example, 56 = (10)(5) + 6

13. 22 ÷ 3 = 7, with 1 in. left over and 17 ÷ 5 = 3, with 2 in. left over. Number of pieces = (7)(3) = 21. The waste is only (1)(2) = 2 sq.in.

14. Let x = cost of n pencils. Then, p/c = n/x. px = cn. Solving, x − cn/p

15. The increase in population is 1200 − 300 = 900. Then, 900/300 = 3 = 300%

TEST 7

DIRECTIONS:
Each question or incomplete statement is followed by several suggested answers or completions. Select the one that *BEST* answers the question or completes the statement. *PRINT THE LETTER OF THE CORRECT ANSWER IN THE SPACE AT THE RIGHT.*

1. If a merchant makes a 20% profit based on the selling price of an article, *what* percent profit does he make on the cost? 1. ...
   A. 15% B. 25% C. 75% D. 300% E. 400%
2. The dial of a meter is divided into equal divisions from 0 to 60. When the needle points to 48, the meter registers 80 amperes. *What* is the *MAXIMUM* number of amperes that the meter will register? 2. ...
   A. 60 B. 92 C. 100 D. 102 E. 120
3. The scale of a certain map is 3/4 inch equals 12 miles. Find, in square miles, the actual area of a park represented on the map by a square whose side is 5/8 inch. 3. ...
   A. $7\frac{1}{2}$ B. 10 C. 40 D. 100 E. None of these
4. Two boys buy a radio for $15 contributing amounts in the ratio of 5:4. Find the *smaller* amount. 4. ...
   A. 4 B. 5 C. 12 D. 6 2/3 E. 1 2/3
5. There are 25 equally placed poles in a row. If the distance from the first to the sixth is 30 feet, find the distance from the first to the twenty-fifth. 5. ...
   A. 120 B. 125 C. 144 D. 150 E. $127\frac{1}{2}$
6. A rectangular room 15' x 19' has a 10' x 10' rug in it. *What* percent of the room is covered? 6. ...
   A. 25 B. 35 C. 45 D. 55 E. 65
7. .8% is the same as one out of 7. ...
   A. 20 B. 40 C. 80 D. 100 E. 125
8. A painted wooden cube whose edge is 3 inches is cut into 27 one-inch cubes. *How many* of these have just two painted sides? 8. ...
   A. 12 B. 18 C. 8 D. 9 E. None of these
9. Four tractors working together can plow a field in 12 hours. *How many* hours will it take 6 tractors to plow the field? 9. ...
   A. 6 B. 9 C. 10 D. 18 E. None of these
10. A company offers a gas range for $63 cash or for $5 down and 10 months payments of $6.50 each. The installment price is, approximately, *what* percent *greater* than the cash price? 10. ...
    A. 7% B. 9% C. 10% D. 11% E. None of these
11. A seesaw 12 feet long is balanced at the middle by a support 3 feet high. If one end of the seesaw is on the ground, *how many* feet above the ground is the other end? 11. ...
    A. 3 B. 6 C. 9 D. 15 E. 18
12. A baseball team won W games and lost L games. *What* fractional part of its games did it win? 12. ...
    A. $\frac{L}{W}$ B. $\frac{W}{L}$ C. $\frac{W-L}{W}$ D. $\frac{W+L}{W}$ E. $\frac{W}{W+L}$

13. A train left A for B, a distance of 290 miles, at 10:10 a.m. The train was scheduled to reach B at 3:45 p.m. If the average rate of the train was 50 m.p.h., it arrived in B 13. ...
   A. 5 minutes *early*
   B. *on time*
   C. 5 minutes *late*
   D. 13 minutes *late*
   E. more than 15 minutes *late*

14. *How many* dollars would it cost to carpet a room r yards long and w feet wide at x cents a square foot? 14. ...
   A. wrx
   B. .03wrx
   C. $\frac{100\ wrx}{3}$
   D. $\frac{100\ wr}{3x}$
   E. $\frac{3wr}{100x}$

15. Find the number of degrees between the hands of a clock at 7:20. 15. ...
   A. 90
   B. 100
   C. 97½
   D. 108
   E. 33 1/3

KEY (CORRECT ANSWERS)

1. B
2. C
3. D
4. D
5. C

6. B
7. E
8. A
9. E
10. D

11. B
12. E
13. D
14. B
15. B

SOLUTIONS TO PROBLEMS

1. Let x = selling price so that .20x = profit. Then, x - .20x = .80x = cost. Percent profit on cost is (.20x/.80x)(100) = 25%

2. Let x = maximum number of amperes. 48/80 = 60/x. Solving, x = 100

3. Let the actual length (or width) of the park = x. Then, $\frac{3}{4}/\frac{5}{8}$ = 12/x. Solving, x = 10. The actual area of the park is 10^2 = 100 square miles.

4. Let 5x and 4x represent the respective amounts. Then, 5x + 4x = 15, so x = $1\frac{2}{3}$. The smaller amount = $(4)(1\frac{2}{3})$ = $6\frac{2}{3}$ dollars.

5. From the 1st pole to the 25th pole represents 24 spaces, so the number of spaces from the 1st pole to the 6th pole is 5. 30 ft. ÷ 5 = 6 ft. = distance between successive poles. Thus, the distance from the 1st pole to the 25th pole is (6)(24) = 144 ft.

6. $10 \times 10 = 100$ and $15 \times 19 = 285$. Then, $\frac{100}{285} \approx .351 \approx 35\%$

7. $.8\% = .008 = \frac{8}{1000} = \frac{1}{125}$ = 1 out of 125

8. The 12 cubes occupying center positions would have only 2 painted sides.

9. The number of tractors is inversely proportional to the number of hours. Let x = required time. 4/6 = x/12, so x = 8 hours.

10. Paying on the installment plan, the cost is 5 + (10)(6.50) = \$70. This represents (70 - 63)/63 × 100 = 11% more than the cash price.

11. 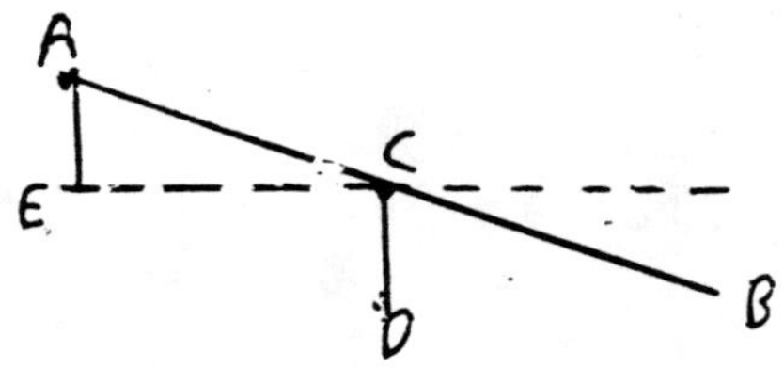

Let CD = 3' support. AC = CB = 6' Now, AE = 3', so point A must be 6' above the ground.

12. Games played = W + L. Fractional part of games won = $\frac{W}{W+L}$

13. Time of travel was $\frac{290}{50}$ = 5.8 hours = 5 hours 48 minutes. Since the train left point A at 10:10 AM, it arrived at point B at 3:58 PM. Thus, it was 13 minutes late.

14. x cents per square foot means 9x cents per square yard = 9x/100 dollars per square yard. The area of the room = (r yards) × ($\frac{w}{3}$ yards) = rw/3 square yards. Total cost to carpet the room = (9x/100)(rw/3) = $\frac{3}{100}$ xrw = .03 wrx dollars.

15. At 7:20, the minute hand is exactly on the numeral 4 and the hour hand lies $\frac{1}{3}$ of the way between the numerals 7 and 8. The distance of $7\frac{1}{3} - 4 = 3\frac{1}{3}$ numerals on the clock is equivalent to $(3\frac{1}{3}/12)(360°) = 100°$.

TEST 8

DIRECTIONS:

Each question or incomplete statement is followed by several suggested answers or completions. Select the one that *BEST* answers the question or completes the statement. *PRINT THE LETTER OF THE CORRECT ANSWER IN THE SPACE AT THE RIGHT.*

1. If both the filling and emptying pipes of a pool are open, the pool fills in 10 hours. If just the filling pipes are open, the pool fills in 4 hours. *How many* hours does it take to empty the pool if only the emptying pipes are open? 1. ...
   A. Less than 5 B. More than 5 C. Exactly 5
   D. More than 6 E. Exactly 6
2. A cylindrical pail 14 inches in diameter and 7 inches high is full of water. The water is poured into a rectangular aquarium 22" long, 21" wide, and 14" high. To *what* depth in inches does the water rise in the aquarium? 2. ...
   A. 2 1/3 B. 9 1/3 C. 5 2/3
   D. $7\frac{1}{4}$ E. None of these
3. A poster is cut down by 10% of its height and 30% of its width. *What* percent of the original area remains? 3. ...
   A. 3 B. 37 C. 70 D. 57 E. 63
4. 4. ...

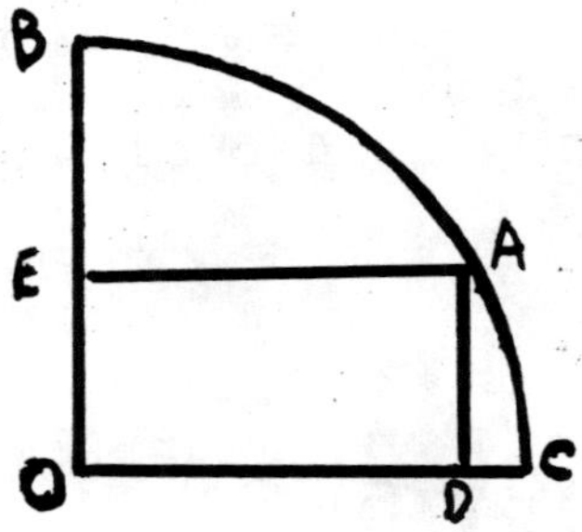

BOC is a quadrant of a circle.
AD = 3 and AE = 4.
Find the length of arc BC.

   A. 5π B. $\frac{5\pi}{2}$ C. 10π D. 12
   E. Cannot be determined from the information given
5. A commuter runs from his house to the station, a distance of 132 feet. It takes him 9 seconds. *What* is his speed in miles per hour? 5. ...
   A. 12 B. 9 C. 8 D. 11 E. 10
6. A swimming pool is 4 yards deep, 6 yards wide, and 8 yards long. If it is filled to one foot from the top, *what* is the volume of water in cubic feet? 6. ...
   A. $24 \cdot 18 \cdot 11$ B. $24 \cdot 18 . 12 - 1$ C. $24 \cdot 18 \cdot 12$
   D. $24 \cdot 18 \cdot 12 - 3$ E. None of these
7. A typist uses lengthwise a sheet of paper 9" x 12". She leaves a 1" margin on each side and a $1\frac{1}{2}$" margin on top and bottom. *What* fractional part of the page is used for typing? 7. ...
   A. $\frac{63}{66}$ B. $\frac{7}{12}$ C. $\frac{5}{9}$ D. 3/4 E. None of these

8. Eight blocks on one side of a scale balance two blocks and a one-pound weight on the other side. *What* is the weight in pounds of *all* ten blocks? 8. ...
   A. 1 B. $1\frac{1}{2}$ C. 1 2/3 D. 2 E. None of these
9. How many numbers between 131 and 259 are divisible by 3? 9. ...
   A. 41 B. 42 C. 43 D. 44 E. None of these
10. The consecutive angles of a quadrilateral are 60, 120, 60, and 120 degrees. If one side is 6 and another is 12, *what* is the perimeter? 10. ...
    A. 18 B. 36 C. $24 + 6\sqrt{3}$
    D. $12 + 6\sqrt{3}$ E. Cannot be determined from the information given
11. Admission tickets for children are 1/3 the price for adults. The price for 3 children and 3 adults is $10.80. *How much* is the price for one adult? 11. ...
    A. $.90 B. $1.20 C. $1.80 D. $2.70 E. $3.00
12. A man walks 100 feet north, 150 feet west, and 100 feet north again. *How many* feet is the distance from where he started to where he finished in a straight line? 12. ...
    A. 350 B. 300 C. 250 D. 200 E. None of these
13. A ferris wheel has a diameter of 60 feet. It makes 3 revolutions per minute. Find the distance in miles that the occupant of one of the cars travels in 5 minutes. ($\pi = \frac{22}{7}$) 13. ...
    A. $\frac{30}{28}$ B. $\frac{15}{28}$ C. $\frac{4}{7}$ D. $\frac{3}{5}$ E. $2\frac{1}{4}$
14. A box contains 2 red balls, 3 blue balls, and 4 white. *What* is the *LEAST* number of balls a blindfolded person must draw to be sure of getting two of the same kind? 14. ...
    A. 2 B. 3 C. 4 D. 5 E. 6
15. If an apple weighs 4/5 of its weight plus 4/5 of an ounce, *what* is its weight in ounces? 15. ...
    A. $3\frac{1}{2}$ B. 1 3/5 C. 4 D. 4 4/5 E. 5

KEY (CORRECT ANSWERS)

1. D
2. A
3. E
4. B
5. E

6. A
7. B
8. C
9. C
10. B

11. D
12. C
13. B
14. C
15. C

SOLUTIONS TO PROBLEMS

1. Let x = time required to empty the pool using only the emptying pipes. Then, $\frac{10}{4} - \frac{10}{x} = 1$. Simplifying, $10x - 40 = 4x$. Solving, $x = 6\frac{2}{3}$ hours, which corresponds to *more than 6*.

2. Volume of pail = $(\pi)(7^2)(7) \approx 1078$ cu.in. Let x = height to which water will rise in aquarium. Then, $1078 = (22)(21)(x)$, so, $x = 2\frac{1}{3}$ in.

3. Let x = original height, y = original width, xy = original area. New height = .9x, new width = .7y, new area = .63xy, which is 63% of the original area.

4. Radius of circle = OA = $\sqrt{3^2 + 4^2} = 5$. Length of arc BC = $(\frac{1}{4})(2\pi)(5) = 5\pi/2$

5. 132 ft. in 9 sec. means $14\frac{2}{3}$ ft. per sec. Since 88 ft. per sec. is equivalent to 60 mph, the commuter's speed in mph = $(60)(14\frac{2}{3}/88) = 10$

6. 6 yds. = 18 ft., 8 yds. = 24 ft., 4 yds. - 1 ft. = 11 ft. The volume, in cubic feet, is $24 \cdot 18 \cdot 11$.

7. The typing section has an area of $(9 - 2)(12 - 3) = 63$ sq.in. The entire sheet of paper has an area of $(9)(12) = 108$ sq.in. Finally, $63/108 = \frac{7}{12}$

8. Let x = weight of each block. Then, $8x = 2x + 1$, so $x = \frac{1}{6}$ lbs. The weight of all ten blocks = $(10)(\frac{1}{6}) = 1\frac{2}{3}$ lbs.

9. The numbers divisible by 3 begin with 132 and end with 258. The total number of these numbers = $(258 - 132)/3 + 1 = 43$

10. Since opposite angles are equal, the given figure must be a parallelogram, wherein opposite sides are also equal. The perimeter = $(2)(6) + (2)(12) = 36$.

11. Let x = admission price per adult, $\frac{1}{3}x$ = admission price per child. $(3)(\frac{1}{3}x) + 3x = 10.80$. Solving, x = \$2.70

12. 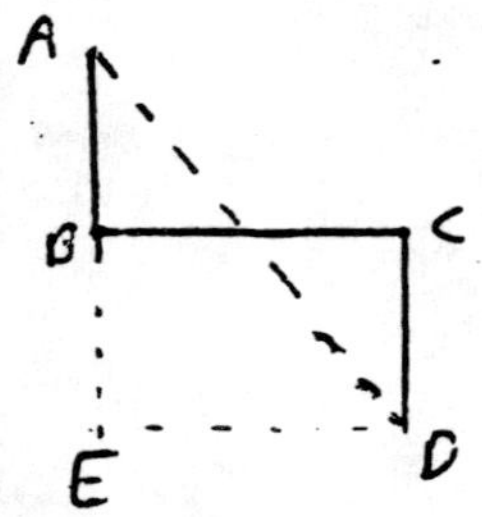

We are seeking the value of DA.
Now, ED = BC = 150 and AE = AB + CD = 200.
Since AED forms a right triangle,
$DA = \sqrt{150^2 + 200^2} = 250$

13. In 1 min., each car of the ferris wheel travels $(\frac{22}{7})(60)(3) =$ 3960/7 ft. In 5 min., this distance = 19,800/7 ft. Since 5280 ft. = 1 mi., the distance traveled in 5 min. becomes $(19{,}800/7) \div 5280 = \frac{15}{28}$ mi.

14. By drawing only 3 balls, the person might get exactly one of each color. However, by drawing 4 balls, at least 2 of them will be the same color.

15. Let x = weight in ounces. Then, $x = \frac{4}{5}x + \frac{4}{5}$.

Solving, x = 4.

EXAMINATION SECTION

TEST 1

DIRECTIONS: Each question or incomplete statement is followed by several suggested answers or completions. Select the one that BEST answers the question or completes the statement. *PRINT THE LETTER OF THE CORRECT ANSWER IN THE SPACE AT THE RIGHT.*

1. John is $\frac{1}{6}$ of his father's age. In 20 years, he will be $\frac{1}{2}$ of his father's age at that time. How old is the father? 1.____
   A. 24 B. 30 C. 36 D. 42 E. 48

2. $(\frac{.7}{.07})(\frac{49}{100}) = 4 + x \quad x =$ 2.____
   A. 4.9 B. .09 C. .9 D. 3.1 E. 3.95

3. Which is the largest? 3.____
   A. $\frac{23}{25}$ B. $\frac{27}{30}$ C. $\frac{15}{16}$ D. $\frac{14}{15}$ E. $\frac{7}{8}$

4. Clyde received a 10% raise in each of the last two years. His present salary is $21,780. What was his starting salary? 4.____
   A. $18,000 B. $19,000 C. $20,000 D. $21,350 E. $26,354

5. At a convention of dentists, 1,000 dentists are from the east coast. One hundred dentists are women; 60 of the women are not from the east coast. How many male dentists are from the east coast? 5.____
   A. 900 B. 850 C. 800 D. 960 E. 940

6. $\frac{1}{3}$ of $\frac{1}{4}$ is what percent of $\frac{5}{12}$? 6.____
   A. .2 B. 5 C. 12 D. 20 E. 500

7. Which line is parallel to the y axis? 7.____
   A. $x = 4y$
   B. $x = \frac{2}{y}$
   C. $x = y + 6$
   D. $xy = 2$
   E. $xy = 2 + 4y^{-1}$

8. The five tires that come with Mary's new car were rotated frequently so that each tire was used for exactly the same amount of time as the others. They were replaced when the odometer read 24,000 miles. How many miles had each been driven? 8.____
   A. 18,000 miles
   B. 30,000 miles
   C. 20,000 miles
   D. 24,000 miles
   E. 19,200 miles

9. $$\begin{array}{r} -(\,7646\,) \\ x \\ \hline 4--- \end{array}$$ What is the smallest number x could be? 9.___

A. 2647 B. 4000 C. 3000 D. 646 E. 3646

10. A bug sits at the edge of a 12 inch (diameter) phonograph record playing at $33\frac{1}{3}$ r.p.m. 10.___
Approximately how fast (in feet/minute) is the bug moving?
A. 3 B. 33 C. 50 D. 100 E. 396

11. An object floats if it weighs less than an equal volume of water. One cc of water weighs 1 gram. Each of the following objects weighs 2 kilograms. 11.___
Which ones float? (All dimensions in cm.)

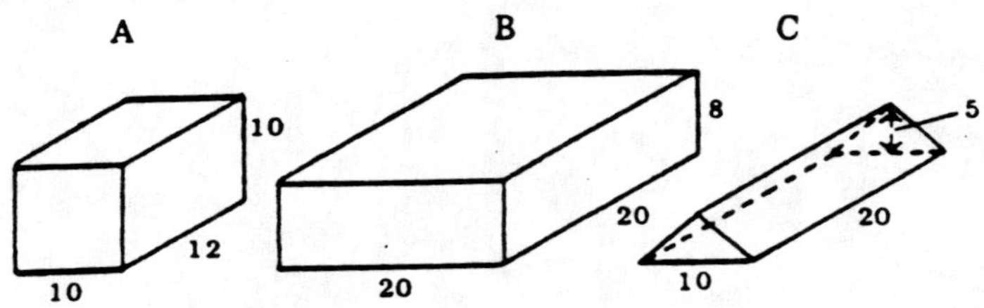

A. A *only* B. B *only* C. C *only* D. B & C E. A & B

12. .04 is 25% of 12.___
A. 0.01 B. 0.16 C. 0.1 D. 1.0 E. 1.6

13. $x^2 + 3x + 2 = 2$, $x < 0$. 13.___
$x =$
A. $\frac{3-\sqrt{8}}{2}$ B. -1 C. -2 D. -3 E. -4

14. If $\frac{3x}{4y} = \frac{1}{8}$, then $\frac{4x}{3y} =$ 14.___
A. $\frac{1}{6}$ B. $\frac{1}{3}$ C. $\frac{2}{3}$ D. 24 E. $\frac{2}{9}$

15. .3% of 25% equals 15.___
A. 7.5 B. .75 C. .075 D. .0075 E. .00075

16. Arrange from least to greatest: 16.___
I. .07 II. $\sqrt{.49}$ III. .075 IV. $(.835)^2$

The CORRECT answer is:
A. I, III, IV, II
B. III, I, IV, II
C. IV, I, II, III
D. I, III, II, IV
E. IV, II, III, I

17. A television set is priced at $490.00. The installment payment contract requires 20% of the price as a down-payment, plus installments of $47.75 per month over a period of 10 months to pay for the set, including interest charges. 17.___

What is the total amount of interest charged?
A. \$83.00 B. \$83.50
C. \$85.50 D. \$85.75
E. \$125.50

18. A florist bought some plants for \$150. He sold enough at 75 cents to meet the cost and had 100 plants left. How many were originally purchased by the florist? 18.___
A. 150 B. 250 C. 300 D. 350 E. 400

19. If 3x + y = 5 and 5x + y = 6, then y = 19.___
A. $\frac{2}{7}$ B. .5 C. 1 D. 2 E. 3.5

20. A purse contains \$3.20 in dimes and quarters. There are 3 less dimes than quarters. How many dimes are there? 20.___
A. 7 B. 10 C. 13 D. 16 E. 20

21. A lawn fertilizer is most effective if 25 pounds is spread over 10,000 square feet. A weed killer must be mixed with the fertilizer but only 3 pounds should be used on every 15,000 square feet. What should the ratio be between the fertilizer and the weed killer when mixed? 21.___
A. 12.5 to 1 B. 3 to 2
C. 8.33 to 1 D. 5.5 to 1
E. 25 to 3

22. If 1 yard = .9 meters, then 1.5 meters = how many yards? 22.___
A. 1.65 B. 1.80 C. 1.60 D. 1.67 E. 1.35

23. ( ) is to 40 as $\frac{x}{5}$ is to ( ). 23.___
A. 4; $\frac{x}{50}$ B. 10; 40x C. 8; x D. 10; 8x E. 5; $\frac{x}{40}$

24. What is the approximate value of $\sqrt{360}$? 24.___
A. 60 B. 18 C. 6 D. 16 E. 19

25. An auto travels at an average of 45 mi/hr for 1 hour and then an average of 60 mi/hr for the next half hour. What is the average speed for the entire time period in miles/hr.? 25.___
A. 47.5 B. 50 C. 52.5 D. 55 E. 62.5

KEY (CORRECT ANSWERS)

1. B	6. D	11. B	16. A	21. A
2. C	7. B	12. B	17. C	22. D
3. C	8. E	13. D	18. C	23. C
4. A	9. A	14. E	19. E	24. E
5. D	10. D	15. E	20. A	25. B

SOLUTIONS TO PROBLEMS

1. Let the father's current age = x and John's current age = $\frac{1}{6}x$.

   In 20 years, their ages will be x + 20 and $\frac{1}{6}x + 20$.

   Then, $\frac{1}{6}x + 20 = \frac{1}{2}(x+20)$, which becomes $\frac{1}{6}x + 20 = \frac{1}{2}x + 10$.

   Solving, x = 30.

2. The left side of this equation becomes (10)(.49) = 4.9
   Now, 4.9 = 4 + x. Solving, x = .9

3. Converting each fraction into a decimal equivalent, we get: .92, .9, .9375, $.9\overline{3}$, and .875, respectively. The largest is .9375 corresponding to $\frac{15}{16}$.

4. Let x = initial salary. With the first 10% raise, his salary is 1.10x. The second 10% raise will bring his salary to (1.10x)(1.10) = 1.21x. Now, 1.21x = \$21,780. Solving, x = \$18,000

5. The number of female dentists from the east coast is 100 - 60 = 40. Thus, the number of male dentists from the east coast must be 1000 - 40 = 960.

6. $\frac{1}{3}$ of $\frac{1}{4}$ means $(\frac{1}{3})(\frac{1}{4}) = \frac{1}{12}$. Then, $\frac{1}{12} \div \frac{5}{12} = \frac{1}{5}$, and $\frac{1}{5} = 20\%$

7. Any line parallel to the y-axis has no slope, and so must be of the form x = c (c is a constant). $x = 2/y^{\circ}$ can be written as x = 2/1 or x = 2.

8. Since only 4 tires are used at the same time, each of the 5 tires will be used $\frac{4}{5}$ or 80% of the elapsed time before replacement. (24,000)(.80) = 19,200.

9. To find the minimum x, we need to find the maximum for the answer (since this is a subtraction). The maximum answer upon subtracting is 4999. Solving, 7646 - x = 4999, we get x = 2647.

10. The circumference = (π)(1 foot) = 3.14 feet (approximately)
    $33\frac{1}{3}$ revolutions = $(33\frac{1}{3})(3.14) = 104\frac{2}{3}$ feet, which is the rate per minute.

11. 2 kilograms = 2000 grams. The only object(s) which float must correspond to more than 2000 cc. Object A has a volume of only 1200 cc. Object B has a volume of 3200 cc. Object C has a volume of only $(\frac{1}{2})(10)(5)(20) = 500$ cc. Object B will float since 3200 cc. of water weighs 3200 grams and $2000 < 3200$. Objects A and C will not float.

12. Solve $.04 = .25x$ to get $x = .16$.

13. Rewrite the equation as $x^2 + 3x = 0$. Then, $x(x+3) = 0$. The two answers are $x = 0$ and $x = -3$. With the restriction $x < 0$, we have $x = -3$.

14. $3x/4y = \frac{1}{8}$. Dividing both sides by $\frac{3}{4}$, we get $\frac{x}{y} = \frac{1}{6}$.

Now, multiply the entire equation $\frac{x}{y} = \frac{1}{6}$ by $\frac{4}{3}$ to get

$4x/3y = (\frac{1}{6})(\frac{4}{3}) = \frac{2}{9}$

15. .3% of 25% becomes $(.003)(.25) = .00075$

16. The equivalent decimals are .07, .7, .075, and .697225. Arranging from least to greatest: .07, .075, .697225, and .7, which correspond to I, III, IV, and II.

17. The actual payments are (.20)($490) + (10)($47.75) = $575.50
Interest amount = $575.50 - $490 = $85.50

18. The number of plants he sold = $150 ÷ $0.75 = 200. Since he had 100 plants left, he originally purchased 200 + 100 = 300 plants.

19. Subtract the first equation from the second to get $2x = 1$. So, $x = .5$. Substitute this x value in either equation. Choosing the first equation, $(3)(.5) + y = 5$. Then, $y = 3.5$

20. Let x = number of dimes, x + 3 = number of quarters. Then, $.10x + .25(x+3) = 3.20$. Simplifying, $.35x + .75 = 3.20$. Finally, $x = 7$

21. For the weed killer, since 3 pounds should be used on 15,000 square feet, this translates into 2 pounds per 10,000 square feet. The ratio on the 10,000 square feet of lawn for fertilizer to weed killer is 25 to 2. This reduces to 12.5 to 1.

22. 1.5 meters = 1.5 ÷ .9 = 1.67 yards

23. Substituting choice C, 8 to 40 = $\frac{1}{5}$ and $\frac{x}{5}$ to $x = \frac{1}{5}$

24. $18^2 = 324$ and $19^2 = 361$. Thus, $\sqrt{360} \approx 19$

25. Total miles = $45 + (\frac{1}{2})(60) = 75$. Total time = $1 + \frac{1}{2} = 1\frac{1}{2}$ hours
Average speed = $75 \div 1\frac{1}{2} = 50$ mi/hr.

—

TEST 2

DIRECTIONS: Each question or incomplete statement is followed by several suggested answers or completions. Select the one that BEST answers the question or completes the statement. *PRINT THE LETTER OF THE CORRECT ANSWER IN THE SPACE AT THE RIGHT.*

1. $\frac{1}{3}$ of 15 = 15% of 1. ____

   A. $\frac{3}{4}$ B. 45 C. 75 D. 5 E. $33\frac{1}{3}$

2. A tree in an apartment building courtyard died, and the cost of cutting down the tree is $350.00. The city will share the cost with the landlord on a 2 to 3 ratio, the landlord paying the larger part. How much will the landlord have to pay? 2. ____
   A. $233.00 B. $175.00
   C. $117.00 D. $150.00
   E. $210.00

3. $\frac{1}{2} + \frac{4}{2x-1} = 6.$ x = 3. ____

   A. $-\frac{1}{2}$ B. $\frac{13}{22}$ C. $\frac{19}{22}$ D. $-\frac{1}{4}$ E. $-\frac{15}{22}$

4. The capacity of a car's cooling system if 17 quarts. $1\frac{3}{4}$ gallons of antifreeze plus 1 pint of rust inhibitor are required to drop the freezing point to -18^0. How much water is required to fill the system to capacity? 4. ____
   A. 21 pints B. 9 pints
   C. 19 pints D. 10 quarts
   E. 18 pints

5. If 1 inch = 2.54 cm., $\frac{3}{4}$ cm. = how many inches? 5. ____

   A. 1.9 B. 3.39 C. .75 D. .19 E. .3

6. A box has the shape of a rectangular solid, with a base measuring 16 inches by 10 inches and a height of 8 inches. What is the approximate length of the sides of a cubic container having the same volume? 6. ____
   A. 9.75 inches B. 10.00 inches
   C. 10.85 inches D. 12.65 inches
   E. 13.15 inches

7. What is a valid formula for the line plotted on the graph? 7. ____
   A. $x = y$
   B. $x = \frac{10}{y}$
   C. $x = 10 - y$
   D. $x = \frac{y}{10}$
   E. $x = y + 10$

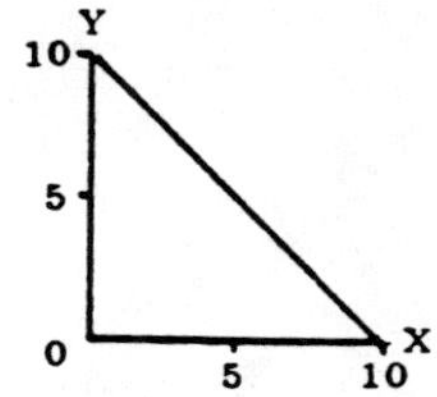

8. In the fraction $\frac{x}{y}$, when 1 is added to the numerator, the fraction equals $\frac{1}{3}$. When 3 is added to the denominator of $\frac{x}{y}$, the fraction equals $\frac{1}{6}$. What is $\frac{x}{y}$? 8.____

A. $\frac{2}{6}$ B. $\frac{2}{3}$ C. $\frac{2}{9}$ D. $\frac{6}{17}$ E. $\frac{2}{12}$

9. What is the *approximate* value of $\frac{(.03)^2(\sqrt{.25} + 3.5)}{.12}$? 9.____

A. .03 B. .36 C. .003 D. 3.0 E. .0036

10. A woman is now three times as old as her son. In four years, the son will be one-half as old as the woman is now. How old is the woman now? 10.____

A. 24 B. 28 C. 30 D. 21 E. 33

11. $\frac{1}{5}$ of 27 = 25% of 11.____

A. $21\frac{3}{5}$ B. 5.4 C. 1.35 D. $\frac{105}{5}$ E. 21.5

12. A rancher had 70 head of cattle. A buyer made four purchases of cattle from the rancher. The rancher now has eighteen cattle remaining. On the average, how many cattle exchanged hands at EACH purchase? 12.____

A. 10.5 B. 13 C. 15 D. 20 E. 52

13. $\sqrt{16 + x} = 4 + 2$. $x =$ 13.____

A. 36 B. 4 C. -10 D. 20 E. 2

14. If 10 cc of 20% acid is mixed with 20 cc of 40% acid, the percentage of acid in the resulting solution is 14.____

A. 50 B. 30 C. $33\frac{1}{3}$ D. 35 E. 60

15. $\frac{5}{6} + \frac{5}{9} - \frac{2}{3} + x =$ a whole number. Then $x = ?$ 15.____

A. $\frac{5}{18}$ B. $\frac{13}{16}$ C. $\frac{17}{18}$ D. $\frac{18}{13}$ E. $\frac{2}{9}$

16. A piece of lumber is 63 inches long. It is to be cut in three pieces. Two pieces are to be of equal length, while the third piece is to be 9 inches longer than each of the other two pieces. How long will the longer piece of lumber be? 16.____

A. 54 inches B. 36 inches
C. 30 inches D. 27 inches
E. 18 inches

17. The sun shining on a tree casts a shadow 45 feet long. A boy five feet tall standing near the tree has a 2 foot 10 inch shadow. How tall is the tree? 17.____

A. 54 feet B. 22.5 feet
C. 37.5 feet D. 79.4 feet
E. 18 feet

18. $\frac{x}{95} = 7.5\%$ x = 18.___

A. 12.7   B. 7.1   C. 8.0   D. 1.26   E. 713

19. A street light shining on a signpost casts a shadow 6 feet long. A child 5 feet tall standing near the signpost casts a shadow 2 feet 3 inches long. How tall is the signpost? 19.___

A. 13.3 feet
B. 6.6 feet
C. 12 feet
D. 20 feet
E. 15.3 feet

20. $\frac{(-2)^{15}}{(-2)^{12}} = ?$ 20.___

A. -4   B. +4   C. -8   D. +8   E. -16

21. Five consecutive whole numbers have a sum of 50. What is the second of the five numbers? 21.___

A. 5   B. 7   C. 9   D. 10   E. 11

22. If z = 35% of w, and y = 15% of z, then y = ___% of w. 22.___

A. 2.33   B. 42.9   C. 5.25   D. 2.25   E. 4.3

23. If $(y + 2)x = \frac{1}{4}$, y = 23.___

A. $\frac{1}{4} - 2x$
B. $\frac{1}{4x} - 2$
C. $\frac{1}{4x+8}$
D. $\frac{x}{4} - 2$
E. $\frac{1-8x}{4}$

24. A set of drill bits are being sold for $200.00. The bits cost the dealer $160.00, plus a $20.00 shipping fee. What percent of the selling price will be profit for the dealer? 24.___

A. 7%   B. 10%   C. 11%   D. 21%   E. 30%

25. Let A be the area of a circle whose diameter is 8. Which of the following numbers is closest to A? 25.___

A. 50   B. 70   C. 100   D. 120   E. 200

KEY (CORRECT ANSWERS)

1. E
2. E
3. C
4. C
5. E
6. C
7. C
8. C
9. A
10. A
11. A
12. B
13. D
14. C
15. A
16. D
17. D
18. B
19. A
20. C
21. C
22. C
23. B
24. B
25. A

SOLUTIONS TO PROBLEMS

1. $\frac{1}{3}$ of 15 = 5. Then, $5 \div .15 = 33\frac{1}{3}$

2. Let 2x = city's cost and 3x = landlord's cost. 2x + 3x = \$350 Solving, x = \$70. Then, landlord's cost is (3)(\$70) = \$210

3. Multiplying the equation by (2)(2x-1), we get (1)(2x-1) + (4)(2) = (6)(2)(2x-1). Simplifying, 2x - 1 + 8 = 24x - 12. This reduces further to 19 = 22x. So, $x = \frac{19}{22}$

4. $1\frac{3}{4}$ gallons = $(1\frac{3}{4})(4)$ = 7 quarts = 14 pints of antifreeze. The capacity of the cooling system = 17 quarts = 34 pints. Since 1 pint of rust inhibitor is needed, the amount of water required is 34 - 14 - 1 = 19 pints.

5. $\frac{3}{4}$ cm = $\frac{3}{4} \div 2.54$ = .295 or about .3 inches

6. The volume of the box = (16)(10)(8) = 1280 cubic inches. If a cubic container has a volume of 1280 cubic inches, each side must be $\sqrt[3]{1280} \approx 10.85$ inches. (Actually, the answer is slightly closer to 10.86)

7. Since the coordinates of the two given points are (10,0) and (0,10), the slope of the line is (10-0) ÷ (0-10) = -1. Y = -1x + B, where B is the y-intercept. Now, B = 10 since (0,10) lies on this line. Y = -1x + 10 is the equation and this can be written as x = 10 - y.

8. From the given information, $(x+1)/y = \frac{1}{3}$ and $x/(y+3) = \frac{1}{6}$

   Rewriting, we have y = 3x + 3 and y = 6x - 3. Adding these equations, 2y = 9x. Thus, $\frac{x}{y} = \frac{2}{9}$.

9. $(.03)^2 = .0009$. $(\sqrt{.25} + 3.5) = 4.0$. The answer becomes (.0009)(4)/.12 = .03. (Change the word *approximate* to *exact*.)

10. Let x = woman's age, $\frac{1}{3}x$ = son's age. Then, $\frac{1}{3}x + 4 = \frac{1}{2}x$.

    This reduces to $\frac{1}{6}x = 4$, so x = 24.

11. $\frac{1}{5}$ of 27 = (.2)(27) = 5.4. Then, 5.4 ÷ .25 = 21.6 = $21\frac{3}{5}$

12. 70 - 18 = 52. Then, 52 ÷ 4 = 13.

13. $\sqrt{16+x} = 6$. Square both sides to get 16 + x = 36. Then, x = 20

14. The amount of acid in the resulting solution is (.20)(10) + (.40)(20) = 10 cc. The solution is 10 + 20 = 30 cc. Percentage of acid is (10/30)(100) = 33 1/3

15. $\frac{5}{6} + \frac{5}{9} - \frac{2}{3}$ = (15 + 10 - 12)/18 = $\frac{13}{18}$. Since choice A is $\frac{5}{18}$,

$\frac{13}{18} + \frac{5}{18} = \frac{18}{18}$ = 1, which is a whole number.

16. Let x = length of each shorter piece and x + 9 = length of the longer piece. x + x + x + 9 = 63. Solving, x = 18. So, the longer piece must be 27 inches.

17. The ratio of the boy's height to his shadow is 60 inches to 34 inches = 30 to 17 (reduced). Let x = height of the tree. Then, x/45 = 30/17. Solving, x ≃ 79.4 feet

18. x/95 = .075. x = (.075)(95) = 7.125 or about 7.1

19. The ratio of the child's height to his shadow is 60 inches to 27 inches = 20 to 9 (reduced). Let x = height of the signpost. Then, x/6 = 20/9. Solving, x - 13.33 or about 13.3 feet.

20. In division, we subtract exponents to get $(-2)^3 = -8$. Of course, the base must remain the same.

21. Let x, x+1, x+2, x+3, x+4 represent the numbers. Then, x + x+1 + x+2 + x+3 + x+4 = 50. Solving, x = 8. The second number must be 9.

22. y = .15z = (.15)(.35)w = .0525w. Thus, y is 5.25% of w.

23. (y+2)(x) = ¼. Dividing both sides by x, we get $y + 2 = \frac{1}{4x}$.

Finally, $y = \frac{1}{4x} - 2$

24. The dealer's total cost is $180 and his profit is $20. The percent profit on the selling price is (20/200)(100) = 10%.

25. $A = (\pi)(4)^2 = 16\pi$ = 50.265 or about 50. Note that the formula is Area = $(\pi)(\text{radius})^2$.

EXAMINATION SECTION

DIRECTIONS: Each question or incomplete statement is followed by several suggested answers or completions. Select the one that BEST answers the question or completes the statement. *PRINT THE LETTER OF THE CORRECT ANSWER IN THE SPACE AT THE RIGHT.*

1. $A = \frac{27}{32}$ in., $B = \frac{7}{8}$ in., $C = \frac{51}{64}$ in., $D = \frac{13}{16}$ in. 1.____

   To arrange the above ruler measurements in order of increasing lengths, the CORRECT arrangement should be
   A. B, D, A, C B. D, C, A, B
   C. C, D, A, B D. C, A, D, B

2. The ratio of 3'6" to 6" is BEST expressed as 2.____
   A. 1 to 7 B. 3.6" to 6"
   C. 6" to 42" D. 7 to 1

3. A layout of a rectangular foundation for a building is drawn to scale. The 72-foot length of the foundation is represented on the drawing by a line 27 inches long. The length, in inches, of the line needed to represent the 45-foot width of the foundation is 3.____

   A. $16\frac{7}{8}$ B. $17\frac{1}{4}$ C. $17\frac{7}{8}$ D. $18\frac{3}{8}$

4. A circle graph is to be made to show the parts of the total city budget allocated to each department; the total budget is 2 billion, 100 million dollars. 4.____
   If 630 million dollars is allocated for education, the number of degrees on the circle graph which would represent the amount for education is *closest to*
   A. 30 B. 54 C. 84 D. 108

5. A sample of brass contained $1\frac{3}{4}$ pounds of copper, $1\frac{1}{4}$ pounds of zinc, and 2 ounces of impurities. 5.____
   The number of pounds of copper in one ton of this type of brass is
   A. 560 B. 800 C. 1080 D. 1120

6. When the temperature drops from 37°F to -8°F, the number of degrees the temperature on the Centigrade scale will fall during the same period is 6.____

   A. $7\frac{2}{9}$ B. 25 C. 49 D. 57

7. The screw which advances the thimble of a micrometer has 40 threads to the inch. If the thimble is turned exactly 3 threads, the micrometer will be opened by ____ inches. 7.____
   A. 0.025 B. 0.075 C. 0.340 D. 0.750

8. A voltmeter scale is divided into 10 major divisions, each of which is divided into five minor divisions. Full scale deflection occurs when 30 volts are across the meter. The number of volts indicated when the needle is on the second minor division beyond the sixth major division is 8.____
   A. 6.4 B. 16.4 C. 18.6 D. 19.2

9. A gear with 48 teeth drives a 64 tooth idler gear which in turn is engaged to a gear with 32 teeth. If the first gear rotates at 1200 rpm, then the last gear rotates, in rpm, at 9.____
   A. 800 B. 900 C. 1600 D. 1800

10. The number of rectangular cards 11 inches long and 8 inches wide that can be cut from a sheet 33 inches long and 27 inches wide with a minimum of waste is 10.____
   A. 6 B. 9 C. 10 D. 12

11. The power used in an electric circuit is proportional to the square of the current flow. If the power used in a circuit is 630 watts when the current is 3 amperes, then the power in watts when the current is 4 amperes will be 11.____
   A. $354\frac{3}{8}$ B. $472\frac{1}{2}$ C. 840 D. 1120

12. The algebraic statement $x^2+y^2=(x+y)^2$ is 12.____
   A. true for all values of x and y
   B. never true
   C. true only if x and/or y equals zero
   D. true only if x equals y

13. If the formula $a = \frac{V-v}{t}$ is solved for v, the expression equivalent to v is 13.____
   A. at−V B. V−at C. $-\frac{at}{V}$ D. $\frac{V}{at}$

14. Of the following four fractions, the one that is *closest* in value to $\sqrt{5}$ is 14.____
   A. $2\frac{1}{10}$ B. $2\frac{1}{5}$ C. $2\frac{1}{8}$ D. $2\frac{1}{2}$

15. During a transfer of oil from one tank to another, $1\frac{1}{2}$ gallons were lost through leaks in the hose. This represented 0.3 percent of the capacity of the first tank. The capacity of this tank in gallons is 15.____
   A. 50 B. 200 C. 450 D. 500

16. In making up a blend containing 45% cotton, 35% dacron, and 20% wool, the formula needed to determine the weight C of cotton needed to mix with D pounds of dacron and W pounds of wool is 16.____

A. $C = \frac{.45(W+D)}{.55}$ B. $C = \frac{.55(W+D)}{.45}$

C. $C = \frac{.35D + .20W}{.45}$ D. $C = .45(.35D + .20W)$

17. A piece of wire $6\frac{1}{4}$ yards long is to be cut into two pieces such that the longer piece is one and one-half as long as the shorter piece. 17.___
The length (in inches) of the *shorter* piece must be
A. 90   B. 100   C. 135   D. 150

18. The number of cc of water that must be added to 75 cc of a 60 percent solution of alcohol and water to change it to a 50 percent solution is *closest to* 18.___
A. 10   B. 15   C. 20   D. 30

19. A small hose can fill a tank with water in two hours while a larger hose can fill the same tank in one hour. The number of minutes it will take for the tank to be filled if both hoses are used at the same time is 19.___
A. 30   B. 40   C. 45   D. 90

20. The volume of an average atom is about 10^{-23} cubic centimeters. The volume of one gene in a human body is about 10^{-17} cubic centimeters. 20.___
Using these figures, we can conclude that the ratio of the volume of a gene to that of an atom is about
A. 60 to 1   B. 1 to 10^{6}
C. 10^{-6} to 1   D. 10^{6} to 1

21. Using six number punches with digits 1, 2, 3, 4, 5, and 6, the number of differently numbered tags that can be made with 3 digit numbers on each tag is 21.___
A. 120   B. 216   C. 278   D. 556

22. In a right triangle, the tangent of either of the acute angles can be found by dividing the lengths of the 22.___
A. opposite leg by the adjacent leg
B. adjacent leg by the opposite leg
C. opposite leg by the hypotenuse
D. hypotenuse by the opposite leg

23. In a right triangle, the cosine of one of the angles is equal to 0.8. The value of the sine of the same angle is 23.___
A. 0.2   B. 0.4   C. 0.6   D. 0.8

24. A sheet metal worker is laying out a pattern for a regular polygon of nine equal sides. The number of degrees in each interior angle of the polygon must be 24.___
A. 40   B. 70   C. 140   D. 160

25. The outside diameter of an automobile's tires is 28 inches. When the wheels are rotating at 720 rpm, the speed of the car (in feet per second) is *closest to* 25.___
A. 30   B. 44   C. 60   D. 88

26. A square peg which measures one inch across the flat sides is to be placed in a round hole. Of the four holes whose diameters in inches are given, which is the *smallest* hole into which the peg will fit? 26.___

A. 1.2 B. 1.3 C. 1.4 D. 1.5

27. The volume in cubic centimeters of a rectangular box 5 inches long, 4 inches wide, and 3 inches deep is *closest to* (one inch is the equivalent of 2.54 cm.) 27.___

A. 4 B. 153 C. 385 D. 1000

28. If a sheet metal storage bin is in the shape of a cube, and has a total surface area of 216 square feet, the volume of the cube (in cubic feet) will be 28.___

A. 216 B. 243 C. 284 D. 312

29. An 8-foot length of steel rod has a circular cross-section whose diameter is one inch. If the weight of 1 cubic inch of steel is $\frac{1}{4}$ pound, then the weight (in pounds) of this piece of rod is *closest to* 29.___

A. 1.6 B. 15.6 C. 18.8 D. 75.2

30. Two solid ball bearings are made of the same material, and the diameter of one bearing is three times that of the other. If the weight of the smaller one is 8 ounces, the weight (in ounces) of the *larger* bearing will be 30.___

A. 24 B. 48 C. 72 D. 216

KEY (CORRECT ANSWERS)

1. C	11. D	21. B
2. D	12. C	22. A
3. A	13. B	23. C
4. D	14. B	24. C
5. D	15. D	25. D
6. B	16. A	26. D
7. B	17. A	27. D
8. D	18. B	28. A
9. D	19. B	29. C
10. B	20. D	30. D

SOLUTIONS TO PROBLEMS

1. Convert all fractions to like denominations: $A = \frac{54}{64}$ in., $B = \frac{56}{64}$ in., $C = \frac{51}{64}$ in., $D = \frac{52}{64}$ in. Thus, in increasing length, the arrangement is C, D, A, B. (Ans. C)

2. Change 3'6" to 42". Then, 42" to 6" = 7 to 1. (Ans. D)

3. Let x = required line. Then, $\frac{27}{x} = \frac{72}{45}$, and $x = 16\frac{7}{8}$ in. (Ans. A)

4. The ratio of 630 million to 2 billion, 100 million is 630 to 2100 = $\frac{3}{10}$. $(\frac{3}{10})(360^\circ) = 108^\circ$. (Ans. D)

5. This sample contains $1\frac{3}{4} + 1\frac{1}{4} + \frac{1}{8} = 3\frac{1}{8}$ lbs. Let x = # of lbs. of copper in 1 ton of the brass sample. $\frac{x}{2000} = \frac{1.75}{3.125}$. Solving by cross-multiplication, x = 1120. (Ans. D)

6. Use $C = \frac{5}{9}(F-32)$. 37°F converts to $2\frac{7}{9}^\circ$C and -8°F converts to $-22\frac{1}{9}^\circ$C. The drop is $24\frac{8}{9}^\circ$ or approximately 25°. (Ans. B)

7. 3 ÷ 40 = .075 inches. NOTE correction of problem. (Ans. B)

8. Each major division is $\frac{30}{10}$ = 3 volts. Each minor division is $\frac{3}{5}$ = .6 volts. 6 major + 2 minor divisions = (6)(3)+(2)(.6)=19.2 volts (Ans. D)

9. Let x = speed of 64 tooth idler. By inverse proportion, $\frac{1200}{x} = \frac{64}{48}$ and x=900. Likewise, if y = speed of last gear, $\frac{900}{y} = \frac{32}{64}$. y = 1800 rpm. (Ans. D)

10. 33 ÷ 11 = 3 columns by 27 ÷ 8 rounded down to 3 rows. (3)(3) = 9. (Ans. B)

11. $P = KC^2$ where P = power, C = current. $630 = (K)(3^2)$ and K=70. Now, $P = 70C^2$. When C=4, $P = (70)(4^2) = 1120$. (Ans. D)

12. Since $(x+y)^2 = x^2+2xy+y^2$, this expression can $= x^2+y^2$ only if $2xy = 0$. This means either x or y or both x,y = 0. (Ans. C)

13. $a = \frac{V-v}{t}$ implies $at = V-v$. Then, $v = V-at$. (Ans. B)

14. $\sqrt{5} = 2.236$ approx. Finding the absolute value of the difference between 2.236 and each of 2.1, 2.2, 2.125 and 2.5 yields .136, .036, .111, and .264, respectively. Thus, 2.2 (or $2\frac{1}{5}$) is closest to $\sqrt{5}$. (Ans. B)

15. Use a proportion: $\frac{1\frac{1}{2}}{x} = \frac{.3\%}{100\%} = \frac{.003}{1}$, where x = capacity of the tank. Solving, x=500. (Ans. D)

16. Since D = .35 (Total Wt.) and W = .20 (Total Wt.), D +W = .55(Total Wt) or Total Wt = (D+W)/.55. Now, C = .45(Total Wt) which by substitution becomes C = .45(D+W)/.55. (Ans. A)

17. Use x for the shorter piece, 1.5x for the longer piece. $x + 1.5x = 6.25$. x = 2.5 yds. = 90 in. NOTE the correction in the wording. (Ans. A)

18. Let x be required number. The original amount of water = (.40)(75) = 30 cc. The new solution will have (30+x)cc of water and (75+x)cc of alcohol and water. Then, we have (30+x)/(75+x) = 50% = .50. Solving, x=15. (Ans. B)

19. Let x = required time operating together (in minutes)

$\frac{x}{120} + \frac{x}{60} = 1$, which yields x=40. Note that $\frac{x}{120}$ represents the fraction of the tank that will be filled by the small hose. (Ans. B)

20. $10^{-17}/10^{-23} = 10^6$ or 10^6 to 1. (Ans. D)

21. Total number of permutations = (6)(6)(6) = 216. (Ans. B)

22. Definition of tangent of an acute angle in a right triangle is (opposite leg)/(adjacent leg). (Ans. A)

23. Cosine = adjacent leg/hypotenuse = $\frac{8}{10}$. Solving for the missing leg as $\sqrt{10^2-8^2} = 6$. Now, sine = opposite leg/hypotenuse $= \frac{6}{10} = .6$. (Ans. C)

24. The sum of all interior angles of any 9-sided polygon = $(7)(180^0) = 1260^0$. If the figure is regular, each interior angle must be $1260 \div 9 = 140^0$. (Ans. C)

25. 1 revolution (in feet) = (28)(3.14) ÷ 12 = 7.33.
720 rpm = 720 ÷ 60 = 12 rev/sec. Since the car travels 7.33 ft. in one revolution, the wheels are moving at (12)(7.33) = 87.96, rounded to 88 ft/sec. (Ans. D)

26. The diagonal of the peg = $\sqrt{2}$ = 1.414 approx. The smallest hole into which it will fit is 1.5. (Ans. D)

27. Volume = (5)(4)(3) = 60 cu.in. Now, 1 cu.in. = $(2.54)^3$ = 16.4 cu.cm. Thus, 60 cu.in. = (60)(16.4) = 984, rounded to 1000 cu.cm. (Ans. D)

28. Each face of the cube = 216/6 = 36 sq.ft. so that each edge = 6 ft. Volume = 6^3 = 216 cu.ft. (Ans. A)

29. Volume = $(3.14)(\text{radius})^2(\text{height})$ = $3.14(.5)^2(96)$ = 75.36 cu.in. Total weight = $(75.36)(\frac{1}{4})$ = 18.84 lbs. (Ans. C)

30. Ratio of radii is 1 to 3. Since volume = $\frac{4}{3}\pi(\text{radius})^3$ for each ball bearing, the ratio of volumes = 1 to 27. The weight of the larger bearing = (8)(27) = 216 ounces. Note that the ratio of radii = ratio of diameters. (Ans. D)

EXAMINATION SECTION

TEST 1

DIRECTIONS: Each question or incomplete statement is followed by several suggested answers or completions. Select the one that BEST answers the question or completes the statement. *PRINT THE LETTER OF THE CORRECT ANSWER IN THE SPACE AT THE RIGHT.*

1. Tom wanted to cut six inches off the end of the board, so he went to the tool chest and took out a 1.___
   A. wrench B. screwdriver C. hammer D. saw

2. Last year, American industry lost a quarter of a billion dollars more from crime than from fire. 2.___
   Any industrialist who feels that fire insurance is a necessary protection cannot afford to overlook the possibility that he also needs protection against
   A. insurance agencies B. labor
   C. government D. crime

3. Jimmie was a little boy who did not want to help his mother or father. 3.___
   Jimmie was
   A. lazy B. strong C. stupid D. kind

4. In areas where wood is widely used for building, there is plenty of work for 4.___
   A. architects B. carpenters C. masons D. electricians

5. The two boys had played together for six years. They did not fight. 5.___
   They were
   A. friends B. cousins C. boys D. enemies

6. Saws driven by gasoline engines cannot be used in areas where a spark or backfire might set off an explosion. 6.___
   Recently, however, power saws operated by compressed air have been designed by German engineers to work in places threatened by
   A. manpower shortages B. enemy attacks
   C. fire hazards D. power cutoffs

7. The speaker's talk was long and dull. It seemed that it would never end. 7.___
   How glad we were when he finally
   A. spoke B. died C. stopped D. clapped

8. I gave the girl twenty cents to buy apples. 8.___
   On the way to the store, she lost the money, so she could not buy the
   A. oranges B. fruit C. candy D. bread

9. The road was built only a few months ago. Already there are cracks in its surface. 9.___
It is too bad that this new road needs to be
A. built B. sold C. widened D. repaired

10. As cities become larger, it is necessary for engineers to seek new sources of water to meet the demands of growing 10.___
A. populations B. children C. gardens D. lakes

11. These mountain peaks will not be conquered easily by a person who lacks climbing experience. 11.___
The Mountain Club advises climbers not to try to scale these until they have
A. become club members
B. climbed other mountains
C. read about climbers
D. joined a party of climbers

12. A girl is reading a book. The book has pictures in it. She shows the pictures to the baby, but all he wants to do is tear the 12.___
A. pages B. rags C. dress D. cloth

13. Jane's favorite TV program is the weekly circus. 13.___
She likes to watch the
A. airplanes B. books C. cars D. clowns

14. In comic strips, people and animals do things that they cannot do in real life. 14.___
Some people can fly without airplanes and some animals can
A. play B. run C. bark D. talk

15. It would be easier to plan the monthly expenses both of business firms and of households is all the months had the same number of 15.___
A. workers B. days C. holidays D. sales

16. It is not only necessary but also enlightening to merely sit, listen, and observe on some occasions. Often it has been said that spectators see more of any athletic contest than anyone else. 16.___
In many situations, in fact, a spectator can usually take note of what is happening as well as, if not better than, one who is
A. paying attention B. actually present
C. involved in the fray D. on the winning team

17. His athletic interests are strong. He enjoys not only baseball and football but almost all 17.___
A. sports B. books C. food D. people

18. Dan got very dirty playing in the yard. Then he went into the house and took a nice warm bath. 18.___
When he stepped out of the tub, he said, *"My, it feels good to be*
A. rich." B. clean." C. tired." D. hungry."

19. The angle that a bomb makes with the horizontal area at the point of impact is called the angle of fall. The degree of penetration of the bomb increases with the size of the angle of fall.
Thus, given an angle of 90 degrees, the amount of penetration will be 19.___
   A. 25% of maximum   B. maximum
   C. unpredictable   D. 50% of maximum

20. The greater part of the world's creative work is done by those who subsist by some other occupation. Science today is vigorous partly because research and teaching go well together. In the fine arts, it is not easy to make a living by really good work, and it is equally as hard to find an occupation that leaves leisure time for creation. Quite likely, this is one reason why art 20.___
   A. appeals to the lazy man
   B. is less flourishing than science
   C. makes such great contributions to our society
   D. is not appreciated by the majority of the people

21. When the driver of the car saw the tree blocking the road, he 21.___
   A. opened the hood   B. went faster
   C. stopped   D. passed it

22. Furniture that is to be left outdoors should be made of materials that will not be ruined by bad 22.___
   A. meals   B. backyards   C. weather   D. children

23. Jane's little kitten cried because it was hungry. It wanted to 23.___
   A. sleep   B. play   C. eat   D. run

24. All the crew bailed out of the plane.
The plane crashed and burned but no lives were 24.___
   A. saved   B. lost   C. rescued   D. parachuted

25. The Chinese philosopher Lao-tse taught his followers to believe in fêng-shui, a mystical spirit connected with the land and giving continuity to the labors of successive generations. The concept of fêng-shui carries with it an admonition to the Chinese farmers that they are merely trustees of the soil that they till, since it belongs not only to them but to all their ancestors and descendants. One practical outcome of this agrarian philosophy is the centuries-old Chinese practice of 25.___
   A. fêng-shuiism   B. soil conservation
   C. feudalism   D. rice cultivation

KEY (CORRECT ANSWERS)

1. D
2. D
3. A
4. B
5. A

6. C
7. C
8. B
9. D
10. A

11. B
12. A
13. D
14. D
15. B

16. C
17. A
18. B
19. B
20. B

21. C
22. C
23. C
24. B
25. B

TEST 2

DIRECTIONS: Each question or incomplete statement is followed by several suggested answers or completions. Select the one that BEST answers the question or completes the statement. *PRINT THE LETTER OF THE CORRECT ANSWER IN THE SPACE AT THE RIGHT.*

1. It seems likely that the word *Gothic* was originally used to describe a type of architecture that suggested barbaric qualities in the nation producing it. It did not indicate that the people of the nation were really descendants of the Goths or that the architecture was originated by the Goths. It only implied that the people and their structures showed 1.___
   A. signs of Gothic influence
   B. a new type of architectural design
   C. trends found only in the art of the Goths
   D. a degree of sternness and rudeness

2. Compulsory retirement provisions in industry give younger men added assurance that new opportunities 2.___
   A. will open up to them
   B. must be sought in new work
   C. are fairly distributed
   D. will help the older workers

3. We planned to drive from New York to Detroit. To decide which highway to follow, we looked at a road 3.___
   A. lane B. builder C. surface D. map

4. Instead of using one word over and over again, a person who has a good vocabulary uses different words with the same 4.___
   A. spelling B. length C. sound D. meaning

5. He could never remember Bill's telephone number. He always had to look it up in the 5.___
   A. almanac B. encyclopedia
   C. telephone directory D. dictionary

6. It is hard to speak properly upon a subject where it is even difficult to convince your hearers that you are speaking the truth. On the one hand, the friend who is familiar with every facet of the story may think that some point has not been set forth with that fullness he wishes and knows it to deserve. On the other hand, he who is a stranger to the matter may be led by envy to suspect exaggeration if he hears anything above his own nature. For men can endure to hear others praised only so long as they can severally persuade themselves of their own ability to equal the actions recounted: when this point is passed, envy comes in and with it 6.___
   A. exaggeration B. false pride
   C. incredulity D. deceit

7. The Spanish settlers of the New World, eager for gold, had little interest in agriculture. 7.____
For many decades, potentially valuable farmland was
A. expensive B. neglected C. demanded D. explored

8. The term *specialization* refers to the system in which each person performs a particular and perhaps different task. This person receives money for his work and with it buys goods and services that others have produced. 8.____
Specialization has thus led to a(n)
A. lower standard of living
B. money economy
C. immobile social structure
D. barter economy

9. The car was stuck in the mud. 9.____
Three men pushed as hard as they could, still the car did not
A. stop B. start C. move D. stall

10. According to T.S. Eliot, *"When a poet's mind is perfectly equipped for its work, it is constantly amalgamating disparate experience: the ordinary man's experience is chaotic, irregular, fragmentary. The latter falls in love, or reads Spinoza, and these two experiences have nothing to do with each other, or with the noise of the typewriter or the smell of cooking; in the mind of the poet, these experiences are* 10.____
A. separately considered."
B. always forming new wholes."
C. contradictory to his philosophy."
D. the bases of artistic work."

11. There were few people at his funeral. 11.____
He had outlived his hundreds of true friends who would have been at the funeral if they
A. had not been so old
B. had known about it
C. could have sent flowers
D. had been alive

12. For expository purposes, the utopias that have been set up thus far may be classified according to their placement on two continua: first, on the continuum extending from chaos to complete harmony, and second, on the continuum extending from behavior ruled by reason to behavior controlled by strict religious axioms. Most utopias that could be classified as showing harmony have been those ruled by fixed precepts. 12.____
There appears to be a(n)
A. direct relationship between chaos and rule by axiom
B. direct relationship between harmony and rule by reason
C. inverse relationship between chaos and rule by axiom
D. circular relationship between chaos and rule by reason

13. Thousands of persons watched the automobile race. Newspapers carried stories and pictures for those who could not 13.___
A. hear B. bet C. go D. drive

14. Fish live in water. They swim and swim all day. They cannot live on land. 14.___
If you take them out of water, they will soon
A. walk B. die C. run away D. get lost

15. In the arena, two gladiators fought each other with short swords. Occasionally, one of the gladiators would be knocked down and would raise a finger to the audience, asking them for mercy. The spectators waved clenched fists to signal that they wished a particular gladiator put to death. 15.___
Other spectators, who favored this fighter, waved open hands, asking that the gladiator be given
A. a defeat
B. a new sword
C. mercy
D. to the lions

16. If the quantity with which a person is concerned is finite, one and one thousand are quite different. But if the quantity under consideration is infinite, one and one thousand are the same. 16.___
Finite quantities can be thought of as equal when
A. compared with each other
B. compared with an infinite quantity
C. regarded as individual cases
D. mathematical principles are ignored

17. Plans for the wolf hunt were being made. The farmers had lost sheep and chickens. The wolves killed their pigs. Even cattle were not 17.___
A. attacked B. safe C. butchered D. hunted

18. The man took his boat out on the lake. 18.___
Black clouds came up in the sky so he had to hurry home before the
A. sun came out
B. lake dried up
C. rain came
D. boat sank

19. Honeybees make honey. They make it from nectar that they get from flowers. 19.___
If there were no flowers, we could not get
A. honey B. roses C. water D. perfume

20. Any proposition that does not involve a contradiction in terms may possibly be true; and if all the circumstances that raise a probability in its favor be stated and enforced, and those which lead to an opposite conclusion be omitted or lightly passed over, it may 20.___
A. properly be declared true
B. be rightly evaluated as false
C. appear to be demonstrated
D. appear ridiculous when actually true

21. Acetylene, a colorless gas, produces a flame whose light penetrates fog and darkness remarkably well. This property, along with the capacity of the acetylene generator to operate without attention for long periods of time, makes the gas valuable for use in 21.___
   A. industrial heating B. mining
   C. lighthouses D. blowtorches

22. Surety bonds covering acceptable completion of the contracts involved in public projects are required by law. One function of these bonds is to insure that the project will be 22.___
   A. finished B. practical C. popular D. inexpensive

23. The mystery writer unfolds his plot in a logical, inexorable sequence. After the first event happens, it seems that the next could not fail to happen. We feel that the incidents follow each other as they do, not because the author planned it so, but because 23.___
   A. we desired it so B. it had to be so
   C. the plot was unique D. it is so in our own lives

24. We didn't have any milk for breakfast because the milkman didn't 24.___
   A. stay B. come C. write D. phone

25. From a purely selfish point of view, it is not advisable to let a person know that you think he is stupid. You might be wrong, in which case he will quite justifiably 25.___
   A. continually ask you for advice
   B. defer to your ability to judge others
   C. concur in your opinion
   D. form the same opinion of you

KEY (CORRECT ANSWERS)

1.	D	11.	D
2.	A	12.	C
3.	D	13.	C
4.	D	14.	B
5.	C	15.	C
6.	C	16.	B
7.	B	17.	B
8.	B	18.	C
9.	C	19.	A
10.	B	20.	C

21. C
22. A
23. B
24. B
25. D

TEST 3

DIRECTIONS: Each question or incomplete statement is followed by several suggested answers or completions. Select the one that BEST answers the question or completes the statement. *PRINT THE LETTER OF THE CORRECT ANSWER IN THE SPACE AT THE RIGHT.*

1. Whether or not this historian will subsist as a standard supreme authority is a question. Wherever and whenever read, he will be read with fascination, with delight, with wonder. And with copious instruction too; but also with copious reserve, with questioning scrutiny, with liberty to reject, and with much exercise of that liberty. The contemporary mind may in rare cases be taken by storm; but posterity, never.
The tribunal of the present is accessible to influence, that of the future is 1.___
   A. incorrupt B. unsympathetic
   C. prejudiced D. predictable

2. Jim knew that morning had not come, for outside it was quite 2.___
   A. dark B. bright C. foggy D. cool

3. In his travels about China as a representative of Kublai Khan, Marco Polo observed that the Chinese were extremely honest.
They left their doors open at night without fear of 3.___
   A. rain B. insects C. cold D. thieves

4. One must be careful about keeping matches out of the reach of 4.___
   A. ladies B. men
   C. young children D. pockets

5. Billy and his friends loved to play cowboys, so his mother bought him a 5.___
   A. tool chest B. cowboy suit
   C. bicycle D. dog

6. A person who enjoys golf will derive more benefit from that sport than from setting-up exercises that he would do with more of a sense of duty than of 6.___
   A. accomplishment B. pleasure
   C. benefit D. determination

7. When we finally reached the cabin, we were very tired. The three-mile walk up the side of the mountain had not been 7.___
   A. interesting B. long C. slow D. easy

8. So numerous, indeed, and so powerful are the causes that serve to give a false bias to the judgment that we, upon many occasions, see wise and good men on the wrong as well as on the right side of questions of the first importance to society. 8.___
This circumstance, if duly attended to by those who are ever so much persuaded of their being in the right in any controversy, would furnish
A. an argument for the opposition
B. a lesson of moderation
C. a change of heart
D. justification of their position

9. The polar bear's sense of smell is very good. 9.___
Though food may be hidden, he is able to
A. want it B. hide it C. see it D. find it

10. At nine o'clock, the school bell rang. 10.___
All the children left the playground and went into the
A. classroom B. office C. park D. store

11. We have solved one long-standing economic problem only to meet another sort of difficulty. For centuries, men tried vainly to supply in sufficient quantity the things that they needed and wanted. Because of recent advances in technology, more goods are available now than are purchased, and this situation will last. 11.___
The new problem is that of
A. reducing production below the desirable level
B. making men want more than enough things
C. equalizing consumption among social classes
D. decreasing the number of luxuries that men want

12. The thermostat is an instrument for automatically adjusting the temperature produced by a heating system. In one type, when the temperature rises to a certain point, it causes a fluid within the thermostat to expand. This expansion activates a mechanism that decreases the amount of fuel supplied. 12.___
When the temperature falls to a certain point, the fluid contracts and activates a mechanism that
A. decreases the temperature
B. restores the system to manual control
C. causes the fluid to expand again
D. supplies more fuel

13. Experts generally agree that the primary cause of war is international competition for economic superiority. Each nation desires to achieve economic advantages equal to those enjoyed by its neighbors, and to attain these a nation may be compelled to add to its territory. Many believe that this struggle for territory is frequently the major cause of war, but I believe that it is only a minor aspect of the greater economic competition. 13.___
Dispute over territory by rival nations is
A. necessary for economic survival
B. the cause of economic struggle

C. the major cause of war
D. necessary for economic survival

14. Long ago in ancient Babylonia, each schoolboy was given a tablet covered with soft clay on which he wrote. When the tablet was filled, he could smooth out the marks with a flat stick, or make himself a new tablet with 14.___
A. bullrushes B. birch bark
C. a fresh ball of clay D. paper

15. The Board of Health is responsible for matters of public health policy and for drafting the city's 15.___
A. traffic regulations B. house numbers
C. tax laws D. sanitary code

16. When he looked at his watch, he began to walk faster. He was afraid he would be 16.___
A. on time B. caught C. late D. slow

17. Until a century or so ago, man was almost immune to scientific investigation. I think that the modern trend is rather clearly revealed by a consideration of the order in which certain natural sciences have become a standard part of most college curricula: first came geology, followed by botany, zoology, and finally psychology. This series seems to suggest an advance by natural science 17.___
A. in usefulness B. in general
C. on man D. on physical science

18. The fat woman tourist sat astride the camel. She tried to smile and look as if she were enjoying her ride, but she really wasn't very 18.___
A. heavy B. foreign
C. rich D. comfortable

19. The shrill note of the referee's whistle told the team that they had broken a 19.___
A. rule B. habit C. record D. leg

20. When life was first coming onto land from the sea, it was washed ashore by one tide and carried back by another. In this way, it could grow used to the land without a 20.___
A. sudden change B. tide
C. success D. gradual change

21. Summer visitors to Niagara Falls cannot imagine that the endless roar of the torrent of rushing water could cease. Were they to return in winter, however, they would find that Nature had silenced the waters by 21.___
A. rechanneling them B. subduing them
C. freezing them D. reducing their volume

22. The couple wanted to dance, but they were so far from the orchestra that they could not 22.___
A. leave the party B. see their friends
C. hear the music D. call the waiter

23. When it began to rain, the children ran into the house so that they would not be 23.___
A. cold B. late C. tired D. wet

24. There was baseball at the Polo Grounds that night. Eight banks of 120 lights, with each light 1500 watts, turned night into 24.___
A. pleasure B. sport C. day D. suspense

25. From the beginning of this self-governing republic, military chieftains have had to lay down their swords before assuming civil offices. Victorious generals in this country, contrary to experience elsewhere in the world, have not used military power to seize 25.___
A. the army and navy B. valuable documents
C. the country's treasury D. political authority

KEY (CORRECT ANSWERS)

1. A
2. A
3. D
4. C
5. B

6. B
7. D
8. B
9. D
10. A

11. B
12. D
13. D
14. C
15. D

16. C
17. C
18. D
19. A
20. A

21. C
22. C
23. D
24. C
25. D

TEST 4

DIRECTIONS: Each question or incomplete statement is followed by several suggested answers or completions. Select the one that BEST answers the question or completes the statement. *PRINT THE LETTER OF THE CORRECT ANSWER IN THE SPACE AT THE RIGHT.*

1. Plants are entirely satisfied with mere existence; lower animals are almost so. Man, as a rule, demands a great deal more from life than sheer being. In fact, one might say that to the degree that a man is content with mere existence, he 1.___
   A. realizes his ambitions B. reflects on his state
   C. is dull and obtuse D. is a sedentary being

2. Many people are killed in automobile accidents by being thrown from the automobile. 2.___
   This could sometimes be prevented if the automobile doors were kept
   A. greased B. locked C. open D. clean

3. Before the Industrial Revolution, each craftsman was forced to keep in his small shop many different kinds of equipment, although he could use only one piece of equipment at a time. 3.___
   Now, in a modern factory, each man is assigned to a machine, and all equipment is
   A. kept repaired B. constantly used
   C. skillfully operated D. elaborately designed

4. Voltaire, probably as much as any other person, popularized Newton's scientific discoveries. It is highly unlikely today that an eminent literary figure would disseminate scientific findings, for the accumulation and complexity of knowledge is such that, to achieve any real understanding, a man must resign himself to 4.___
   A. specificity of inquiry
   B. knowing nothing
   C. taking a graduate degree
   D. lack of scientific knowledge

5. Since the queen bee is an autocrat, there is room in each hive for only one queen. 5.___
   When a strange queen bee wanders into a hive that already has a queen, there is
   A. room for her
   B. no disturbance in the hive
   C. a royal reception
   D. a battle for power

6. I am amazed, therefore, that none have yet found out the secret of flattering the worthless, and yet of preserving a safe conscience. 6.___
I have often wished for some method by which a man might do himself and his deceased patron justice without being under the hateful reproach of
   A. self-conviction
   B. sincere flattery
   C. his admiring friends
   D. envious rivals

7. Even primitive man found it necessary to have a home of some kind to protect himself from changes in the weather. Since he had no tools for constructing such a shelter, he had to live in 7.___
   A. caves
   B. cabins
   C. cottages
   D. houses

8. Fire irons do not rust when they are used constantly. They are kept dry by the 8.___
   A. light
   B. danger
   C. heat
   D. color

9. According to modern modes of thought, elements of nature are not to be considered resources until there is some use for them in our technology. 9.___
Thus, if, for some reason, zinc were no longer necessary in our civilization, no matter how little there was in the country, we would say that
   A. there could never be a scarcity of zinc
   B. there was a scarcity of the natural resource mentioned
   C. as far as technology is concerned, there was a scarcity of zinc
   D. there was not a scarcity of the natural resource zinc

10. The boxer lay on the floor of the ring while the referee counted to ten. His fans were disappointed. Now he would no longer be 10.___
   A. champion
   B. tired
   C. alive
   D. out

11. The art of executing a design in color on textiles, or batik, is as difficult as etching or painting. It is practically impossible to correct a mistake in drawing or color after it has been made on cloth. 11.___
Truly, this is no art for those who work by
   A. dependence on vision alone
   B. dim illumination
   C. trial-and-error methods
   D. hand rather than with tools

12. There are several types of human blood. The blood given in a transfusion must match the patient's blood. If the transfused blood is of a different type from the patient's blood, blood clotting and death will result. 12.___
When a patient is given a transfusion, his very life is dependent on the
   A. amount of blood available
   B. anesthetic administered
   C. surgical skill of the doctor
   D. type of the transfused blood

13. The wolf's footsteps showed that it had been prowling around outside the hut during the night, and the broken-down door showed that it had found an 13.___
A. escape B. entrance C. animal D. enemy

14. The atmosphere is saturated with change. It has the light-headed going around in fantastic circles, and even the most level-headed are filled with a sense of 14.___
A. optimism B. satisfaction C. permanency D. insecurity

15. Although installation of dial phones has replaced many thousands of telephone operators, the total number of persons employed in this industry has continued to rise. This fact should help destroy the myth that 15.___
A. dial phones can never entirely replace switchboards
B. employment depends upon machinery
C. machinery increases unemployment
D. employment and mechanization go hand in hand

16. The public imagination was stirred by the effrontery of this colorful swindler whom the newspapers referred to as a modern 16.___
A. prophet B. pirate C. kidnaper D. knight

17. Death, other conditions remaining the same, is more profoundly affecting in summer than in other parts of the year. There is an antagonism between the tropical redundancy of life in summer and the frozen sterilities of the grave. 17.___
The summer we see, the grave we haunt with our thoughts; the glory is around us, the darkness is within us; and, summer and death coming into collision,
A. we comprehend the inevitable pattern of life and death
B. each exalts the other into stronger relief
C. the summer becomes meaningless and is forgotten
D. the beauty of one eases the pain of the other

18. They had to wade across the stream, for at the point where they wished to cross there was no 18.___
A. ford B. water C. bridge D. bank

19. Man is inconsistent in his likes and dislikes. What he loves at twenty, he hates at forty, but this inconsistency speaks well of his ability to profit from experience. 19.___
If he never changed his attitudes, he would be marked as
A. a wise man B. true to himself
C. unable to learn D. preferring simple things

20. One of the great needs of utopias, which usually have inefficient methods of obtaining food and other necessities, is a large percentage of workers per number of members. 20.___
This might be achieved, in the very short run, by
A. outlawing marriage and children
B. modernizing farming techniques
C. encouraging marriage
D. adopting infants

21. Leaders seem to operate on the theory that pity is a powerful force that can overcome even the jealousy of their followers. 21.___
Leaders loudly complain about pressure and overwork merely to
   A. deplore the suffering of the great
   B. abate the edge of envy
   C. increase their range of sentiments
   D. make their prestige more obvious

22. Most of the prehistoric reptiles were unable either to adapt to the ice that eventually covered their accustomed habitat or to migrate to 22.___
   A. warmer zones B. Canada
   C. modern countries D. frozen lands

23. Serfs were not bought and sold; rather, they were transferred with the land upon which they worked. 23.___
The essential economic characteristic of serfdom was bondage to
   A. labor B. masters C. soil D. chains

24. In India, actors in the early days of the theater were among the lower class of a rigid society. 24.___
Parents feared that their children might take up dramatic careers, for the theater through the years had supported only
   A. drama critics B. trained performers
   C. vagabonds and profligates D. amateurs

25. The Indians had eaten little for many months. 25.___
Only the strongest people of the tribe remained alive, and now they were weak from
   A. war B. cold C. hunger D. sorrow

KEY (CORRECT ANSWERS)

1. C
2. B
3. B
4. A
5. D

6. A
7. A
8. C
9. D
10. A

11. C
12. D
13. B
14. D
15. C

16. B
17. B
18. C
19. C
20. A

21. B
22. A
23. C
24. C
25. C

LOGICAL REASONING

EVALUATING CONCLUSIONS IN LIGHT OF KNOWN FACTS

EXAMINATION SECTION

DIRECTIONS: For the following questions, select the letter before the statement below which BEST expresses the relationship between the facts and the conclusion.
Mark your answer:
A. The facts prove the conclusion; or
B. The facts disprove the conclusion; or
C. The facts neither prove nor disprove the conclusion.
PRINT THE LETTER OF THE CORRECT ANSWER IN THE SPACE AT THE RIGHT.

1. FACTS: Andy types half as fast as Bill. Bill types twice as slow as Charlie. Bill types 60 words a minute. 1.___

CONCLUSION: Charlie types 30 words a minute.

2. FACTS: If Albert gets traded to the Cubs, Chris will have to be traded to the Padres. Albert will avoid being traded only if he hits a home run in his turn at bat. If Chris goes to the Padres, Dave will be traded to the Dodgers. Albert strikes out in this crucial at-bat. 2.___

CONCLUSION: Dave gets traded to the Dodgers.

3. FACTS: All beads are forms of jewelry. All jewelry is expensive. Everyone loves expensive beads. 3.___

CONCLUSION: All beads are expensive.

4. FACTS: No shrimp are mussels. Mussels are bivalves. All mussels have shells. 4.___

CONCLUSION: Therefore, no shrimp have shells.

5. FACTS: On their latest diet, Abby, Bea, Celia, and Donna lost a combined total of 260 pounds. Abby lost twice as much as Celia. Celia lost half as much as the woman who lost the most. Donna lost 80 pounds. 5.___

CONCLUSION: Abby lost 100 pounds; Bea, 30; Celia, 50; and Donna, 80.

6. FACTS: Ann's office is two floors above Brenda's. Brenda's office is one floor below the only woman in the building whose birthday is today. Sally's office is on the third floor. Ann's office is on the fourth floor. 6.___

CONCLUSION: Today is Ann's birthday.

7. FACTS: Douglas Ave. is perpendicular to Bates St. Bates St. is parallel to Adams Ave. Douglas Ave. is parallel to Charles St. Evans Ave. is parallel to the streets that are perpendicular to Bates St. 7.___

CONCLUSION: Evans Ave. is perpendicular to Douglas Ave.

8. FACTS: There's one out, and Bill is the runner on third base. If Arnie hits the ball hard, Bill will run, but so slowly that he will be out at home plate. The team captain, on second base, will not run unless Arnie hits the ball hard. The captain runs. 8.___

CONCLUSION: Bill is safe.

9. FACTS: Some members of this genus are members of that species. All members of that species are butterflies. Some butterflies are different from others. 9.___

CONCLUSION: Some members of this genus are butterflies.

10. FACTS: Some woodwinds are clarinets. Flutes are not clarinets. All clarinets are beautiful things. 10.___

CONCLUSION: Therefore, all beautiful things are woodwinds.

11. FACTS: Using a grid exactly like the one below, Joe Genius filled in the numbers 1 through 9 in the boxes. Each horizontal, vertical, and diagonal row added up to 15. A different number went in each box. 11.___

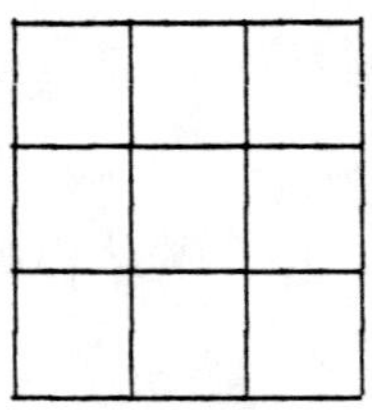

CONCLUSION: The number Joe put in the middle box was 6.

12. FACTS: Max, Nick, Pete, and Ollie all bought different colored suits: grey, green, blue, and brown, but not necessarily respectively. Max paid less for his green suit than Nick paid for his suit. Ollie paid twice what Pete paid. Pete paid the same as the man who bought the grey suit. Ollie bought the brown suit. 12.___

CONCLUSION: Ollie paid the most.

13. FACTS: Four people (Alice, Bob, Carol, and Dave) are sitting at a square table, discussing their favorite sports. Bob sits directly across from the jogger. Carol sits to the right of the basketball player. Alice sits across from Dave. The golfer sits to the left of the tennis player. A man sits on Dave's right. 13.___

CONCLUSION: Dave plays golf.

14. FACTS: An employer decided to offer a job to everyone who scored higher than 50 on an exam. Alice scored 20. Betty scored lower than Carol, but more than twice as high as Alice. 14.___

CONCLUSION: Of the three women, only Carol was offered the job.

15. FACTS: If Camille's squirrel has rabies and the squirrel bites Casey's cat, the squirrel will have to be caught and the cat will get rabies. If the cat has had rabies shots within the last two years, the cat will not get rabies. Casey's cat did not get rabies. 15.___

CONCLUSION: Casey's cat has had rabies shots within the last two years.

16. FACTS: Sally will file a grievance only if Bill fires her. If Laura tells Frank the whole story, Frank will tell it to Bill. If Bill hears the whole story, he will not fire Sally. Laura tells Fred the whole story. 16.___

CONCLUSION: Sally files a grievance.

17. FACTS: If Alice leaves work early, Barb has to work late, and Barb wants to go to the game tonight. The singing of the National Anthem always precedes the game. Carl calls Alice and asks her out to dinner. Due to a thunderstorm, the singing of the National Anthem gets delayed. If Alice goes out to dinner with Carl, she will have to leave work early so she can go home and turn off her crockpot. Alice accepts Carl's invitation. 17.___

CONCLUSION: Barb misses the first inning of the game.

18. FACTS: Earl thinks of any whole number from 1 through 10. Because she is using the most efficient system, Eva absolutely guarantees Earl that she can correctly guess the number he's thinking of in five questions or less. Eva asks Earl a series of *yes/no* questions and guesses the number in five questions or less every time. Earl and Eva agree to play the game again in the exact same way, except that he will think of a whole number from 1 through 6. 18.___

CONCLUSION: Using the same system, four is the absolute highest number of *yes/no* questions that Eva will need to ask in order to guess the number that Earl is thinking of this time.

19. FACTS: Lois will cook dinner today only if Ted, Robbie, and Jennifer are all home by 6 P.M. Robbie will come home by 6 P.M. only if band practice ends early. If Ted plays softball after work, he will take Jennifer with him, and they will not be home by 6 P.M. Band practice ends early today. 19.___

CONCLUSION: Lois cooks dinner today.

20. FACTS: Three card players each start with $10. Each round they play has two losers and one winner. The losers in each round have to give the winner $2 apiece. Chuck wins the first and third rounds; Bruce wins the second. At the end of the third round, Artie proposes that they change the rules so that the losers each have to give the winner half their accumulated money. They agree, play one more round, and Artie wins it. 20.___

CONCLUSION: At the end of the fourth round, Chuck has less money than Artie.

21. FACTS: No part-time workers at this plant get paid vacations. All cleaners at this plant are part-time workers. Joe gets a paid vacation. 21.___

CONCLUSION: All cleaners at this plant get paid vacations.

22. FACTS: If Myles breaks the lamp, Lucy will scream. If Tom finds Rachel spraying Windex into the cat's dish, he'll scream. If Geoffrey doesn't hear from the French soon, he'll scream. Tom screams. 22.___

CONCLUSION: Myles broke the lamp.

23. FACTS: If Tina goes to the store, Ike will go with her. If Ike goes to the store, he will buy doughnuts. If Dick cleans the house, Sally will go to the store. If Sally goes to the store, Tina will go with her. Dick cleans the house. 23.___

CONCLUSION: Ike buys doughnuts.

24. FACTS: If Joe passes the test, Jill won't apply for the job. If Jill applies for the job, she'll get it. If Jill doesn't apply for the job, Jeanne will be annoyed. Joe passes the test. 24.___

CONCLUSION: Jeanne gets annoyed.

25. FACTS: Mary, Debbie, May, and Joan are the only people waiting for the photocopier to be fixed. When it's fixed, Debbie has to use it first because she's doing work for the boss. Joan has to use it right after the person who's been waiting the longest. The person who has the most work to copy gets to use the machine second. May has been waiting the longest. The person who has been waiting longest is not the person who has the most work to copy. 25.___

CONCLUSION: Joan gets to use the photocopier third.

KEY (CORRECT ANSWERS)

1. B
2. A
3. A
4. C
5. C

6. B
7. B
8. B
9. A
10. C

11. B
12. A
13. A
14. C
15. C

16. C
17. C
18. A
19. C
20. A

21. B
22. C
23. A
24. A
25. B

LOGICAL REASONING
EVALUATING CONCLUSIONS IN LIGHT OF KNOWN FACTS
EXAMINATION SECTION

COMMENTARY

This section is designed to provide practice questions in evaluating conclusions when you are given specific data to work with.

We suggest you do the questions three at a time, consulting the answer key and then the solution section for any questions you may have missed. It's a good idea to try the questions again a week before the exam.

In the validity of conclusion type of question, you are first given a reading passage which describes a particular situation. The passage may be on any topic, as it is not your knowledge of the topic that is being tested, but your reasoning abilities. The passage is likely to detail several proposed courses of action and factors affecting these proposals. The reading passage is followed by a conclusion based on the facts in the passage, or a description of a decision taken regarding the situation. The conclusion is followed by a number of statements which have a possible connection to the conclusion. For each statement, you are to determine whether:

A. The statement proves the conclusion.
B. The statement supports the conclusion but does not prove it.
C. The statement disproves the conclusion.
D. The statement weakens the conclusion but does not disprove it.
E. The statement has no relevance to the conclusion.

Remember that the conclusion after the passage is to be accepted as the outcome of what actually happened, and that you are being asked to evaluate the impact each statement would have had on the conclusion.

Questions 1-8 are based on the following paragraph.

In May of 1993, Mr. Bryan inherited a clothing store on Main Street in a small New England town. The store has specialized in selling quality men's and women's clothing since 1885. Business has been stable throughout the years, neither increasing nor decreasing. He has an opportunity to buy two adjacent stores which would enable him to add a wider range and style of clothing. In order to do this, he would have to borrow a substantial amount of money. He also risks losing the goodwill of his present clientele.

CONCLUSION: On November 7, 1993, Mr. Bryan tells the owner of the two adjacent stores that he has decided not to purchase them. He feels that it would be best to simply maintain his present marketing position, as there would not be enough new business to support an expansion.

A. The statement proves the conclusion.
B. The statement supports the conclusion but does not prove it.
C. The statement disproves the conclusion.
D. The statement weakens the conclusion.
E. The statement is irrelevant to the conclusion.

1. A large new branch of the county's community college holds its first classes in September of 1993. 1.___

2. The town's largest factory shuts down with no indication that it will reopen. 2.___

3. The 1990 United States Census showed that the number of children per household dropped from 2.4 to 2.1 since the 1980 census. 3.___

4. Mr. Bryan's brother tells him of a new clothing boutique specializing in casual women's clothing which is opening soon. 4.___

5. Mr. Bryan's sister buys her baby several items for Christmas at Mr. Bryan's store. 5.___

6. Mrs. McIntyre, the President of the Town Council, brings Mr. Bryan a home-baked pumpkin pie in honor of his store's 100th anniversary. They discuss the changes that have taken place in the town, and she comments on how his store has maintained the same look and feel over the years. 6.___

7. In October of 1993, Mr. Bryan's aunt lends him $50,000. 7.___

8. The Town Council has just announced that the town is eligible for funding from a federal project designed to encourage the location of new businesses in the central districts of cities and towns. 8.___

Questions 9-18 are based on the following paragraph.

A proposal has been put before the legislative body of a small European country to require air bags in all automobiles manufactured for domestic use in that country after 1999. The air bag, made of nylon or plastic, is designed to inflate automatically within a car at the impact of a collision, thus protecting front-seat occupants from being thrown forward. There has been much support of the measure from consumer groups, the insurance industry, key legislators, and the general public. The country's automobile manufacturers, who contend the new crash equipment would add up to $1,000 to car prices and provide no more protection than existing seat belts, are against the proposed legislation.

CONCLUSION: On April 21, 1994, the legislature passed legislation requiring air bags in all automobiles manufactured for domestic use in that country after 1999.

A. The statement proves the conclusion.
B. The statement supports the conclusion but does not prove it.
C. The statement disproves the conclusion.
D. The statement weakens the conclusion.
E. The statement is irrelevant to the conclusion.

9. A study has shown that 59% of car occupants do not use seat belts. 9.___

10. The country's Department of Transportation has estimated that the crash protection equipment would save up to 5,900 lives each year. 10.___

11. On April 27, 1993, Augusta Ranconi was named head of an advisory committee to gather and analyze data on the costs, benefits, and feasibility of the proposed legislation on air bags in automobiles. 11.___

12. Consumer groups and the insurance industry accuse the legislature of rejecting passage of the regulation for political reasons. 12.___

13. A study by the Committee on Imports and Exports projected that the sales of imported cars would rise dramatically in 1999 because imported cars do not have to include air bags, and can be sold more cheaply. 13.___

14. Research has shown that air bags, if produced on a large scale, would cost about $200 apiece, and would provide more reliable protection than any other type of seat belt. 14.___

15. Auto sales in 1991 have increased 3% over the previous year. 15.___

16. A Department of Transportation report in July of 2000 credits a drop in automobile deaths of 4,100 to the use of air bags. 16.___

17. In June of 1994, the lobbyist of the largest insurance company receives a bonus for her work on the passage of the air bag legislation. 17.___

18. In 2000, the stock in crash protection equipment has risen three-fold over the previous year. 18.___

Questions 19-25 are based on the following paragraph.

On a national television talk show, Joan Rivera, a famous comedienne, has recently insulted the physical appearances of a famous actress and the dead wife of an ex-President. There has been a flurry of controversy over her comments, and much discussion of the incident has appeared in the press. Most of the comments have been negative. It appears that this time she might have gone too far. There have been cancellations of two of her five scheduled performances in the two weeks since the show was televised, and Joan's been receiving a lot of negative mail. Because of the controversy, she has an interview with a national news magazine at the end of the week, and her press agent is strongly urging her to apologize publicly. She feels strongly that her comments were no worse than any other she has ever made, and that the whole incident will *blow over* soon. She respects her press agent's judgment, however, as his assessment of public sentiment tends to be very accurate.

CONCLUSION: Joan does not apologize publicly, and during the interview she challenges the actress to a weight-losing contest. For every pound the actress loses, Joan says she will donate $1 to the Cellulite Prevention League.

A. The statement proves the conclusion.
B. The statement supports the conclusion but does not prove it.
C. The statement disproves the conclusion.
D. The statement weakens the conclusion.
E. The statement is irrelevant to the conclusion.

19. Joan's mother, who she is very fond of, is very upset about Joan's comments. 19.___

20. Six months after the interview, Joan's income has doubled. 20.___

21. Joan's agent is pleased with the way Joan handles the interview. 21.___

22. Joan's sister has been appointed Treasurer of the Cellulite Prevention League. In her report, she states that Joan's $12 contribution is the only amount that has been donated to the League in its first six months. 22.___

23. The magazine receives many letters commending Joan for the courage it took for her to apologize publicly in the interview. 23.___

24. Immediately after the interview appears, another one of Joan's performances is cancelled. 24.___

25. Due to a printers strike, the article was not published until the following week. 25.___

Questions 26-30 are based on the following paragraph.

The law-making body of Country X must decide what to do about the issue of videotaping television shows for home use. There is currently no law against taping shows directly from the TV as long as the videotapes are not used for commercial purposes. The increasing popularity of pay TV and satellite systems, combined with the increasing number of homes that own videocassette recorders, has caused a great deal of concern in some segments of the entertainment industry. Companies that own the rights to films, popular television shows, and sporting events feel that their copyright privileges are being violated, and they are seeking compensation or the banning of TV home videotaping. Legislation has been introduced to make it illegal to videotape television programs for home use. Separate proposed legislation is also pending that would continue to allow videotaping of TV shows for home use, but would place a tax of 10% on each videocassette that is purchased for home use. The income from that tax would then be proportionately distributed as royalties to those owning the rights to programs being aired. A weighted point system coupled with the averaging of several national viewing rating systems would be used to determine the royalties. There is a great deal of lobbying being done for both bills, as the manufacturers of videocassette recorders and videocassettes are against the passage of the bills.

CONCLUSION: The legislature of Country X rejects both bills by a wide margin.

A. The statement proves the conclusion.
B. The statement supports the conclusion but does not prove it.
C. The statement disproves the conclusion.
D. The statement weakens the conclusion.
E. The statement is irrelevant to the conclusion.

26. Country X's Department of Taxation hires 500 new employees to handle the increased paperwork created by the new tax on videocassettes. 26.___

27. A study conducted by the country's most prestigious accounting firm shows that the cost of implementing the proposed new videocassette tax would be greater than the income expected from it. 27.___

28. It is estimated that 80% of all those working in the entertainment industry, excluding performers, own videocassette recorders. 28.___

29. The head of Country X's law enforcement agency states that legislation banning the home taping of TV shows would be unenforceable. 29.___

30. Financial experts predict that unless a tax is placed on videocassettes, several large companies in the entertainment industry will have to file for bankruptcy. 30.___

Questions 31-38.

DIRECTIONS: The following questions 31 through 38 are variations on the type of question you just had. It is important that you read the question very carefully to determine exactly what is required.

31. In this question, select the choice that is most relevant to the conclusion. 31.___
1. The Buffalo Bills football team is in second place in its division.
2. The New England Patriots are in first place in the same division.
3. There are two games left to play in the season, and the Bills will not play the Patriots again.
4. The New England Patriots won ten games and lost four games, and the Buffalo Bills have won eight games and lost six games.

CONCLUSION: The Buffalo Bills win their division.

A. The conclusion is proved by sentences 1-4.
B. The conclusion is disproved by sentences 1-4.
C. The facts are not sufficient to prove or disprove the conclusion.

32. In this question, select the choice that is most relevant to the conclusion. 32.___
1. On the planet of Zeinon there are only two different eye colors and only two different hair colors.
2. Half of those beings with purple hair have golden eyes.
3. There are more inhabitants with purple hair than there are inhabitants with silver hair.
4. One-third of those with silver hair have green eyes.

CONCLUSION: There are more golden-eyed beings on Zeinon than green-eyed ones.

A. The conclusion is proved by sentences 1-4.
B. The conclusion is disproved by sentences 1-4.
C. The facts are not sufficient to prove or disprove the conclusion.

33. In this question, select the choice that is most relevant to the conclusion. 33.___
John and Kevin are leaving Amaranth to go to school in Bethany. They've decided to rent a small truck to move their possessions. Joe's Truck Rental charges $100 plus 30¢ a mile. National Movers charges $50 more but gives free mileage for the first 100 miles. After the first 100 miles, they charge 25¢ a mile.

CONCLUSION: John and Kevin rent their truck from National Movers because it is cheaper.

A. The conclusion is proved by the facts in the above paragraph.
B. The conclusion is disproved by the facts in the above paragraph.
C. The facts are not sufficient to prove or disprove the conclusion.

34. For this question, select the choice that supports the information given in the passage. 34.___

Municipalities in Country X are divided into villages, towns, and cities. A village has a population of 5,000 or less. The population of a town ranges from 5,001 to 15,000. In order to be incorporated as a city, the municipality must have a population over 15,000. If, after a village becomes a town, or a town becomes a city, the population drops below the minimum required (for example, the population of a city goes below 15,000), and stays below the minimum for more than ten years, it loses its current status, and drops to the next category. As soon as a municipality rises in population to the next category (village to town, for example), however, it is immediately reclassified to the next category.

In the 1970 census, Plainfield had a population of 12,000. Between 1970 and 1980, Plainfield grew 10%, and between 1980 and 1990 Plainfield grew another 20%. The population of Springdale doubled from 1970 to 1980, and increased 25% from 1980 to 1990. The city of Smallville's population, 20,283, has not changed significantly in the last twenty years. Granton had a population of 25,000 people in 1960, and has decreased 25% in each ten year period since then. Ellenville had a population of 4,283 in 1960, and grew 5% in each ten year period since 1960.

In 1990,

A. Plainfield, Smallville, and Granton are cities
B. Smallville is a city, Granton is a town, and Ellenville is a village
C. Springdale, Granton, and Ellenville are towns
D. Plainfield and Smallville are cities, and Ellenville is a town

35. For this question, select the choice that is most relevant to the conclusion. 35.___

A study was done for a major food distributing firm to determine if there is any difference in the kind of caffeine containing products used by people of different ages. A sample of one thousand people between the ages of twenty and fifty were drawn from selected areas in the country. They were divided equally into three groups.

Those individuals who were 20-29 were designated Group A, those 30-39 were Group B, and those 40-50 were placed in Group C.
It was found that on the average, Group A drank 1.8 cups of coffee, Group B 3.1, and Group C 2.5 cups of coffee daily. Group A drank 2.1 cups of tea, Group B drank 1.2, and Group C drank 2.6 cups of tea daily. Group A drank 3.1 8-ounce glasses of cola, Group B drank 1.9, and Group C drank 1.5 glasses of cola daily.

CONCLUSION: According to the study, the average person in the 20-29 age group drinks less tea daily than the average person in the 40-50 age group, but drinks more coffee daily than the average person in the 30-39 age group drinks cola.

A. The conclusion is proved by the facts in the above paragraph.
B. The conclusion is disproved by the facts in the above paragraph.
C. The facts are not sufficient to prove or disprove the conclusion.

36. For this question, select the choice that is most relevant to the conclusion. 36.___
1. Mary is taller than Jane but shorter than Dale.
2. Fred is taller than Mary but shorter than Steven.
3. Dale is shorter than Steven but taller than Elizabeth.
4. Elizabeth is taller than Mary but not as tall as Fred.

CONCLUSION: Dale is taller than Fred.

A. The conclusion is proved by sentences 1-4.
B. The conclusion is disproved by sentences 1-4.
C. The facts are not sufficient to prove or disprove the conclusion.

37. For this question, select the choice that is most relevant to the conclusion. 37.___
1. Main Street is between Spring Street and Glenn Blvd.
2. Hawley Avenue is one block south of Spring Street and three blocks north of Main Street.
3. Glenn Street is five blocks south of Elm and four blocks south of Main.
4. All the streets mentioned are parallel to one another.

CONCLUSION: Elm Street is between Hawley Avenue and Glenn Blvd.

A. The conclusion is proved by the facts in sentences 1-4.
B. The conclusion is disproved by the facts in sentences 1-4.
C. The facts are not sufficient to prove or disprove the conclusion.

38. For this question, select the choice that is most relevant to the conclusion. 38.___

1. Train A leaves the town of Hampshire every day at 5:50 A.M. and arrives in New London at 6:42 A.M.
2. Train A leaves New London at 7:00 A.M. and arrives in Kellogsville at 8:42 A.M.
3. Train B leaves Kellogsville at 8:00 A.M. and arrives in Hampshire at 10:42 A.M.
4. Due to the need for repairs, there is just one railroad track between New London and Hampshire.

CONCLUSION: It is impossible for Train A and Train B to follow these schedules without colliding.

A. The conclusion is proved by the facts in the above paragraph.
B. The conclusion is disproved by the facts in the above passage.
C. The facts are not sufficient to prove or disprove the conclusion.

KEY (CORRECT ANSWERS)

1. D	11. C	21. D	31. C
2. B	12. C	22. A	32. A
3. E	13. D	23. C	33. C
4. B	14. B	24. B	34. B
5. C	15. E	25. E	35. B
6. D	16. B	26. C	36. C
7. B	17. A	27. B	37. A
8. A	18. B	28. E	38. B
9. B	19. D	29. B	
10. B	20. E	30. D	

ANSWER SHEET

TEST NO. ____________ PART ______ TITLE OF POSITION ______________________
(AS GIVEN IN EXAMINATION ANNOUNCEMENT - INCLUDE OPTION, IF ANY)

PLACE OF EXAMINATION ______________________ ______________________ DATE ____________
(CITY OR TOWN) (STATE)

RATING

USE THE SPECIAL PENCIL. MAKE GLOSSY BLACK MARKS.

1	A B C D E	26	A B C D E	51	A B C D E	76	A B C D E	101	A B C D E
2	A B C D E	27	A B C D E	52	A B C D E	77	A B C D E	102	A B C D E
3	A B C D E	28	A B C D E	53	A B C D E	78	A B C D E	103	A B C D E
4	A B C D E	29	A B C D E	54	A B C D E	79	A B C D E	104	A B C D E
5	A B C D E	30	A B C D E	55	A B C D E	80	A B C D E	105	A B C D E
6	A B C D E	31	A B C D E	56	A B C D E	81	A B C D E	106	A B C D E
7	A B C D E	32	A B C D E	57	A B C D E	82	A B C D E	107	A B C D E
8	A B C D E	33	A B C D E	58	A B C D E	83	A B C D E	108	A B C D E
9	A B C D E	34	A B C D E	59	A B C D E	84	A B C D E	109	A B C D E
10	A B C D E	35	A B C D E	60	A B C D E	85	A B C D E	110	A B C D E

Make only ONE mark for each answer. Additional and stray marks may be counted as mistakes. In making corrections, erase errors COMPLETELY.

11	A B C D E	36	A B C D E	61	A B C D E	86	A B C D E	111	A B C D E
12	A B C D E	37	A B C D E	62	A B C D E	87	A B C D E	112	A B C D E
13	A B C D E	38	A B C D E	63	A B C D E	88	A B C D E	113	A B C D E
14	A B C D E	39	A B C D E	64	A B C D E	89	A B C D E	114	A B C D E
15	A B C D E	40	A B C D E	65	A B C D E	90	A B C D E	115	A B C D E
16	A B C D E	41	A B C D E	66	A B C D E	91	A B C D E	116	A B C D E
17	A B C D E	42	A B C D E	67	A B C D E	92	A B C D E	117	A B C D E
18	A B C D E	43	A B C D E	68	A B C D E	93	A B C D E	118	A B C D E
19	A B C D E	44	A B C D E	69	A B C D E	94	A B C D E	119	A B C D E
20	A B C D E	45	A B C D E	70	A B C D E	95	A B C D E	120	A B C D E
21	A B C D E	46	A B C D E	71	A B C D E	96	A B C D E	121	A B C D E
22	A B C D E	47	A B C D E	72	A B C D E	97	A B C D E	122	A B C D E
23	A B C D E	48	A B C D E	73	A B C D E	98	A B C D E	123	A B C D E
24	A B C D E	49	A B C D E	74	A B C D E	99	A B C D E	124	A B C D E
25	A B C D E	50	A B C D E	75	A B C D E	100	A B C D E	125	A B C D E

ANSWER SHEET

TEST NO. ______ PART ______ TITLE OF POSITION ______
(AS GIVEN IN EXAMINATION ANNOUNCEMENT - INCLUDE OPTION, IF ANY)

PLACE OF EXAMINATION ______ (CITY OR TOWN) ______ (STATE) DATE ______

RATING

USE THE SPECIAL PENCIL. MAKE GLOSSY BLACK MARKS.

1	A	B	C	D	E	26	A	B	C	D	E	51	A	B	C	D	E	76	A	B	C	D	E	101	A	B	C	D	E
2	A	B	C	D	E	27	A	B	C	D	E	52	A	B	C	D	E	77	A	B	C	D	E	102	A	B	C	D	E
3	A	B	C	D	E	28	A	B	C	D	E	53	A	B	C	D	E	78	A	B	C	D	E	103	A	B	C	D	E
4	A	B	C	D	E	29	A	B	C	D	E	54	A	B	C	D	E	79	A	B	C	D	E	104	A	B	C	D	E
5	A	B	C	D	E	30	A	B	C	D	E	55	A	B	C	D	E	80	A	B	C	D	E	105	A	B	C	D	E
6	A	B	C	D	E	31	A	B	C	D	E	56	A	B	C	D	E	81	A	B	C	D	E	106	A	B	C	D	E
7	A	B	C	D	E	32	A	B	C	D	E	57	A	B	C	D	E	82	A	B	C	D	E	107	A	B	C	D	E
8	A	B	C	D	E	33	A	B	C	D	E	58	A	B	C	D	E	83	A	B	C	D	E	108	A	B	C	D	E
9	A	B	C	D	E	34	A	B	C	D	E	59	A	B	C	D	E	84	A	B	C	D	E	109	A	B	C	D	E
10	A	B	C	D	E	35	A	B	C	D	E	60	A	B	C	D	E	85	A	B	C	D	E	110	A	B	C	D	E

Make only ONE mark for each answer. Additional and stray marks may be counted as mistakes. In making corrections, erase errors COMPLETELY.

11	A	B	C	D	E	36	A	B	C	D	E	61	A	B	C	D	E	86	A	B	C	D	E	111	A	B	C	D	E
12	A	B	C	D	E	37	A	B	C	D	E	62	A	B	C	D	E	87	A	B	C	D	E	112	A	B	C	D	E
13	A	B	C	D	E	38	A	B	C	D	E	63	A	B	C	D	E	88	A	B	C	D	E	113	A	B	C	D	E
14	A	B	C	D	E	39	A	B	C	D	E	64	A	B	C	D	E	89	A	B	C	D	E	114	A	B	C	D	E
15	A	B	C	D	E	40	A	B	C	D	E	65	A	B	C	D	E	90	A	B	C	D	E	115	A	B	C	D	E
16	A	B	C	D	E	41	A	B	C	D	E	66	A	B	C	D	E	91	A	B	C	D	E	116	A	B	C	D	E
17	A	B	C	D	E	42	A	B	C	D	E	67	A	B	C	D	E	92	A	B	C	D	E	117	A	B	C	D	E
18	A	B	C	D	E	43	A	B	C	D	E	68	A	B	C	D	E	93	A	B	C	D	E	118	A	B	C	D	E
19	A	B	C	D	E	44	A	B	C	D	E	69	A	B	C	D	E	94	A	B	C	D	E	119	A	B	C	D	E
20	A	B	C	D	E	45	A	B	C	D	E	70	A	B	C	D	E	95	A	B	C	D	E	120	A	B	C	D	E
21	A	B	C	D	E	46	A	B	C	D	E	71	A	B	C	D	E	96	A	B	C	D	E	121	A	B	C	D	E
22	A	B	C	D	E	47	A	B	C	D	E	72	A	B	C	D	E	97	A	B	C	D	E	122	A	B	C	D	E
23	A	B	C	D	E	48	A	B	C	D	E	73	A	B	C	D	E	98	A	B	C	D	E	123	A	B	C	D	E
24	A	B	C	D	E	49	A	B	C	D	E	74	A	B	C	D	E	99	A	B	C	D	E	124	A	B	C	D	E
25	A	B	C	D	E	50	A	B	C	D	E	75	A	B	C	D	E	100	A	B	C	D	E	125	A	B	C	D	E